DEAD ON ARRIVAL

POLITICS AND SOCIETY IN TWENTIETH-CENTURY AMERICA

Series Editors

WILLIAM CHAFE, GARY GERSTLE, LINDA GORDON, AND JULIAN ZELIZER

A list of titles in this series appears at the back of the book

DEAD ON ARRIVAL

THE POLITICS OF HEALTH CARE
IN TWENTIETH-CENTURY AMERICA

Colin Gordon

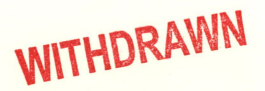

PRINCETON UNIVERSITY PRESS   PRINCETON AND OXFORD

Copyright © 2003 by Princeton University Press
Published by Princeton University Press, 41 William Street,
Princeton, New Jersey 08540
In the United Kingdom: Princeton University Press, 3 Market Place,
Woodstock, Oxfordshire OX20 1SY

Library of Congress Cataloging-in-Publication Data
Gordon, Colin, 1962–
Dead on arrival : the politics of health care in twentieth-century America / Colin Gordon.
p. cm. — (Politics and society in the twentieth-century America)
Includes bibliographical references and index.
ISBN 0-691-05806-7 (alk. paper)
1. Medical policy—United States. 2. Medical care—Political aspects—United States—
I. Title. II. Series.
RA395.A3 G67 2003
362.1' 0973—dc21   2002072257

British Library Cataloging-in-Publication Data is available

This book has been composed in New Baskerville

Printed on acid-free paper. ∞

www.pupress.princeton.edu

Printed in the United States of America

10 9 8 7 6 5 4 3 2 1

For Susan

Contents

Acknowledgments

Like the health care system it describes, this book reflects a tangle of material, intellectual, and political influences. For the book at least, the intervention of these third parties has been most welcome. I can offer only the "UCR" (usual, customary, reasonable) reimbursement of this prefatory note, and the assurance that, however widely the credit is shared, I assume sole liability for the results. First (as in the health care system), the money: the University of British Columbia and the University of Iowa provided wonderful institutional support. The research was underwritten by a major grant from the Social Sciences and Humanities Research Council of Canada, and smaller grants from the Truman and Roosevelt presidential libraries. Finishing the manuscript was made possible by a three-semester Faculty Scholarship from the University of Iowa.

The assistance and patience of archivists were crucial to this project. Special thanks to Bob McCown at the University of Iowa, Tab Smith at the National Archives, and Michael Nash at the Hagley Museum and Library. David Colman, Nora Jaffary, Jennifer Peters, Eric Roberson, and Diane Wadden provided invaluable research assistance.

Over the past few years, my understanding of the American health care system has been sharpened by a range of conversations, conferences, and correspondence. For their contributions (and sometimes skepticism), I would especially like to thank Thomas Clark, Alan Derickson, Milton Fisk, Linda Gordon, Marie Gottschalk, Beatrix Hoffman, Roger Horowitz, Ira Katznelson, Jennifer Klein, Nelson Lichtenstein, Marc Linder, Cathie Jo Martin, Edie Rasell, Leslie Reagan, Joel Rogers, and Landon Storrs. My colleagues at UBC and Iowa have offered practical support, intellectual support, and—most important—the example of serious scholarship. Special thanks on this score to Doug Baynton, Ken Cmiel, Jeff Cox, Bill French, Bob Jefferson, Paul Krause, Maureen McCue, Mac Rohrbough, Johanna Schoen, Leslie Schwalm, Allen Steinberg, Shel Stromquist, and Allan Tully.

At the Press, thanks to Brigitta van Rheinberg for her editorial guidance (and patience), Jonathan Hall for his help with the last-minute details, and Elizabeth Gilbert for her deft red pencil.

Some of the material on the 1940s (from a number of chapters) was previously published as "Why No Health Insurance in the United States? The Limits of Social Provision in War and Peace, 1941–1948," *Journal of Policy History* 9:3 (1997): 277–310. Some of the material on the 1990s previously appeared in "Dead on Arrival: Health Care Reform in the

United States," *Studies in Political Economy* 39 (Autumn 1992): 141–158; "Dead on Arrival: The Past and Future of American Health Care," *Open Magazine*, 1995, 1–30; "Cosmetic Surgery: Health Care the Corporate Way," *The Nation* 252 (25 Mar. 1991): 376–380; and "The American Politics of Canadian Health Care," *Canadian Dimension* (Sept. 1992): 17–20.

Abbreviations

AAAPSS	*Annals of the American Academy of Political and Social Science*
AALL	American Association for Labor Legislation
AAMA	American Automobile Manufacturers Association
ACW	Amalgamated Clothing Workers
AFDC	Aid to Families with Dependent Children
AFFFHW	American Federation of Full-Fashioned Hosiery Workers
AFHW	American Federation of Hosiery Workers
AFL	American Federation of Labor
AFSCME	American Federation of State, County, and Municipal Employees
AHA	American Hospital Association
AJPH	*American Journal of Public Health*
AMA	American Medical Association
AMPAC	American Medical Political Action Committee
BCA	Blue Cross Association
BHM	*Bulletin of the History of Medicine*
BMSJ	*Boston Medical and Surgical Journal*
BW	*Business Week*
CCMC	Committee on the Costs of Medical Care
CES	Committee on Economic Security
CHIP	Comprehensive Health Insurance Plan (1970s)
CHIP	Children's Health Insurance Plan (1990s)
CHP	Clinton health plan
CHTF	Clinton Health Care Task Force
CIO	Congress of Industrial Organizations
CNH	Committee for the Nation's Health
CNHI	Committee for National Health Insurance
DLC	Democratic Leadership Council
DNC	Democratic National Committee
EMIC	Emergency Maternity and Infant Care program
ERISA	Employment and Retirement Income Security Act
FASB	Federal Accounting Standards Board
FDRPL	Franklin D. Roosevelt Presidential Library
FHIP	Family Health Insurance Plan
FSA	Farm Security Administration (1935–1945)
FSA	Federal Security Agency (1945–1950)
FTC	Federal Trade Commission
GCF	General Classified Files (HEW Records)

GDP	Gross domestic product
GHAA	Group Health Association of America
HA	*Health Affairs*
HAUC	Health and Accident Underwriters Conference
HBR	*Harvard Business Review*
HEW	Department of Health, Education, and Welfare
HIAA	Health Insurance Association of America
HIP	Health Insurance Plan of New York
HIPPA	Health Insurance Portability and Accountability Act
HMO	Health maintenance organization
HSAC	Health Security Action Coalition
HSTPL	Harry S. Truman Presidential Library
ICHWA	Interdepartmental Committee on Health and Welfare Activities
IES	Insurance Economics Society
IJHS	*International Journal of Health Services*
ILGWU	International Ladies Garment Workers' Union
ILRR	*Industrial and Labor Relations Review*
IRD	Industrial Relations Department (NAM)
JAH	*Journal of American History*
JAMA	*Journal of the American Medical Association*
JHPPL	*Journal of Health Politics, Policy, and Law*
JNMA	*Journal of the National Medical Association*
LBJPL	Lyndon Baines Johnson Presidential Library
MBA	Mutual benefit association
MLR	*Monthly Labor Review*
MMFQ	*Milbank Memorial Fund Quarterly*
MSA	Medical savings account
NAACP	National Association for the Advancement of Colored People
NABSP	National Association of Blue Shield Plans
NAM	National Association of Manufacturers
NEC	National Education Campaign (1950)
NEJM	*New England Journal of Medicine*
NFIB	National Federation of Independent Business
NICB	National Industrial Conference Board
NMA	National Medical Association
NPC	National Physicians Committee
NRPB	National Resources Planning Board
NWLB	National War Labor Board
NYT	*New York Times*
OASI	Old Age Security Income (Social Security pensions)
OH	Oral history

PCHCA	Physician's Committee for Health Care for the Aged
PCHNN	President's Commission on the Health Needs of the Nation
PHS	Public Health Service
PNHP	Physicians for a National Health Program
POF	President's Official File (Roosevelt and Truman papers)
PPF	President's Personal File (Roosevelt and Truman papers)
PSF	President's Secretary's File (Roosevelt and Truman papers)
RNC	Republican National Committee
SCHIP	State Children's Health Insurance Plan
SHSW	State Historical Society of Wisconsin
SSA	Social Security Administration
SSB	Social Security Board
SSC	Secretary's Subject Correspondence (HEW Records)
SSF	Secretary's Subject Files (HEW Records)
UAW	United Auto Workers
UAW-SSD	United Auto Workers Social Security Department
UCR	Usual, customary, and reasonable (billing)
UMW	United Mine Workers
USCCR	United States Commission on Civil Rights
USW	United Steel Workers
VA	Veterans Administration
WBGH	Washington Business Group on Health
WFM	Western Federation of Miners
WHCF	White House Central File (Nixon and Johnson papers)
WHSF	White House Special File (Nixon Papers)
WMD	Wagner-Murray-Dingell bill
WSJ	*Wall Street Journal*

DEAD ON ARRIVAL

Introduction

Why No National Health Insurance in the United States?

W HY, alone among its democratic capitalist peers, does the United States not have national health insurance? This question, or variations of it, has invited a range of replies, some focusing on specific historical episodes, others invoking broad political or cultural or economic explanations for the peculiar trajectory of American social policy. At the same time, the explanatory laundry list is profoundly unsatisfying. Historical accounts often have trouble climbing from narrative to explanation; little of the episodic scholarship on the failure of health reform contributes to our larger sense of the American welfare state and its limits. And theoretical accounts often stumble on the descent to historical context; the debate between state-centered and economic explanations, for example, rests largely on abstractions (capitalism, industrialism, democracy) that are neither unique to the American setting nor offered in such a way that they make sense in specific historical contexts.[1] In explaining this hole in the American welfare state, we must consider both the relative success of other American social programs during the years in which health insurance was beating at the door and, at least implicitly, the relative success of health insurance in other national settings. Our understanding of the politics of American health care must explain both the exceptional character of the American welfare state and the distinct trajectory of health policy within it. And we must consider the absence of national health insurance in light of public support for reform. As one observer asks: "In effect a powerful army sits before an undefended goal but fails to move. Why?"[2]

The answer rests on the privileged status enjoyed by economic interests in American politics. In health politics, the nature and the alignment of economic or class interests defy easy theoretical categorization. In some respects, the health debate reflects the larger confrontation between labor and capital: employers and insurers have drawn on their control over private investment and economic growth and their com-

---

[1] Ira Katznelson, "Rethinking the Silences of Social and Economic Policy," *Political Science Quarterly* 101:2 (1986): 307–325.

[2] Daniel Greenberg, "National Health Insurance—Forever Imminent?" *NEJM* 293:9 (28 August 1975): 461.

mand of day-to-day political resources to shape public policy. At the same time, the uneasy relationship between health provision and private production has often confounded expectations and found labor clamoring for private coverage or employers looking to public solutions. In turn, doctors—the most prominent "health interest"—derive their status less from control over "production" than from their social origins, professional training, professional organization, and impressive command of political resources. And attention to conventional class forces tends to obscure the reasons why the United States is alone among its democratic capitalist peers in resisting national health care. For these reasons, I trace the influence of doctors, employers, insurers, and others less as *structural* interests whose mere presence discourages reform than as *instrumental* interests whose political stakes and political clout (vis-à-vis the state or each other) are unique to the American setting.[3]

The clout of private interests has been magnified in health politics—the only arena of social provision in which private providers, private consumers, and private intermediaries were well ensconced before national reforms were contemplated. This circumstance exaggerated the influence of economic interests and their stakes in reform. The ability and willingness of economic interests to shape health policy eroded an already fragile sense of universal social provision and encouraged the growth of private, employment-based benefits as an alternative. Such alternatives, in turn, reflected and reinforced long-standing patterns of racial and sexual discrimination in such a way that, over time, even reformers rarely challenged the family-wage or Jim Crow premises of private and public social policy. I am interested, in this sense, both in the influence of health interests over the course of the twentieth century and in the consequences of that influence in public and private patterns of health provision, the politics and political culture of health policy, and the broader limits and dilemmas of the American welfare state.

Competing Explanations

Some explanations for American health policy tackle the "why no health insurance" question head on; others collapse health policy into the larger development of the American welfare state; still others offer essentially descriptive explanations in the course of narrating a particular epi-

---

[3] Robert Alford, *Health Care Politics: Ideological and Interest Group Barriers to Reform* (Chicago, 1976), 13–17; John Myles and Adnan Turegun, "Comparative Studies in Class Structure," *Annual Review of Sociology* 20 (1994): 110–11; Vicente Navarro, *Medicine under Capitalism* (New York, 1976), 138–43.

sode or debate. These explanations, in turn, employ a variety of comparative, narrative, and theoretical approaches: some draw loosely on the theoretical literature in order to make sense of historical events; others draw loosely on the historical literature in order to advance theoretical claims about American political development. My own interests and purposes lie somewhere in between. I recognize the importance of building theoretical bridges between academic disciplines and across national boundaries, but I also recognize the difficulty of fitting a past reconstructed from primary sources into neat theoretical boxes. In exploring this scholarship, I am less interested in building up and knocking down straw figures than in scavenging for insights and suggesting the constraints and limits of other explanations. Broadly speaking, these explanations fall into three categories, each of which—in its own way—touches upon the particular absence of health insurance and the broader exceptionalism of the American experience.

The Liberal or Pluralist View

Perhaps the most persistent explanation for health care exceptionalism is the liberal or pluralist view. In this view, the welfare state is a response to the demographic, economic, and political demands of industrialization—reflecting not the demands of labor or capital, but a brokered consensus. This view attributes the failures of health reform in the United States to a popular or cultural faith in private solutions and a corresponding distrust of "radical" political solutions. The United States lacks national health insurance, as Eli Ginzburg argues, because such a policy "runs counter to long-standing American attitudes towards government and deep-seated beliefs . . . in the efficacy of market solutions to social problems." In contrast to Britain and Canada and others, the United States boasts "a more fragmented polity, a fluid class structure, and a narrower range of ideological debate." Such explanations generally assume that the American people were naturally receptive to the arguments made by opponents and naturally leery of those made by reformers. As Daniel Fox argues, the latter undermined their chances by refusing to compromise on "practical" or piecemeal reforms and polarizing the debate in such a way that "arguments about proper policy were conducted as holy wars."[4] And such explanations generally dismiss

---

[4] James Morone, *The Democratic Wish: Popular Participation and the Limits of American Government* (New York, 1990), 257–65; Paul Starr, *The Social Transformation of American Medicine* (New York, 1982); Monte Poen, *Harry Truman versus the Medical Lobby* (Columbia, Mo., 1979); Daniel M. Fox, *Health Policies, Health Politics: The British and American Experi-*

the "why no national health insurance" question as irrelevant or ahistorical, preferring instead to focus on the incremental reforms enacted in its place.[5]

There are a number of problems with this view. It often takes for granted the causal importance of ideas and language. Although charges of socialized medicine and the like shaped and chilled social policy debates, scholars too often exaggerate the sincerity of such ideas, underplay the ways in which they were contested, and ignore the ways in which opponents of reform were able to turn liberal politics to conservative ends.[6] Indeed, the American welfare state has been constructed on quite elastic cultural grounds: much of our current policy would be considered beyond the pale by nineteenth-century standards, just as the contemporary backlash might seem an unusual retreat from the vantage of 1948 or 1968. Reliance on "liberal values" to explain the absence of national health insurance cannot account for either the parallel success of other social programs or the failure of health insurance despite persistent popular support.[7] Finally, this view is largely indifferent to the material advantages and political institutions that privilege some ideas over others. Other countries with professional medical associations and liberal political cultures, after all, emerged from the middle years of the twentieth century with some form of national health insurance. The influence of the American Medical Association (AMA) and others in the American setting reflected not the natural resonance of their message but the immense resources that they brought to bear on politics and public debate.[8]

---

ence, 1911–1965 (Princeton, N.J., 1986), 11–14, 47–51, 79–83, 89–93 (quoted at 3–4, 51). For a critical summary of this view, see Walter Korpi, "Power, Politics, and State Autonomy in the Development of Social Citizenship: Social Rights during Sickness in Eighteen OECD Countries since 1930," *American Sociological Review* 54 (1989): 311–12; Ginzberg quoted in Vicente Navarro, "Why Some Countries Have National Health Insurance, Others Have National Health Services, and the United States Has Neither," *IJHS* 28 (1989): 383–84.

[5] Daniel M. Fox, "The Decline of Historicism: The Case of Compulsory Health Insurance in the United States," *BHM* 57 (1983): 609.

[6] Robert Westbrook, "Fighting for the American Family: Private Interests and Political Obligation in World War II," in *Power as Culture*, ed. T. J. Jackson Lears and Richard Wightman Fox (New York, 1993): 135–60; Gary Gerstle, "The Protean Character of American Liberalism," *American Historical Review* 99:4 (1994): 1045–47.

[7] Katznelson, "Rethinking the Silences of Social Policy," 310; Sven Steinmo and Jon Watts, "It's the Institutions Stupid! Why Comprehensive National Health Insurance Always Fails in America," *JHPPL* 20:2 (1995): 331–32; Navarro, "Why Some Countries Have National Health Insurance," 383–35.

[8] Navarro, "Why Some Countries Have National Health Insurance," 384; David Wilsford, *Doctors and the State: The Politics of Health Care in France and the United States* (Durham, N.C., 1991): 84–117, 181–220.

The Institutionalist View

A state-centered or institutional account has recast our understanding of American exceptionalism by focusing on the autonomy and capacity of the state. Recognizing that American welfare policy diverged from that of its democratic peers *despite* common intellectual traditions and the shared experience of industrialization, the institutional account turns its attention to differences in political structure—arguing, most broadly, that the weakness of national political institutions and the absence of programmatic party competition after 1896 made it impossible for reformers to transform a relatively generous Civil War pension system into a lasting welfare state. This institutional vacuum invited private alternatives and enabled conservatives to use both a fragmented state and its attendant political culture to frustrate reform. Although this scholarship has focused on programs other than health policy, its implications for our understanding of the latter are clear: institutions matter, and the trajectory of social reform will usually reflect the capacity of those institutions to accommodate new demands. National health insurance, in this view, made little headway because "American political institutions are structurally biased against this kind of comprehensive reform."[9]

This view too has a number of problems. Most important, it dismisses or distorts the influence of economic interests. In part, this reflects an explanatory strategy that combines a devastating critique of crude Marxist state theory with an uncritical deference to traditional political history.[10] In part, this reflects an assumption that elements of political or institutional weakness are static background conditions—and not themselves consequences of the efforts of economic interests to shape or limit state power. And in part, this reflects an eagerness to interpret frustration

---

[9] Theda Skocpol, *Protecting Soldiers and Mothers: The Political Origins of American Social Policy* (Cambridge, Mass., 1992); Ann Orloff, "The Political Origins of America's Belated Welfare State," in *The Politics of Social Policy in the United States*, ed. Margaret Weir, Ann Orloff, and Theda Skocpol (Princeton, N.J., 1988), 37–80; Theda Skocpol and John Ikenberry, "The Political Formation of the American Welfare State in Historical and Comparative Perspective," *Comparative Social Research* 6 (1983): 91; Ann Orloff and Theda Skocpol, "Why Not Equal Protection? Explaining the Politics of Public Social Spending in Britain, 1900–1911, and the United States, 1880s–1920s," *American Sociological Review* 49 (1984): 728–29; Steinmo and Watts, "It's the Institutions Stupid!" 330–68 (quoted at 330); Theda Skocpol, "Is the Time Finally Ripe? Health Insurance Reforms in the 1990s," *JHPPL* 18 (1993): 536–37.

[10] Theda Skocpol, "Political Response to Capitalist Crisis: Neo-Marxist Theories of the State and the Case of the New Deal," *Politics and Society* 10 (1982): 155–201.

with political outcomes as evidence of the independence or autonomy of the state—rather than as a reflection of the diverse and often contradictory political demands made by different economic interests. Eagerness to "bring the state back in" is often accompanied by a tendency to usher all other factors out—a tactic that confuses the insight that "institutions matter" with the implausibility that "only institutions matter."[11] Institutionalists have accordingly retreated from a state-centered focus on administrative capacities to a broader, polity-centered consideration of the capacities of both state institutions and political interests.[12] But such assessments typically consider economic interests alongside all other potential political actors without any allowance for their disproportionate stake in political outcomes or their disproportionate command of political resources.

In turn, the institutionalist account underplays the influence of race and gender, and accommodates only their institutional reflections (the relative clout of women's organizations or the unusual congressional clout of southern Democrats, for example). Generally, this view acknowledges the important fact that some women worked for, and others were the target of, maternal health programs, but overlooks the ways in which private and public family-wage assumptions shaped the form and function and legitimacy of all aspects of social provision. Distinctions between deserving and undeserving recipients fragmented any sense of universalism even as they sought to create an entering wedge for state welfare. And the confinement of health care to either private consumption or workplace provision marked less an institutional distinction between public and private responsibility than the prevailing assumption that dependency on the state was a temporary interruption of, or unhappy alternative to, dependence on men.[13] Similarly, racial assumptions and interests were far more pervasive than the influence of southerners in Congress or the Democratic Party. While Southerners ensured that federal social policy not trespass on the deeply racialized political economy

[11] Jill Quadagno, "Theories of the Welfare State," *Annual Review of Sociology* 13 (1987): 118–25; Linda Gordon, "Gender, State, and Society: A Debate with Theda Skocpol," *Contention* 2:3 (Spring 1993): 143; Frances Fox Piven and Richard Cloward, *Regulating the Poor: The Functions of Public Welfare*, rev. ed. (New York, 1993): 433–40.

[12] Skocpol, *Protecting Soldiers and Mothers*, 47–54.

[13] Gordon, "Gender, State, and Society," 143–55; William Forbath, *Law and the Shaping of the American Labor Movement* (Cambridge, Mass., 1991): 25–29; Nancy Fraser and Linda Gordon, "Contract vs. Charity: Why Is There No Social Citizenship in the United States?" *Socialist Review* (1992): 45–46, 47, 52–53; Gwendolyn Mink, "The Lady and the Tramp: Gender, Race, and the Origins of the American Welfare State," in *Women, the State, and Welfare*, ed. Linda Gordon (Madison, Wis., 1990): 92–93, 99; Carol Pateman, "The Patriarchal Welfare State," in *Democracy and the Welfare State*, ed. Amy Gutmann (Princeton, N.J., 1988): 238–50.

of the South, the construction of the "deserving citizen" as a white male industrial worker was rooted in ideas and practices reaching far beyond sectional politics.[14]

Finally, the institutional account is peculiarly ill equipped to explain the divergent paths of health insurance and the other Social Security programs. In terms of raw administrative capacity (especially between 1935 and 1950), the employment-based programs that succeeded (pensions and unemployment insurance) effectively started from scratch, while the program that failed (health insurance) rested on a substantial and diverse foundation of private and public expenditures and programs (including the Veterans' Administration, the Children's Bureau, and extensive public health programs). Economic interests were willing to accommodate the socialization of pensions and unemployment insurance in 1935 but proved unwilling, largely because both private provision and private financing were at stake, to do the same for health insurance. The absence of national health insurance, in short, is precisely opposite the result one would expect from state-centered explanation of the late bloom of American social policy.

The Radical View

Radical scholars have explained American health policy (or its absence) as a reflection of class politics, stressing both the influence of economic interests and the relative weakness of the working class. In some versions, health policy simply reflects the instrumental or structural interests of capital, pressing medicine into a for-profit market mold or responding in a Bismarckian fashion to social unrest. In other versions, the United States is portrayed as a social democratic laggard, and the absence of national health insurance as yet another facet of the failure of socialism in the American setting. Such accounts typically incorporate a particularly damning portrait of both the AMA and the repressive liberalism of American political culture. In sharp contrast to the liberal view, radical scholars argue that politics have frustrated, rather than reflected, popular aspirations and values.[15]

---

[14] Eileen Boris, "The Racialized Gendered State: Constructions of Citizenship in the United States," *Social Politics* (Summer 1995); Robert Lieberman, "Race, State, and Inequality in the United States, Great Britain, and France" (unpublished, ms., 1999); Robert Lieberman, *Shifting the Color Line: Race and the American Welfare State* (Cambridge, Mass., 1998); Michael Brown, *Race, Money, and the American Welfare State* (Ithaca, N.Y., 1999).

[15] Korpi, "Power, Politics, and State Autonomy in the Development of Social Citizenship," 311–12; David Himmelstein and Steffie Woolhander, "The Corporate Compromise: A Marxist Interpretation of the American Health Care System," *Monthly Review* (May 1990): 22–23; Navarro, "Why Some Countries Have National Health Insurance," 383–404.

There is much to recommend this view. It is appropriately dismissive of claims about a liberal consensus or the conservatism of American workers, and it is attentive to the economic incentives and interests underlying both health politics and the institutional setting in which they have played out. But this view, like others, has its shortcomings. Such accounts are maddeningly vague as historical explanations, often relying upon functional or teleological assumptions about the behavior of capital or the goals of social policy.[16] Such accounts cannot explain why the American experience departs so markedly from that of its capitalist peers, except by falling back on an exceptionalist argument based on often-dubious causal and comparative premises.[17] And this view tends to collapse the politics of race and gender into the larger riddle of class politics, assuming that "natural" solidarities cut across historical divisions within the working class and obscuring the ways in which some workers proved the fiercest defenders of both the family wage and white privilege. Finally, this view underestimates the importance of diverse and often contradictory class interests. The driving force behind American health politics is not so much the political advantages enjoyed by health interests but the political disarray of those interests—especially when political solutions divided important constituencies or threatened to satisfy one at the expense of another. [18] Health interests shared a general contempt for state intervention and a common language for responding to its threat, but the state was also an arena in which they competed fiercely for political advantage and a tool they would not hesitate to use when it suited their purposes.

Speculations and Considerations

Although none of these explanations are entirely sufficient or satisfactory, this bathwater contains its share of babies and it makes little sense to discard it all. Ideas matter. Political choices are shaped, and often whittled away, by the ideological or linguistic tools at hand. Institutions matter. Political choices are often shaped, and in some cases created, by the political setting within which they play out. And interests matter.

---

[16] Skocpol, "Political Response," 155–67.

[17] Alan Dawley, "Farewell to American Exceptionalism: A Comment," in *Why Is There No Socialism in the United States?* ed. Jean Heffer and Jeanine Rovet (Paris, 1988): 311; Michael Zuckerman, "The Dodo and the Phoenix: A Fable of American Exceptionalism," in *American Exceptionalism? U.S. Working Class Formation in International Context,* ed. Rick Halpern and Jonathan Morris (New York, 1997): 14–35.

[18] Colin Gordon, "Why No Corporatism in the United States? Business Disorganization and Its Consequences," *Business and Economic History* 27:1 (1998): 29–46.

Political choices are peculiarly responsive to, and sometimes made directly by, those who command the lion's share of political and material resources. The question is not which of these explanations is the right one, but how they relate to one another. How can we construct an explanation in which causes can be distinguished from consequences and vice versa? How can we weave together a multicausal or multilayered account without overdetermining the outcome—without rendering the historical goal of national health insurance not only elusive but implausible? In the chapters that follow, I explore the twentieth-century health debate through a series of thematic narratives. This explanatory strategy is intended not only to draw out the importance of particular issues, arguments, and constraints over time but to avoid the tendency of chronological narratives to offer discrete and contingent explanations. I sketch the history of the health debate in chapter 1, an overview that serves as both a summary account of modern American health politics and a narrative baseline for the thematic chapters that follow.

The most direct and tangible consequence of interest-driven health policy, as I trace in chapter 2, was the growth of private benefits. The establishment of a private welfare state reflected the ability of employers to shape social policy and encouraged workers to turn from national political solutions to the promise of the bargaining table. I trace the rise (and fall) of the private welfare state and suggest the ways in which workplace benefits distracted, shaped, and trumped public programs. My goal here is to assess the experience of private social policy, plumb the motives of business and labor as they bargained over the terms and scope of private social provision, and suggest the ways in which private benefits not only filled a gap in the famously backward American welfare state but also undermined the pursuit of universal benefits and directed social policy away from those who needed it the most.

As private benefits emerged as a surrogate for public policy, health policy was distorted and distracted by the emergence of a peculiarly American system of social insurance. As I argue in chapter 3, reformers and opponents alike tried to fit health insurance into a social insurance mold despite the fact that health care was not simply an extension of the employment relationship, and could not be plausibly organized around the idea of "contributory" entitlement. In turn, the boundaries of social policy debated through the early decades of the century—some reflecting the efforts of reformers to get a foot in the door, some reflecting the efforts of conservatives to close the door—gradually hardened into distinctions between deserving and undeserving citizens, and between employment-based contributory programs and stigmatized public assistance. Chapter 4 expands upon this by tracing the broader political culture of the health debate, including the famously hysterical antiradicalism of the AMA and others, the ritual demonization of other national health systems, and the profound (if often contradictory) influence of market assumptions on health provision and politics.

Doubts about universal provision and fascination with the contributory principle reflected and reinforced broader limits to the very notion of social citizenship in the United States. Perhaps the most fundamental of these limits, as I suggest in chapter 5, was race. From the earliest considerations of national health policy, race was a central, if often unspoken, consideration. Racial assumptions shaped health policy in part because they shaped local and national understandings of public health. White southerners shaped national health policy by maintaining segregated professions and institutions, and by digging in (in national and state politics) against public programs that threatened to upset Jim Crow. In turn, African Americans and Latinos were largely left behind by job-based social insurance and half-heartedly targeted (and whole-heartedly stigmatized) by penurious and locally administered social assistance programs.

Gender shaped the health insurance debate as well, and although the United States was clearly not exceptional in this regard, the combination of national political weakness and private provision did affect American women and men in exceptional ways—especially in the persistent distinction between private contractual benefits organized around a family-wage ideal and public charitable benefits aimed at women and children. In the former, women are considered dependents, and even working women have claimed only token citizenship in the private welfare state. Such assumptions shaped the ways in which women participated—as reformers and as recipients—in the development of American social policy. I come back to the deeply gendered premises of health provision at a number of points: in chapter 2, I suggest the ways in which private coverage both sorted beneficiaries by gender and incorporated the ideology of the family wage; in chapter 3, I suggest the ways in which the politics of social insurance were imbued with the logic of the family wage, and the ways in which maternalism—as a strategy for identifying "deserving citizens"—served as both an opportunity and an obstacle; in chapter 4, I suggest the ways in which the broader political culture of health care was organized, in part, around the idea that public coverage threatened masculine independence.

In chapter 6, I turn to patterns of influence in health politics, devoting particular attention to the shifting terms of a corporate compromise among employers, doctors, and insurers. Although the motives and relative influence of these interests changed over time, their ability and willingness to shape health policy proved distressingly consistent. This chapter offers both a case study of the close relationship between economic and political power in the United States and an explanation for the limits of health politics outlined in the other chapters. The flip side of this story, of course, is that reform interests—working through the state, the Democratic Party, professional associations, and the labor movement—were weak and fragmented. In chapter 7, I show how reformers were persistently outmaneuvered and outspent by their opponents, and how this monotonous disadvantage whittled reform initiatives down to a pattern of incremental change and half-hearted compromise. In this respect, the history of health policy underscores the importance of economic interests in American politics, not only for their direct influence in particular reform episodes but for their ability to maintain an institutional setting that invited their influence and discouraged others.

Though teased out separately, these themes—the emergence of a private welfare state, the politics and political culture of social insurance, the intersection of race and social policy, the influence of health interests, the disarray of reform interests—are closely intertwined. The political clout of economic interests reflected both immediate and relative material advantages and their ability, over time, to undermine social democratic organization and the emergence of autonomous state interests. The elaboration of health care's corporate compromise not only drove health provision away from the state and into private bargaining, but also justified that choice by leaning heavily on the political, intellectual, and psychological framework of social insurance. Private bargaining, in turn, was shaped by the influence of race and gender both on labor markets and on the peculiarly American construction of social citizenship. Labor's notorious voluntarism underscored the ability of economic interests to turn the state against labor (and labor against the state), and the invocations to "manly independence" and "whiteness" woven through the history of American trade unionism. And the very necessity of distinguishing between the deserving and the undeserving in a climate of less-than-universal provision reflected the unwillingness or inability of labor and others to pursue broadly social democratic alternatives.

1

The Political Economy of American Health Care: An Overview, 1910–2000

THE contours of the American health debate emerge most clearly in six historical moments. Between 1915 and 1920, Progressive reformers pressed unsuccessfully for state legislation mandating health insurance for industrial workers. In 1934–35, architects of Social Security toyed with the inclusion of health coverage alongside pension, unemployment, public assistance, and public health programs. In the next decade, New Dealers floated various proposals for adding health coverage, an effort that ultimately failed in 1949. After 1949, reformers retreated to the idea of offering coverage to those already eligible for Social Security, an effort that won the passage of Medicare and Medicaid in 1965. Almost immediately, the question of more expansive coverage became entangled with spiraling costs and the competitive implications of employment-based coverage. Such concerns shaped the last two episodes in reform: a tug-of-war between the Nixon administration and congressional liberals in the early 1970s, and the debacle of the Clinton proposal twenty years later.

Health Care and the Search for Order, 1910–1933

From 1914 to 1920 the American Association for Labor Legislation (AALL) promoted a model state bill for employment-based sickness insurance. Like other Progressives, AALL reformers were primarily interested in the impact of industrialization; they proposed insuring wages lost due to illness rather than the costs of care and confined their attention to industrial employees earning less than $1,200 a year. The AALL bill was introduced in three state legislatures in 1916 and eleven more in 1917; it came close to adoption in New York (where it passed the Senate but not the Assembly) and it was defeated by referendum in California in 1918. The AALL attracted a peculiar array of support and opposition. The American Medical Association initially blessed it, although many state medical societies were leery and the support of organized medicine would not last. Although the AALL plan echoed notions of efficiency championed by some business interests, it was condemned by all the important business associations. And while many union locals and state federations threw themselves behind the plan, the leadership of the American Federation of Labor (AFL) dismissed it. Most important, the plan was scored by the insurance industry, largely because it threatened to displace the lucrative market in private burial insurance.[1]

The debate was sharpened by American's entry into the war in 1917. Reformers drew upon the dismal rate of draft deferrals and suggested that "our *laissez faire* industrial policy has been at least partly responsible for the fact that half of our young men cannot qualify physically when the army calls." Opponents countered that health insurance was "a dangerous device, invented in Germany, announced by the German emperor from the throne the same year he started plotting and preparing to conquer the world." By 1919, opponents had largely succeeded in portraying health reform (in the words of one New York doctor) as "Un-American, Unsafe, Uneconomic, Unscientific, Unfair, and Unscrupulous" and attributing its support to "Paid Professional Philanthropists, busybody Social Workers, Misguided Clergymen and Hysterical Women."[2]

As the AALL effort faltered, Progressives did win the passage of a federal initiative in maternal health, the Sheppard-Towner Act of 1921. While the AALL proposals were shaped by concern for the productivity and security of male breadwinners, maternal health programs were shaped by a maternalist strain of social intervention that aimed to both mother the poor and Americanize them. Unlike the social insurance programs floated by the AALL, maternal health coverage (in the eyes of opponents) also threatened to undermine the family wage by allowing

[1] John Andrews, "Progress towards Health Insurance" (1917), reel 62, American Association for Labor Legislation [AALL] Papers (microfilm), Ronald Numbers, "The Specter of Socialized Medicine," in *Compulsory Health Insurance: The Continuing American Debate,* ed. Ronald Numbers (Westport, Conn., 1982), 5–6; "Report of the Committees on Social Insurance" (1918), reel 63, AALL Papers.

[2] Forrest Walker, "Compulsory Health Insurance: 'The Next Great Step in Social Legislation,' " *JAH* 56 (1969): 290–304; Ronald Numbers, "The Third Party: Health Insurance in America," in *The Therapeutic Revolution: Essays in the Social History of American Medicine,* ed. Charles Rosenberg and Morris Vogel (Philadelphia, 1979), 177–81 (N.Y. doctor quoted at 180); "Memorandum re Doctors" (1918), reel 63, AALL Papers; Testimony of Arthur Broughton (1916), reel 62, AALL Papers; "Standards of Sickness Insurance," (1914), reel 62, AALL Papers; Charles Mayo [AMA] address (1917), reel 62, AALL Papers; "Business Men on Health Insurance," *Survey* 37 (24 Feb. 1917); "The National Civic Federation on Compulsory Health Insurance" handwritten notes, Box 209, Edwin Witte Papers, State Historical Society of Wisconsin [SHSW], Madison, Wis.; Ronald Numbers, *Almost Persuaded: American Physicians and Compulsory Health Insurance, 1912–1920* (Baltimore, 1978); "The Draft and Health Insurance," *Survey* 39 (2 Mar. 1918): 608.

the state to displace the father. Sheppard-Towner counted uneven success. Funds were limited, and (at the insistence of organized medicine) Congress appropriated money for public health education but not the provision of care. Still, in many settings local health activists accomplished a great deal with limited resources and beneath the professional radar of the medical associations. But conservatives hammered away at the program through the 1920s, eroding federal appropriations and undermining state participation. Supporters went back to Congress in 1926 but won only a two-year funding extension that phased out the entire program in 1929.[3] Beyond Sheppard-Towner, the 1920s saw no significant health reform proposals. Republican administrations pressed voluntarist solutions through organizations like the American Child Health Association or events like the 1930 White House Conference on Child Health and Protection and otherwise devoted their attention to an ultimately futile effort to reorganize federal health programs around a new Public Health Service (PHS). Private foundations took the lead in efforts to address issues of public health, research, and access to health services. Doctors only sporadically conceded the limits of private medicine and offered no meaningful solutions.[4]

While political attention waned, the problems identified by Progressive reformers and public health officials did not go away. Opponents argued that voluntary solutions be given a chance, but private coverage was paltry. As other welfare capitalist programs flourished, employers rarely offered work-based medical coverage. Insurance offered by commercial insurers, fraternal orders, firms, and trade unions touched only a fraction of the population and, as one observer noted in 1917, "the great mass of the poorly paid workers are in large measure automatically shut out." Insurers viewed the moral hazard of individual coverage as insurmountable and insisted that "assurance of stipulated sum during sickness can only safely be transacted, and then only in a limited way, by fraternal organizations having a perfect knowledge of and complete

[3] Douglas Parks, "Expert Inquiry and Health Care Reform in New Era America: Herbert Hoover, Ray Lyman Wilbur, and the Travails of the Disinterested Experts" (Ph.D. diss., University of Iowa, 1994), 90–94; "House Amendments" (21 Nov. 1921), Box 233, Central File, 1921–1924, and "Extension" files (1930–1932), Box 422, Central File, 1929–1932, both in RG 102, Records of the Children's Bureau, National Archives, College Park, Md.; Molly Ladd-Taylor, *Mother-Work: Women, Child Welfare, and the State, 1890–1930* (Urbana, Ill., 1994), 167–90; Robyn Muncy, *Creating a Female Dominion in American Reform, 1890–1935* (New York, 1991), 93–157.

[4] Parks, "Expert Inquiry and Health Care Reform," 22–193; James Rorty, "The Case of John A. Kingsbury," *The Nation* 142 (24 June 1936); "Health Insurance," *BMSJ* 193:12 (17 Sept. 1925): 577–78.

supervision over the individual members." Although (as one observer noted of New York City alone) there were "literally thousands of petty health insurance funds," these routinely failed through adverse selection or employed "numerous masked technicalities" to avoid paying benefits. And such coverage was not really health insurance, but a combination of wage replacement and death benefits; this was "not a provision for a rainy day," as one reformer lamented, "but a provision for meeting a single contingent expense, viz, the cost of burying the dead."[5] Not surprisingly, there remained a close correlation—measured by per capita doctor's visits, hospitalization, immunization, or any of the conventional mortality indices—between income and access to health. In spite of sliding-scale fees and an oft-cited tradition of charity care, nearly one-half of those who earned less than $2,000 a year received no care of any kind. Of the $3,565 million spent on care annually (1929 figures), over 80 percent was spent directly by patients, about 15 percent by governments, and the rest by philanthropies and private industry.[6]

The wage and productivity losses cited by the AALL and others increasingly paled beside the rising costs of care—prompting reformers and academics to put together a Committee on the Costs of Medical Care (CCMC) to study the problem. Between 1928 and 1932 the CCMC published no fewer than twenty-seven book-length research reports, five of which detailed and applauded experiments in cooperative medicine or group practice. Although the CCMC promised to "refrain from arriving at conclusions regarding remedy," many of its members were determined to build a case for group insurance. In the CCMC's early deliberations, battle lines emerged between medical and reform interests. Its final report, which cautiously endorsed group practice and prepayment, was accompanied by a blistering minority report (signed by eight doctors) that condemned any departure from individual, fee-for-service practice. The CCMC reports (published in the depths of the Depression) had little impact, except as a warning shot across the bow of both organized medicine and the New Deal.[7]

---

[5] U.S. Department of Labor, *Proceedings of the Conference on Social Insurance*, Bureau of Labor Statistics Bulletin 212 (Washington, D.C., 1917), 540; Edgar Sydenstriker, "Existing Agencies for Health Insurance in the United States," in *Proceedings of the Conference on Social Insurance*, 430, 433, 438–52, 470–71; Rufus Potts, "Joint-Stock Company Health Insurance," in *Proceedings of the Conference on Social Insurance*, 512–15.

[6] Paul Starr, *The Social Transformation of American Medicine* (New York, 1982), 242; CCMC, *Medical Care for the American People* (Chicago, 1932), 6–9, 14.

[7] Starr, *Transformation of American Medicine*, 258–64; "American Association for Labor Legislation" (1940?), reel 63, AALL Papers; Parks, "Expert Inquiry and Health Care Reform," 203–9, 284–394; CCMC, *Medical Care for the American People*, 44–55; "Provision of

What Kind of Welfare State? Health Care and the New Deal, 1934–1945

The Depression recast the politics of health, both by challenging the charity tradition among financially strapped providers and by introducing an array of federal health programs.[8] The idea of national health insurance resurfaced during the 1934–35 debate over Social Security. Armed with the CCMC research and Depression conditions, the Committee on Economic Security (the administration's task force on social security legislation) initially viewed health insurance not just as "equally important" (alongside pensions and unemployment insurance) but as "the most immediately practicable and financially possible form of economic security." For the CES, the logic of national health insurance was unassailable. Private insurance was "totally inadequate to meet the needs of the population and [held] no promise of being much more effective in the near future."[9] At the same time, national health insurance would (unlike other Social Security programs) simply rearrange private expenditures and accomplish universal coverage with little public burden.[10] The CES proposed combining wage-loss and maternity benefits with a separate system of service benefits—all to be financed by a combination of payroll taxes and general revenues. This was a timid step for a nation which, as one reformer noted, boasted 1934 appropriations of under

Means for the Payment of Medical Care" (Nov. 1930), Box J8:6, Walton Hamilton Papers, Rare Books and Manuscripts, Tarlton Law Library, University of Texas, Austin, Tex.

[8] Roy Lubove, "The New Deal and Health," *Current History* 45:264 (Aug. 1963): 79–81; R. C. William, "The Medical Care Program for Farm Security Administration Borrowers," *Law and Contemporary Problems* 6:4 (Winter 1939): 583–89; Michael Grey, "Poverty, Politics and Health: The Farm Security Administration Medical Care Program, 1935–1945," *Journal of the History of Medicine and Allied Sciences* 44:3 (July 1989): 320–30.

[9] "Minutes of the Meeting of the Executive Committee" (27 Sept. 1934), Box 1, Committee on Economic Security [CES] Records, RG 47, Social Security Administration, National Archives; Witte to Epstein (28 Sept. 1934), Box 56, CES Records; Committee on Medical Care Meeting (26 Sept. 1934), and Executive Committee Meeting (27 Sept. 1934), both in Box 65, Witte Papers; "Plan for the Study of Economic Security" (1934), President's Official File 1086, Franklin D. Roosevelt Papers, Franklin D. Roosevelt Presidential Library [FDRPL], Hyde Park, N.Y.; *The Nation* 139 (12 Dec. 1934), 664; David Rothman, "A Century of Failure: Health Care Reform in America," *JHPPL* 18:2 (1993): 271–85; Daniel Hirshfeld, *The Lost Reform: The Campaign for Compulsory Health Insurance in the United States from 1932 to 1943* (Cambridge, Mass., 1970); CES, "Risks to Economic Security Arising out of Ill Health," Box 2, CES Records.

[10] "Preliminary Draft Abstract of a Program for Social Insurance against Illness" (1934), Box 2, CES Records; Medical Advisory Board [CES], Minutes of Meetings (29 Jan. 1935), p. 119, Box 67, Witte Papers; "Abstract of a Program for Social Insurance against Illness" (1935), pp. 83–85, Box 67, Witte Papers; CES, "Interim Report for Consideration at Meetings" (Jan. 1935), Box 5, CES Records.

$150,000 for the Women's Bureau, under $350,000 for the Children's Bureau, and over $400,000 for the eradication of hog cholera.[11]

But the CES retreated and ultimately proposed little more than scattered public health spending. By late 1934 CES staff observed glumly that "this Committee and the Administration have lost interest in the subject of health insurance." The CES was persistently anxious about the reaction of doctors and spent nearly as much time assuaging their fears as it did considering program details. CES staffers admitted privately that their reports were "weak on the question of provision for medical care," that "extreme care is necessary to avoid the organized opposition of the medical profession," and that "there is not a very great chance for the adoption of legislation at this Session on the subject."[12] When the time came to present the committee's final report, some CES members urged the inclusion of health insurance, hoping that by raising the issue they might lay the ground for future efforts. But those who feared that controversy over health insurance would doom the whole bill won out and the health title was dropped.[13]

The exclusion of health insurance in 1935 was softened by the promise of further study—a strategy endorsed by opponents seeking to stall reform, by politicians eager to express concern without confronting medical interests, and by reformers hoping to keep the issue alive. In 1936 the administration created an Interdepartmental Committee on Health

[11] Jennifer Klein, "Managing Security: The Business of American Social Policy, 1910s–1960" (unpublished ms., 2000), 261–62; CES, "Risks to Economic Security Arising out of Ill Health," Box 2, CES Records; CES Preliminary Reports (1935) in Box 6, CES Records; "Abstract of a Program for Social Insurance against Illness" (1935), pp. 90–94, Box 67, Witte Papers; Witte to Cohen (14 Dec. 1934), Box 17, CES Records.

[12] (Quote) Witte to Bruce (10 Dec. 1934), Box 2, CES Records; "Preliminary Report of the Committee on Economic Security" (1934), p. 9, Box 65, Witte Papers; Witte, "The Health Insurance Study of the Committee on Economic Security" (Dec. 1934), Box 5, CES Records; Medical Advisory Board, Minutes of Meetings (30 Jan. 1935), p. 220, Box 67, Witte Papers; "Preliminary Report of the Staff of the CES" (Sept. 1934), pp. 67–70, "Confidential Report of the Advisory Council" (18 Dec. 1934), and CES, "Report to the President" (Jan. 1935), all in Box 1 (Mss WP), Arthur J. Altmeyer Papers, SHSW; Starr, *Transformation of American Medicine*, 266–67; "Abstract of a Program for Social Insurance against Illness" (1935), pp. 49–50, Box 67, Witte Papers; *Report to the President of the Committee on Economic Security* (Washington, D.C., 1935), p. 6, Box 65, Witte Papers; Myers to Williams (1 May 1935) and "Suggestions for a Long-Time and an Immediate Program" (1934), both in Box 48, Harry Hopkins Papers, FDRPL.

[13] Edwin Witte, *The Development of the Social Security Act* (Madison, Wisc., 1963), 187–88; "Minutes of the Meetings of the Technical Board," Box 65, Witte Papers; Medical Advisory Board, Minutes of Meetings (29 Jan. 1935), p. 2, Box 67, Witte Papers; CES Minutes (4 Dec. 1934), p. 8, in Box 65, Witte Papers; Arthur J. Altmeyer, *The Formative Years of Social Security* (Madison, Wis., 1966), 57–58; Sydenstriker to Witte (24 Oct. 1934), Box 42:231, Series II, Isidore Falk Papers, Sterling Library, Yale University, New Haven, Conn.; Michael Brown, *Race, Money, and the American Welfare State* (Ithaca, N.Y., 1999), 31–47, 56–62.

and Welfare Activities (ICHWA) "to survey the whole range of government relationship to the health and medical care activities of the United States." Like the CCMC a decade earlier, the ICHWA became both an opportunity for reformers to make their case and a lightning rod for opposition. The ICHWA assumed widespread support for national health insurance, reiterated the argument that it would simply reorganize private spending, and sought to add health coverage to Social Security's social insurance (job-based) and social assistance (welfare) tracks.[14] In response, medical interests replayed their response to the CCMC, arguing that the Committee's findings had been "cooked" by a cadre of radicals. The administration was lukewarm, especially in the wake of the 1938 elections, and offered little more than increased federal hospital funding.[15] Reformers turned their attention to Congress and persuaded Senator Robert Wagner (D-N.Y.) to incorporate the ICHWA recommendations into what would, for the next decade, become an annual event: the Wagner-Murray-Dingell (WMD) health bill. First introduced in late 1939, WMD proposed to expand Social Security's public health and maternal health programs and launch new grant-in-aid programs to assist states with hospital construction, indigent care, and disability insurance. Although its congressional sponsors considered the 1939 bill little more than an opening gambit, reformers were optimistic. "Unless the United States is drawn actively into the war," wrote Michael Davis in late 1939, "legislative action on medical care, federally and in many states, seems certain to take place."[16]

[14] Memorandum Regarding the National Health Program (Dec. 1938), President's Secretary's File [PSF] 137, FDR Papers; Falk, "Report of the Technical Committee on Medical Care" (July 1938), Box 11, Decimal 025, Social Security Board [SSB] Records, Office of the Commissioner, SSA Records; "Report of the Technical Committee" (1938), and "Report and Recommendations on National Health by the Interdepartmental Committee to Coordinate Health and Welfare Activities" (1939) in *President's Annual Message on Health Security*, H. Doc. 120 (76/1: Jan. 1939); "A National Health Program," reprinted in *JAMA* 111:5 (30 July 1938): 432–54; Memorandum to the President Regarding the National Health Program (12 Oct. 1938), Box 11, Records of the Interdepartmental Committee to Coordinate Health and Welfare Activities [ICHWA], FDRPL; draft "The Nation's Health" (1938), Box 10, ICHWA Records; ICHWA, "Report and Summary" (Jan. 1939), Box 3, Altmeyer Papers; ICHWA, "Draft Report and Recommendations on National Health" (Jan. 1939), Box 5, Oscar Chapman Papers, Harry S. Truman Presidential Library [HSTPL], Independence, Mo.; Report of Proceedings before the ICHWA (18 July 1938), pp. 319–53, Box 29, ICHWA Records.

[15] Altmeyer, *Formative Years of Social Security*, 95–96, 117; Starr, *Transformation of American Medicine*, 276–77; Meeting of the Interdepartmental and Technical Committees (19 Dec. 1939), Box 3, Altmeyer Papers.

[16] Statement of Senator Wagner (28 Feb. 1939), Box 32, ICHWA Records; Falk to Roche (20 Dec. 1938), Box 11, Decimal 025, SSB Records, Office of the Commissioner, SSA Records; "Senator Wagner Introduces Health Program Legislation," *JAMA* 112:9 (1939): 846; "The Wagner Bill," *JAMA* 112:10 (1939): 999–1002; Falk, "Some Alternatives in the Health

World War II pushed the health debate in a number of directions, some unexpected, some contradictory. For reformers, the democratic rhetoric of the war, the federal role in wartime mobilization, and the index of national health provided by the draft hastened the urgency and possibility of national health insurance.[17] Reformers retooled the WMD bill as an "American Beveridge Plan" (after war-era British reforms) offering broader Social Security coverage, public employment offices, disability benefits, and health insurance.[18] Opponents drew very different conclusions, arguing that expansive welfare programs were the province of the war's fascist villains, that benefits could be provided through private employment, and that federal health programs should be confined to the especially deserving case of military service. Such mixed feelings were evident in the National Resources Planning Board 1942 report *Security, Work, and Relief Policies* (which argued that full employment might be sufficient social insurance) and in the administration, which publicly supported WMD but privately sought to dampen the enthusiasm of its proponents.[19] While WMD lay dormant, the war shaped health policy in other ways. War-era regulations clamped down on wage bargaining but allowed employers to offer insurance and pension benefits and granted such benefits favorable tax treatment. The result, although its importance was barely noted at the time, was a profusion of employment-based health insurance plans. In turn, a combination of long-standing deficiencies and exceptional wartime demands increasingly pressed the federal government to focus its attention and resources on hospital construction (the 1946 Hill-Burton Act) and coverage for veterans.[20]

Program" (5 Dec. 1939), Box 14, Decimal 026, SSB Records, Office of the Commissioner, SSA Records; Davis Memo (Dec. 1939), Box 140, Morris Cooke Papers, FDRPL.

[17] Senate Committee on Education and Labor, Press Release (4 Jan. 1945), President's Official File [POF] 103:2, FDR Papers; Senate Subcommittee on Wartime Health and Education, *Interim Report* (S. 74), Washington, D.C., 1944, pp. 1–2, 17–19; Draft: Social Security and Social Services (1943), PSF 165, FDR Papers; National Congress of Parents and Teachers to FDR (11 Oct. 1941), POF 1710:4, FDR Papers.

[18] Edward Berkowitz, *Mr. Social Security: The Life of Wilbur J. Cohen* (Lawrence, Kans., 1995), 51–52; "The Wagner-Murray-Dingell Social Security Plan," *JAMA* 122:9 (1943): 609; Rose Ehrlich and Michael Davis, "Four National Health Bills Compared" (Oct. 1945), Box 210, Witte Papers.

[19] Alan Brinkley, *The End of Reform: New Deal Liberalism in Recession and War* (New York, 1995), 154–64, 250–58; NRPB, "Security, Work and Relief Policies" (1942), POF 1092:6, FDR Papers; The Twentieth Century Fund, "A Postwar Budget for America" (1942), Box B:8 William Davis Papers, SHSW; Altmeyer to Corning (23 Feb. 1968); Altmeyer to Poen (10 Apr. 1957), Box 5 (Mss 400), Altmeyer Papers; Altmeyer to Rosenman (6 Sept. 1944); "Suggested Draft of President's Message on Social Security (25 Aug. 1942), Box 3 (Mss WP), Altmeyer Papers.

[20] Beth Stevens, "Complementing the Welfare State: The Development of Private Pension, Health Insurance and Other Employee Benefits in the United States" International Labour Office, Labour-Management Relation Series no. 65 (Geneva, 1986); Chamber of

The Postwar Moment: Public Policy and Private Alternatives, 1945–1950

In the flush of postwar optimism, the Truman administration threw its support behind WMD. The 1945 version offered grants for hospital construction and public health, indigent care, nationalized unemployment insurance, and social insurance health coverage—the latter financed by an 8 percent payroll tax. Congressional Republicans responded with a raft of alternatives, the most prominent of which was the Taft bill (after Ohio senator Robert Taft), which combined means-tested assistance with deference to medical control. Reformers were horrified both by the paucity of the Taft bill and by its direct threat (via the means test) to the principle of social insurance. At the same time, some reformers were distressed by an administration bill that fell far short, in their eyes, of "the simplicity, objectivity, and certainty" of national health insurance. Hearings opened to a combination of high drama and low comedy (Taft stormed out on the first day when his effort to raise the specter of socialized medicine was cut short), and the bill died quietly on the desks of the Senate Finance and House Ways and Means committees.[21]

Although the administration continued to work with congressional liberals after 1946, both also labored to make the endlessly redrafted WMD bill more palatable to medical conservatives by offering up paeans to patient choice and provider autonomy. Congressional Republicans persisted with spare, means-tested alternatives, which, as one observer noted, "leave the bulk of the population—the middle-income groups—as they find them, with little or no opportunity to get medical and hospital care at rates of payment within their own resources except as they may be pushed into the assistance group by the costs of expensive or chronic illness." And moderates in both parties floated compromises—including a version of the old AALL bill, the establishment of local nonprofit insurance pools, and subsidies for the purchase of private insurance.[22]

Commerce, *War Service Bulletin* (7 Oct. 1942), Box I:17, Chamber of Commerce Papers, Hagley Museum and Library, Wilmington, Del.; Edwin Amenta and Theda Skocpol, "Redefining the New Deal: World War II and the Development of Social Provision in the United States," in *The Politics of Social Policy in the United States*, ed. Margaret Weir, Ann Orloff, and Theda Skocpol (Princeton, N.J., 1988), 82.

[21] "The Wagner-Murray-Dingell Bill," *JAMA* 128:5 (1945): 369–72; Statement of Senator Wagner (19 Nov. 1945), Box 3, Altmeyer Papers; "The Taft-Smith-Donnel Bill," *JAMA* 133:12 (1947): 868; (quote) Rufus Miles to Elmer Staats (26 Nov. 1947), POF 419F, Box 1262, Harry S. Truman Papers, HSTPL; Falk to C. Winslow (31 Dec. 1946), Box 3, Decimal 11.1, Division of Research and Statistics, SSA Records; Monte Poen, *Harry Truman versus the Medical Lobby* (Columbia, Mo., 1979), 60–61, 88–90.

[22] "Statement by the President" (2 Sept. 1948), POF 103, Box 575, Truman Papers; Speeches and messages file, Box 3 (Mss WP), Altmeyer Papers; Poen, *Truman versus the*

The postwar debate ended in 1949 with an unprecedented flurry of lobbying and spending by medical interests. The AMA raised a war chest of over a million to fight the public relations battle and was largely successful in making health policy a theater of the cold war. But unlike the failures of 1915 or 1935, the 1940s debate was accompanied by important secular changes in the organization of medical care. Rather than simply being swept off the table, the battle for national health insurance was trumped by the emergence of private alternatives. Employment-based health insurance grew in response to the threat and reality of unionization, to federal incentives (especially during the war), and to the persistent failure of health legislation.[23]

Steady growth in private coverage distracted reform. In 1935 hospitalization, surgical, and medical insurance each covered about two million persons; by 1950 hospital insurance reached fifty-five million, surgical insurance reached thirty-nine million, and medical insurance reached seventeen million. Before the war, employment-based health plans were relatively rare (surveys found only fourteen such plans in 1926 and only forty-eight in 1939) but by the late 1940s over half of firms employing under 250 persons and over two-thirds of firms employing over 250 offered some form of health insurance. "History may show what that we saw this year was a race between social security developments under collective bargaining and under the Social Security Act," lamented Social Security pioneer I. S. Falk in 1949. "It may have been a great misfortune that the issues came to a head in coal and steel before Congress could complete action on [SSA] amendments." When the Truman administration deferred national health insurance to yet another committee for further study in 1952, it did so against the backdrop of an emerging corporate compromise in medical care. Future reform efforts would be pressed by the persistent inadequacy of care but reduced to mopping up around employment-based care, whether that meant giving employers incentives to offer coverage, making private insurance accessible to those who fell outside "insurable" employee groups, or picking up responsibility for those who were out of the private labor market altogether.[24]

Medical Lobby, 96, 98–99; (quote) J. Donald Kingsley to Sen. Elbert Thomas (20 May 1949), Box 211, Witte Papers; "Comparison of Three Major Health Bills," Box 211, Witte Papers; Ewing, FSA notes for State of the Union Address (31 Oct. 1947), POF 419F, Box 1262, Truman Papers; Starr, *Transformation of American Medicine,* 285.

[23] "Comparison of Three Major Health Bills," Box 211, Witte Papers; NPC, "Compulsion: The Key to Collectivism" (1949), p. 75, SHSW Pamphlets; "U.S. Medicine in Transition," *Fortune* 30:6 (Dec. 1944), 157; *BW* (11 July 1942), 17; *BW* (23 Apr. 1949), 114–15.

[24] (Quote) "Developments, Trends, and Outlook in Collective-Bargaining Welfare Plans" (Nov. 1949), Box 77:839, Series II, Falk Papers; "Position on National Health Insurance" (Jan. 1950) and Wood to Ewing (20 Jan. 1950), both in Box 45, Decimal 011.4, Federal Security Agency [FSA], Office of the Administrator, General Classified Files [GCF], 1944–

The Long Road to Medicare, 1950–1967

Although its mandate resembled that of the ICHWA a decade earlier, the 1952 President's Commission on the Health Needs of the Nation (PCHNN) never raised its sights above the task of mollifying the medical profession. Its report, released against the backdrop of the Korean War, had more to say about military preparedness than it did about health insurance, and its recommendations were modest: more hospital construction, more medical education, more "encouragement" of private plans.[25] This too, was the tone struck by the Eisenhower administration. Private insurance is "a sound and effective method of meeting unexpected hazards," argued the new president, "in the best tradition of vigorous and imaginative American enterprise." Or as one advisor put it more bluntly: "President Eisenhower is flatly opposed to the socialization of medicine and believes that the greatest bulwark against it is to be found in furthering the progress already made by voluntary health insurance plans." Although many Republicans accepted the basic premises of Social Security, their fiscal anxieties and close political relationship with organized medicine precluded serious consideration of health reform.[26]

Aside from dispensing funds for programs such as Hill-Burton, the administration's only foray into health policy was the idea of federal reinsurance of private health plans. Under such a program, the federal government would effectively insure the insurers, with the goal of securing existing coverage and encouraging insurers to offer policies to more marginal risks. Reinsurance would "demonstrate the concern of the Administration," hoped Health, Education, and Welfare (HEW) officials, "and at the same time, make clear the will of Congress that voluntary health insurance be the mechanism for helping the great bulk of our people to help themselves . . . thereby closing the gaps in voluntary cover-

---

1950), Records of the Department of Health, Education, and Welfare [HEW], RG 235, National Archives; Raymond Munts, *Bargaining for Health: Labor Unions, Health Insurance, and Medical Care* (Madison, Wis., 1967), 3–80; Health Insurance Statements, Box 57, Records of the President's Commission on the Health Needs of the Nation [PCHNN], HSTPL.

[25] Poen, *Truman versus the Medical Lobby,* 186–93; "Report of the PCHNN" (1952), Box 5, Decimal 011, GCF (1951–1955), HEW Records.

[26] (Quote) "Health Message—Jan. 24 Draft" (24 Jan. 1955), Box 235, Decimal 901, GCF (1951–1955), HEW Records; (quote) Chester Keefer to Anthony Novicki (22 Dec. 1954), Box 235, Decimal 901, GCF (1951–1955), HEW Records; Poen, *Truman versus the Medical Lobby,* 212–18; "Material for Meetings: Admin. Hobby's Advisory Committee" (Mar.–June 1953), Box 5 (Mss WP), Altmeyer Papers; Daniel Fox, *Health Policies, Health Politics: The British and American Experience, 1911–1965* (Princeton, N.J., 1982), 188–206; Alvin David, "Old-Age, Survivors, and Disability Insurance: Twenty-Five Years of Progress," *ILRR* 14:1 (Oct. 1960): 13–14.

age and making passage of a compulsory health insurance bill politically impossible." But the idea had few admirers. The very concession that reinsurance was necessary undermined assurances that private insurance could do the job. Many were leery of subsidizing private insurers when it seemed that "at the most, the bill might provide a motivation for some indemnity plans to extend their present benefits for longer periods and costlier ('catastrophic') illnesses—but at correspondingly higher premium costs." The proposal was even scorned by the very interests it aimed to please. The AMA was leery of a program so likely to fall short of expectations and invite further meddling. Commercial insurers, though interested in public subsidies, saw the precedent of federal intervention as too high a price.[27]

Reinsurance failed in 1954 and in 1956. The administration responded with a range of lesser initiatives (including federal insurance of hospital mortgages and tax incentives) but few, including those at HEW, took these proposals seriously. The hospital mortgage bill was drafted by officials at Kaiser (a company that had pioneered employment-based group practice plans at its West Coast shipyards in the 1940s), who had to plead with congressional staffers not to dub it the "Kaiser Bill." The AMA opposed the plan, fearing it would lead to more plans along the Kaiser model. And few saw much promise in tax incentive plans, arguing that there was "little or no tax-saving incentive for those in most need of protection" and that such plans would amount to "allowing public funds to be privately administered." Proponents acknowledged that any tax-based plan would secure existing coverage rather than expand it and worried that the "reinsurance bill and tax device, particularly if packaged together, could be charged as 'health for the wealthy.' "[28] As the administration toyed with these proposals, reformers devoted their attention to the prospect of adding health coverage for Social Security pensioners.

[27] Statement of Ovetta Hobby (11 Mar. 1954), Box 88, Henry J. Kaiser Papers, Bancroft Library, University of California, Berkeley; Bradshaw Mintener to Herbert Nelson (9 Nov. 1954), Box 235, Decimal 901, GCF (1951–1955), HEW Records; Poen, *Truman versus the Medical Lobby*, 210–11; (quote) Committee for the Nation's Health, "Health Service Prepayment Plan Reinsurance Act" (Mar. 1954), Box 67:654, Series II, Falk Papers; George McCoy to Nelson Rockefeller (2 Dec. 1954), Box 235, Decimal 901, FSA, Office of the Administrator, GCF (1951–1955), HEW Records; Edwin Faulkner, "Why Federal Reinsurance Is Not the Answer," *JAMA* 156:16 (1954): 1508.

[28] "Reinsurance of Health Service Prepayment Plans" (Apr. 1955), Box 9, Decimal 011, GCF (1951–1955), HEW Records; *BW* (6 Apr. 1957): 151; "Health Legislation" folder (1953), Box 77, and Coke to Calhoun (7 Feb. 1955), Box 165, Henry J. Kaiser Papers; (quote) Snyder to Murray (30 June 1949), Box 45, Decimal 011.4, GCF (1994–50); "Income Tax Allowance for National Health Insurance" (1949), Box 45, Decimal 011.4, GCF (1944–1950), and (quote) "Tax Exemptions" (9 Apr. 1954), Box 235, Decimal 901, GCF (1951–1955), HEW Records.

For some, this was another foot in the door strategy: by identifying an especially needy or deserving fragment of the population, they hoped to establish the precedent and practicality of public health insurance. For others, public responsibility for the health of retirees would supplement the norm of family-wage, employment-based provision. All agreed that the elderly were the one group that was at once in need of coverage, deserving of public assistance, and left behind by private insurance.[29]

Serious consideration of what would become Medicare began in the late 1950s, a point at which another decade of private insurance had failed to incorporate the elderly and both Democrats and Republicans were looking to the 1960 elections. The 1958 Forand bill promised a range of medical care to Social Security pension (Old Age Security Income, or OASI) beneficiaries, administered by either a federal agency or nonprofit Blue Cross plans and financed by a small increase in OASI taxes.[30] Though neither designed nor destined for passage in 1958, the Forand bill cut the template for the health debate of the early 1960s by confining its attention to post-employment hospitalization coverage. While the logic of extending health coverage to OASI recipients seemed straightforward, there remained confusion on a number of points. It was not clear whether health coverage fit the social insurance model—not only because health benefits followed medical need rather than past contributions but because, at least at the program's inception, the costs would be borne by current workers (tantamount to arguing, as Chicago Blue Cross director Robert Evans put it, that "every son should support a father, not necessarily his own"). Reformers hoped to trade on the popularity of Social Security's contributory programs; opponents argued for a means-tested alternative. In turn, it was not clear whether public retiree care was a boon or a threat to private insurance. Although insurers conceded privately that Forand would either pick up risks that private insurers had long avoided or relieve those who did offer post-65 coverage, most health interests (and the administration) worried that the pro-

[29] PCHNN, "Working Draft: Health of the Aging" (20 May 1952), pp. 2–3, Box 74, Witte Papers; Health Insurance Statements, Box 57, PCHNN Records; Oscar Ewing OH, pp. 195–96, HSTPL; PCHNN, "First Draft: Health of the Aging" (26 June 1952), pp. 2–3, 13–14, Box 74, Witte Papers; Witte to Falk (4 June 1952) and Witte to Breslow (6 July 1952), Box 74, Witte Papers; Wilbur Cohen, "Reflections on the Enactment of Medicare and Medicaid," *Health Care Financing Review,* Supp. (1985): 4; Edward Berkowitz, *America's Welfare State* (Baltimore, 1991), 164; Herman Somers and Anne Somers, *Medicare and the Hospitals: Issues and Prospects* (Washington, D.C., 1967), 6–7; Wilbur Cohen OH [85–59], p. 4, Lyndon Baines Johnson Presidential Library [LBJPL], Austin, Tex.; Edwin Witte, "Economic Aspects of the Health Problems of the Aging" (1952), Box 74, Witte Papers.

[30] Theodore Marmor, *The Politics of Medicare* (Chicago, 1970), 14–23, 31; "Background on Medical Care Needs of and Health Insurance for the Aged" (2 Dec. 1959), Box 225, Decimal 900.1, Secretary's Subject Correspondence [SSC], (1956–1974), HEW Records.

posal would "sound the death knell for voluntary effort in the field of basic hospitalization insurance for the aged" or (as the AMA put it) invite "the camel's nose of socialized medicine" inside the tent.[31]

The administration scrambled to offer something without retreating from its essential faith in private insurance and private medicine. Through 1958 and 1959, it considered a range of alternatives, including subsidies for private insurance, tax deductions for medical expenses or premiums, some form of catastrophic coverage, and a means-tested program of public coverage. Reformers were quick to point out the combination of limited coverage and administrative complexity inherent in all of these proposals, and even administration officials conceded privately that these were political and not practical alternatives. When the administration finally presented its Medicare response to congressional reformers in May of 1960, the proposal, as *Business Week* noted dryly, "set some sort of record for unpopularity."[32]

Through 1960 debate increasingly focused on the option of a state-based program of indigent care—essentially the same program floated by congressional Republicans in the 1940s. "After tossing the potato back and forth throughout 1960," one observer noted, "Congress, deciding that it was far too hot to handle in an election year, dropped it, and instead, passed the Kerr-Mills bill[,] which provided for welfare aid rather than an insurance program." Kerr-Mills raised the federal contribution to state programs for indigent care and established a new program of matching funds for medical assistance to the aged. For opponents of OASI-based coverage, means-testing promised to weed out those

[31] Robert Cunningham III and Robert M. Cunningham, Jr., *The Blues: A History of the Blue Cross and Blue Shield System* (De Kalb, Ill., 1997), 119; "Meeting with Consultant on Health Insurance" (20 Nov. 1959), Box 225, Decimal 900.1, SSC (1956–1974), HEW Records; "Comments on Budget Bureau Analysis" (Dec. 1959), Box 225, Decimal 900.1, SSC (1956–1974), HEW Records; "Notes on the Forand Bill" (9 Feb. 1960), Box 1, Part I, Series I, Records of the United Auto Workers Social Security Department [UAW-SSD], Archives of Labor History and Urban Affairs, Wayne State University, Detroit, Mich.; *BW* (16 Apr. 1960), 184; "Tomorrow's Meeting on Health Care for the Aged" (17 Nov. 1959) , Box 225, Decimal 900.1, SSC (1956–1974), HEW Records.

[32] "Tomorrow's Meeting on Health Care" (17 Nov. 1959) , Box 225, Decimal 900.1, SSC (1956–1974), HEW Records; Flemming to Folsom (10 Nov. 1959), Box 124, Decimal 900.1, Secretary's Subject Files [SSF] (1955–1975), HEW Records; "Consideration of Plan for 100% Tax Deduction" (Apr. 1960), Box 225, Decimal 900.1, SSC (1956–1974), HEW Records; "Summary of Alternatives" (21 Dec. 1959), Box 225, Decimal 900.1, SSC (1956–1974), HEW Records; "Replies," Box 51, Decimal 011, SSF (1955–1975), HEW Records; "Draft Cabinet Paper: Background on Medical Care Needs of and Health Insurance for the Aged (2 Dec. 1959), Box 225, Decimal 900.1, SSC (1956–1974), HEW Records; "Political implications of the Administration's activities" (4 Jan. 1960), Box 225, Decimal 900.1, SSC (1956–1974), HEW Records; "Inherent Defects . . ." (12 May 1960), Box 1, Part I, Series I, UAW-SSD; *BW* (21 May 1960), 200.

who could pay—an approach, as one HEW official put it, "likely to have the support of the insurance industry, and probably organized medicine and hospital associations." Although reformers objected to both state control and means testing, they found it difficult to attack a program whose benefits (if only for the indigent) were more expansive than those offered by Forand. It was a compromise, as the *Nation* concluded, which "smelled of political expediency." And it was a compromise that did more to underscore the problem than to address it. "The blunt truth," as Senator Pat McNamara (D-Mich.), noted at the time, "is that it would be the miracle of the century if all the states—or even a sizable number—would be in a position to provide the matching funds to make the program more than just a plan on paper." By 1963 only thirty-two states had established Kerr-Mills programs, and five populous northern states claimed 90 percent of the federal matching funds.[33]

Despite anticipation of the election and the compromises cobbled together in its shadow, the politics of health did not change dramatically in 1961. The Kennedy administration embraced the "politics of growth" and the view that health provision was a responsibility best met by full employment. Congressional turnover in 1960 was not as dramatic as many had expected, and congressional efforts continued to be shaped by the choice between sending meaningful legislation to certain death in southern-dominated committees or settling for meager alternatives. Real progress would come only after a combination of social unrest and congressional turnover (in 1962 and 1964) made substantive reform necessary and possible. But even then health care was the stepchild of the Great Society; "at a time of expansive reform," Paul Starr has noted, "[reformers] continued to back a measure framed in the more conservative 1950s."[34] The administration supported a watered-down version (dubbed the King-Anderson bill after its congressional sponsors) that offered OASI coverage of hospital and nursing home costs financed by a small increase in Social Security taxes. But few saw any prospect of getting King-Anderson out of the hands of Ways and Means chair Wilbur Mills, and the administration proved willing to trade health reform for congres-

---

[33] (Quote) Richard Harris, "Annals of Legislation: Medicare," *New Yorker* (16 July 1966), 36; " 'Medicare,' the Cure That Could Cause a Setback," *Fortune* 67:5 (May 1963): 167; Berkowitz, *America's Welfare State*, 168–69; "Summary of Alternatives" (21 Dec. 1959), Box 225, Decimal 900.1, SSC (1956–1974), HEW Records; Marmor, *Politics of Medicare*, 34–37 (McNamara quote at 36).

[34] Gareth Davies, *From Opportunity to Entitlement: The Transformation and Decline of Great Society Liberalism* (Lawrence, Kans., 1996), 26–29; Ira Katznelson, "Was the Great Society a Lost Opportunity?" in *The Rise and Fall of the New Deal Order*, ed. Gary Gerstle and Steve Fraser (Princeton, N.J., 1989), 185–211; Brown, *Race, Money, and the American Welfare State*, 256; (quote) Starr, *Transformation of American Medicine*, 369.

sional cooperation on tax legislation in 1961 and a reciprocal trade bill in 1962. While some in Congress and the White House hoped to bring Mills around, the administration moved cautiously: in an effort to mollify fiscal conservatives and doctors, its 1963 proposal allowed for private intermediaries and retreated to basic hospitalization coverage. In turn, strategists in HEW and Congress toyed with tax incentives and federal subsidies that might make King-Anderson more palatable, but made little progress.[35]

Opponents, meanwhile, did what they could to derail reform—including an effort to cut off funding for King-Anderson by raising Social Security benefits and taxes. At stake, clearly, was not only the share of Social Security contributions necessary to fund Medicare but the relationship between the established pension program and the proposed medical program: reformers wanted to ride the popularity of Social Security, opponents wanted to portray medical coverage as a threat to its solvency. By late summer, Johnson's advisors concluded, "we should allow the proposed Social Security benefit increase to die, because if the increase becomes operative Medical Care is lost for all time." In the conference committee charged with sorting this out, House members held out for a benefit increase without medical coverage while the Senate conferees (working closely with the administration) voted to reject any bill that did not include Medicare. Mills conceded that many of his Democratic colleagues would have voted for the bill had it escaped committee, but that "they felt their chances for re-election would be enhanced if the bill did not come to the House floor and were preserved as an issue." In the White House, the electoral implications were even clearer. "I don't think *you* should be kicking Goldwater," one aide advised Johnson, "but this is a great opportunity for us to beat him to death among these older people if we play it right."[36]

[35] "1963 Legislative Program" (n.d.), Box 84, Joseph Califano Papers, LBJPL; Wilbur Cohen OH [72–26], p. 2:2; Marmor, *Politics of Medicare*, 39–49, 53–54; Jim Akin to the Secretary (17 Jan. 1962): Box 137, Decimal 011, SSC (1956–1974), HEW Records; "The 1962 Legislative Outlook," *The Nation* 194 (6 Jan. 1962), 12–13; Javits, "Health Care Insurance Act of 1964" (Jan. 1964), Box 5, Physicians Committee on Health Insurance for the Aged Papers, SHSW; Wilbur Cohen to Clinton Anderson (22 Dec. 1964), Box 292, Commissioner's Correspondence (1936–1969), HEW Records; Memorandum Re: Baker Proposal Regarding Deduction (July 1963), Box 166, SSC (1956–1974), HEW Records; Rashi Fein, *Medical Care, Medical Costs: The Search for a Health Insurance Policy* (Cambridge, Mass., 1989), 62.

[36] Ribicoff to LBJ (20 July 1964), White House Central File [WHCF] LE/IS 75, Lyndon B. Johnson Papers, LBJPL; Manatos to O'Brien (14 Aug. 1964), WHCF LE/IS 75, LBJ Papers; "1964 Legislative Program" (n.d.), Box 84, Califano Papers; Manatos to O'Brien (14 Aug. 1964), WHCF LE/IS 75, LBJ Papers; Wilson to O'Brien (20 Apr. 1964), Box 3, Office Files of Henry Wilson, LBJPL; Moyers to LBJ (2 Sept. 1964) WHCF LE/IS 75, LBJ Papers.

Legislative progress after 1964 was dramatic. A redrafted King-Anderson again focused on hospitalization in order to avoid the wrath of the doctors. The AMA responded with Eldercare, a more expansive but means-tested alternative. And other congressional and health interests offered numerous compromises. In previous sessions, this blizzard of options would have been enough to bury the issue. But at the urging of Wilbur Cohen and others, Mills assembled all of the proposals together into a single bill—the famous "three-layer cake" composed of Medicare Part A (OASI hospitalization insurance), Medicare Part B (voluntary, supplemental OASI coverage of doctor's charges), and Medicaid (an expansion of Kerr-Mills). By accommodating opponents' concerns, reformers won passage of a bill that was both enormously complex and "unassailable politically from any serious Republican attack."[37] The combination of coverage for the elderly and means testing buttressed private insurance by picking off its poorest risks. The federal government deferred day-to-day administration to private providers and intermediaries in such a way, as one critic noted, that it "surrendered direct control of the program and its costs." Doctors won the distinction between hospitalization and medical insurance, and pressed Congress and HEW to adopt a "usual, customary, and reasonable" (UCR) reimbursement policy that lifted the burden of charity care. Medicare and Medicaid marked an incremental victory and a larger defeat: by peeling off yet another fragment from the universal pool, it eroded much of the remaining sentiment for national health insurance; and by setting up the government as a third-party payer, it spurred an ongoing anxiety about health care costs that would press many to conclude that health care was simply too expensive to fix. In the eyes of Johnson's economic advisors, the "shotgun marriage" of 1965 was "politically astute" but also created a program that was "twice as difficult to administer as it needed to be" and "almost guaranteed [to be] highly inflationary."[38]

[37] Wilson, "1964 Legislative Proposals" (n.d.), Box 3, Office Files of Henry Wilson; "1965 Legislative Program" (n.d.), Box 84, Califano Papers; O'Brien to LBJ (27 January 1964), WHCF LE/IS 75, LBJ Papers; Wilbur Cohen, "Hospital Insurance for the Aged" (2 Mar. 1963), WHCF LE/IS 75, LBJ Papers; Fein, *Medical Care, Medical Costs*, 62–65; Marmor, *Politics of Medicare*, 59–68; Cohen, "Reflections on the Enactment of Medicare and Medicaid," 3, 9; James Malloy and David Skinner, "Medicare on the Critical List," *HBR* 62:6 (Nov.–Dec. 1984): 123; Berkowitz, *Mr. Social Security*, 227–38; "Mr. Mills's Elder-medi-bettercare," *Fortune* 71:6 (June 1965): 167; "Specifications for a Three Part Health Plan" (3/3/65), WHCF LE/IS 75, LBJ Papers.

[38] Report of the 1964 Task Force on Health (Nov. 1964), Box 1, Task Force Reports, LBJPL; (quote) Starr, *Transformation of American Medicine*, 375; "Mr. Mills's Elder-medi-bettercare," 166–67; "Medicare: The Major Defects," *The Nation* 200 (28 June 1965): 698; *BW* (17 Jan. 1970): 51; Theodore Marmor, "Coping with a Creeping Crisis: Medicare at Twenty," in *Social Security: Beyond the Rhetoric of Crisis*, ed. Theodore Marmor and Jerry Mas-

After 1965 the budgetary damage done by the war in Vietnam stalled innovation and imposed new fiscal pressures. The administration devoted little attention to new health programs and struggled to keep Medicare and Medicaid under control (Medicare ran well ahead of its projected costs, and the generosity of some states sent the federal share of Medicaid spiraling out of control). The administration toyed with the idea of "kiddycare," which would pull Social Security's maternal health (Title V) programs and Medicaid into comprehensive coverage for maternity and early childhood, but as a 1967 Health Task Force concluded, "rising costs and present budget constraints" kept it off the table. Increasingly, the administration floated little more than proposals to "extend expiring programs or recommend repackaging of existing laws" and focused its efforts on supply-side reforms (including "reimbursement incentives" and other alternatives to UCR billing) that might rein in health inflation and federal spending.[39]

Private and public health coverage continued to grow between 1950 and 1965, although it is difficult—given uneven reporting, overlapping coverage, and a bewildering array of group plans and forms of coverage—to offer anything but rough estimates. Hospitalization benefits for workers were, by the mid-1960s, matched by surgical and medical coverage, and all benefits were routinely extended to workers' dependents. Coverage by private hospitalization insurance grew from 49 percent of the workforce in 1950 to nearly 70 percent in 1965, surgical insurance grew from 35 percent to 65 percent, and basic medical coverage grew from 18 percent to over 60 percent. Virtually all of this growth occurred in employment-based group insurance pioneered by Blue Cross and Blue Shield and then picked over by commercial insurers.[40] Insurers contin-

---

haw (Princeton, N.J., 1988), 178–84; Fein, *Medical Care, Medical Costs,* 115; Sven Steinmo and Jon Watts, "It's the Institutions Stupid! Why Comprehensive National Health Insurance Always Fails in America," *JHPPL* 20:2 (1995): 350–53; Kermit Gordon OH, pp. 4:16–17, LBJPL.

[39] George Silver, "Recommended Maternal and Child Health Care Programs for Fiscal Year 1968" (Oct. 1966), Box 61, Califano Office Files, LBJPL; Walter Heller, "What Price Great Society?" (21 Dec. 1965), Confidential File WE 9, LBJ Papers; "Social Security Amendments of 1967," Box 51, Califano Office Files; Cater to LBJ (10 Sept. 1966), Box 15, Douglas Cater Office Files; LBJPL; Report of the 1965 Task Force on Health (Nov. 1964), Box 1, Task Force Reports, LBJPL; (quotes) Report of the 1967 Task Force on Health, Box 33, Califano Office Files, LBJPL; Califano to LBJ (1 Oct. 1965), Schultze to Califano (27 Sept. 1965), both in WHCF FG 364, LBJ Papers; Califano to Gardner (21 Aug. 1967), Box 33, Califano Office Files, Box 33; 1968 Task Force notes in Box 220, Gaither Office Files, LBJPL; (quote) HEW SSA Administrative History, Box 9, Part 18, p. 106, LBJPL.

[40] Margaret Klem, "Voluntary Medical Care Insurance," *AAAPSS* 273 (1951): 99; Louis Reed, "Employee Health Benefits Programs," *Public Health Reports* 72:12 (Dec. 1957): 1080; Brown, *Race, Money, and the American Welfare State,* 179–80; FSA, "Background Statement on Old-Age and Survivors Hospitalization Insurance" (25 June 1951), Box 211, Witte Papers;

ued to avoid "the aged, those employed in groups to small to be insured, the self employed, the rural population, the physically substandard, those uninsured because of termination of the insurance coverage, and certain dependents of insured persons." Access to group coverage remained more dependable for higher-income groups, and this advantage actually grew through the 1950s. Although private insurance reached nearly three-quarters of the population by 1964, it reached barely a third of those with incomes under $2,000 a year, barely half of those over sixty-five, and less than half of the nonwhite population. As a group-based employment benefit, health insurance echoed the disparities of private labor markets: it was most commonly claimed by salaried or unionized white male workers in northern industrial states. Before and after the reforms of 1965, rates of utilization, illness without medical attendance, and health expenditure continued to vary directly with income, occupation, race, and region.[41]

The costs and benefits of coverage varied widely, a problem routinely obscured, one observer noted, "by outpourings from the insurance carriers about the growing percentage of the population 'protected' by voluntary health insurance—where 'protected' means anything embraced by the ownership of any kind of health-insurance policy or certificate, however small or limited the insurance it provides." Nearly half of all private carriers in 1960 did not even meet the standards for membership in the Health Insurance Association of America (HIAA). Although rates of coverage grew steadily, the insured share of the nation's health bill grew more modestly. In 1950 insurance met only about 11 percent of health expenditures. This share doubled in the early 1950s but then grew more slowly, leveling off at about one-third in the mid-1960s. Indeed, when the AMA (in the shadow of Medicare) claimed that 65 percent of seniors were covered, critics were quick to point out how little such "coverage" meant. "I am reminded of the story about the horse-rabbit stew that was

Edmund Whitaker, "Experience of the Commercial Insurance Companies," in American Management Association, "Company Experience with Major Medical Expense," *Insurance Series* 105 (1954): 3–10; Chamber of Commerce, *Employee Benefits Historical Data, 1951–1979* (Washington, D.C., 1981), 27, 32; Clifford Staples, "The Politics of Employment-Based Insurance in the United States," *IJHS* 19:3 (1989): 425; Department of Labor, *Health, Insurance, and Pension Plans in Union Contracts,* Bulletin 1187 (1955); NICB, "Trends in Company Group Insurance Programs," *Studies in Personnel Policy* 159 (1957): 8–12.

[41] Anne Somers, "Some Basic Determinants of Medical Care and Health Policy," *MMFQ* 46:1 (Jan. 1968): 25; (quote) "Blueprint of Proposed Industry Program" (Oct. 1956), Box 18, Orville Grahame Papers, University of Iowa Special Collections, Iowa City, Iowa; Cecil Sheps and Daniel Drosness, "Prepayment for Medical Care," *NEJM* 264:9 (2 Mar. 1961): 444–45; Stevens, "Complementing the Welfare State," 24–26; SSB, Bureau of Research and Statistics, "Need for Medical-Care Insurance" (Apr. 1944), pp. 9–11, Box 206, Witte Papers.

advertised as half-and-half," Representative Albert Ullman (D-Ore.) noted. "When pinned down, it was one horse and one rabbit, so I think we should know what we are talking about when we discuss coverage." And while Medicare brought coverage rates for the elderly over 80 percent, public and private insurance together still met only a third of the elderly's health bill.[42]

Insurance addressed the financial consequences of ill health but not access to services (a problem underscored by the task of implementing Medicare and Medicaid in a segregated southern hospital system). And the 1965 reforms accelerated an inflationary crisis. Changing patterns of medical practice and new technologies had always pressed health costs ahead of general inflation. The innovation of third-party payment and service benefits increased not only costs but pressure for more expansive insurance against them. Medicare and Medicaid made things worse by opening the federal coffers to providers on terms heretofore enjoyed only by defense contractors, and by sticking public programs with the most expensive risks. Although all OASI programs suffered from the growing gap between current contributors and current beneficiaries, Medicare was plagued by rising costs as well. And while all welfare programs suffered the presumptive illegitimacy of charitable assistance, Medicaid was further undermined by rising costs and the recalcitrance of many providers.[43]

Health Care and Economic Decline, 1968–1990

The question of expanding coverage after 1965 was increasingly trumped by inflationary fears. Reformers still hoped to extend Medicare, Medicaid, and private insurance into a universal system and remained surreally optimistic that the time for national health insurance had arrived. It was at the convergence of these contradictory efforts—to control health

---

[42] (Quote) I. S. Falk, "Medical Care: Its Social and Organizational Aspects," *NEJM* 270:1(2 Jan. 1964): 23–24; Stanley Olson, "Health Insurance for the Nation," *NEJM* 284:10 (11 Mar. 1971), 526; Max Seham, "The Failure of Voluntary Health Insurance," *The Progressive* 27:9 (1958): 18; Franz Goldmann, "Which Way Voluntary Health Insurance?" *NEJM* 272:14 (8 Apr. 1963): 722; Somers, "Some Basic Determinants of Medical Care and Health Policy," 25; Wilbur Cohen, "Current Problems in Medical Care," *NEJM* 281:4 (24 July 1969): 194; Ulman quoted in Harris, "Annals of Legislation: Medicare," 71; Anne R. Somers and Herman Somers, "Health Insurance: Are Cost and Quality Controls Necessary?" *ILRR* 13:4 (1960): 582–83.

[43] Sheps and Drosness, "Prepayment for Medical Care," 393; Malloy and Skinner, "Medicare on the Critical List," 123–26.

spending on the one hand, and to maintain the momentum of 1965 on the other—that the reform efforts of the early 1970s were forged. The Nixon administration, the last to preside over the era of postwar growth and the first to confront the challenge of economic decline, was torn. Though less fiscally conservative than its Republican predecessors and less socially conservative than its Republican successors, the administration clearly felt its role was to check congressional enthusiasm. "In terms of an overall strategy to counter the Democratic push for a compulsory national health insurance scheme," suggested one advisor in 1969, "would it be credible to propose a reform of Medicare and Medicaid, emphasizing the improvement of the health care delivery system, and oppose any compulsory national health insurance plan on the grounds that they [*sic*] would: (1) necessitate a large increase in taxes, (2) endanger existing private health plans, and (3) based on the experience of countries like England and Canada, be likely to lead to a deterioration in health care?"[44]

Though determined to "let sleeping dogs lie," the administration was forced to respond to the "Health Security" plan drafted by the Committee for National Health Insurance (CNHI) and sponsored in Congress by Senator Edward Kennedy (D-Mass.) and Representative Martha Griffiths (D-Mich.). John Ehrlichman blasted the plan as "a demagogic ploy since we can neither afford such a program nor would it be a good thing for the practice of medicine in this country." The administration cobbled together cost estimates that vastly inflated the plan's budgetary impact (a tack that forced it to argue simultaneously that its own programs were conquering health inflation and that the CNHI was underestimating future inflation) and directed HEW to look into subsidizing private insurance, but otherwise rested on its conviction that "the status of health in this country is so disputed—whether there is a crisis, if so what kind of crisis, and how to approach it—that it is difficult to even get a starting point for discussion of alternatives." Administration officials argued that they should "focus nationwide attention on the President's concern, . . . inform the country that we made a proposal and it was the Congress who failed to act, . . . block the Kennedy plan . . . [and] ensure that the administration receives credit for what is enacted."[45]

[44] Collins, *More*, 68–131; James Morone, *The Democratic Wish: Popular Participation and the Limits of American Government* (New York, 1990), 268–85; (quote) "Questions the President Should Ask" (1971), Box IS:1, White House Special File (Confidential Files) [WHSF], Richard M. Nixon Papers, National Archives.

[45] (Quote) Dwight Chapin to Bryce Harlow (27 May 1969), Box IS:2, WHSF, Nixon Papers; (quote) Ehrlichman to Ed Morgan (17 Dec. 1969), Box 36, File IS:1, WHSF, Nixon Papers; Max Fine to [CNHI] Executive Committee Members (28 Sept. 1970), Box 110, Part II, Series VI, UAW-SSD Records; Arthur Hess (HEW) to Altmeyer (21 Feb. 1970), Box

In early 1971 public support ran 2–1 in favor of national health insurance, a majority in Congress favored one of the major proposals, and even Ways and Means chair Mills assumed that some version would pass. The Health Security Act proposed universal coverage of physicians' services and hospitalization alongside limited mental health, dental, and prescription drug benefits, financed by a combination of payroll taxes and general revenues. Proponents (again) argued that the plan could cover "the entire population for a cost no greater than that actually expended to provide fragmentary service for fewer" and that it could relieve employers of the uneven burden of work-based benefits and states of the uneven burden of Medicaid.[46] The administration's response was a piecemeal proposal to patch over gaps in coverage: a mandate of employment-based coverage, a means-tested Family Health Insurance Plan (FHIP) for families with children not covered by the mandate, and pared-back Medicare and Medicaid coverage for everyone else. Like other facets of Nixonian social policy, this marked an effort to shift attention and resources from the urban underclass to uninsured, blue-collar, "silent majority" workers. Critics blasted the proposal, pointing out that benefits under FHIP were better than those specified by the employer mandate but less generous than those offered by Medicaid. And the administration found it difficult both to justify peeling off families with children into a separate program and to establish a threshold for FHIP eligibility that was high enough to make the program worthwhile but not so high as to step on the toes of private insurers or subject "self-sustaining" families to a means test. In the end, the administration conceded privately that FHIP amounted to little more than "stretching present Medicaid money over twice as many people."[47]

3, Altmeyer add.; "Confidential Memorandum on Paying Medical Bills" (25 Jan. 1971), Box IS:2, WHSF, Nixon Papers; (quote) "Health Options, 1971" (13 July 1970), Box IS:1, WHSF, Nixon Papers; Meeting of the Domestic Council Health Subcommittee (11 Dec. 1970), Box HE:1, File 7, WHCF, Nixon Papers; (quote) "Proposed Health Game Plan" (12 Mar. 1971), Box IS:1, WHSF, Nixon Papers.

[46] "Americans Now Favor a National Health Plan," *NYT* (9 Aug. 1971); Herman Somers and Anne Somers, "Major Issues in National Health Insurance," *MMFQ* 50 (Apr. 1972), 179–180; CNHI, "Statement of Principles" (Nov. 1968), Box 3, Altmeyer add.; "Six Major Health Plans," Box 3, Altmeyer add.; Summaries of 1970 and 1971 Proposals in Box 4, Altmeyer add.; "National Health Insurance Act of 1971," "American Hospital Association," "Health Care Insurance Act of 1971," "National Health Insurance Improvements Act of 1971," "Health Security Act of 1971," all in Box 198:1, Wilbur Cohen Papers, SHSW; CNHI, "Health Security Program" (undated draft), Box 3 (Mss 400), Altmeyer Papers.

[47] Ehrlichman to Nixon (10 Nov. 1970), Box IS:1, WHSF, Nixon Papers; Brown, *Race, Money, and the American Welfare State*, 295–97, 307–9; "National Health Insurance Act of 1971," Box 198:1, Cohen Papers; (quote) Glasser to Jeffrey (2 July 1970), Box 105, Part II, Series VI, UAW-SSD Records; Health Insurance Q&A (1970), Box HE:1, WHCF, Nixon Papers; "Confidential Memorandum on Paying Medical Bills" (25 Jan. 1971), Box IS:2,

The most important of the alternative proposals was the AMA's Medicredit bill, a combination of tax credits against the costs of insurance and insurance vouchers for those with little or no taxable income. The HIAA's National Health Care Act proposed a three-tiered system of private insurance built around private coverage for employee groups, tax incentives for "self-sustaining" individuals, and subsidized private coverage for the poor. The American Hospital Association (AHA) weighed in with a proposal for nonprofit health care corporations that would pool and administer both employment-based care and federally subsidized indigent care. Others options included a universal plan with limited coverage, and a measure favored by some moderate Republicans that would have crept toward universal coverage by expanding Medicaid to all those without stable access to employment-based group coverage.[48] Not surprisingly, the legislative cacophony (fourteen different bills) yielded volumes of congressional testimony but little else. While legislation stalled, reformers and opponents converged on the idea of mandated employment-based care as a logical starting point. For insurers and doctors, this was one way of conceding the importance of expanding coverage while ensuring that new coverage ran in private channels. For some employers, this seemed the only way of evening out health costs across competitive markets and escaping a system that passed the costs of treating the uninsured onto employers anyway. For some reformers, expanding employment-based care was the next-best thing to displacing it. Indeed, the CNHI considered but dismissed a combination of mandated employment coverage and government insurance pools (virtually identical to the 1992 Clinton plan), because it doubted "that this sort of plan would float politically—it would look too much like a gimmick."[49]

The interested parties recast their proposals through 1973–74 but, disappointed by their failure in the previous session, reformers gave the most ground. "Health Security" reappeared under the joint sponsorship of Kennedy and Wilbur Mills—retreating slightly on benefits, allowing private insurers to act as intermediaries, and relying on a combination of

WHSF, Nixon Papers; "Report of the Domestic Council Health Policy Review Group" (8 Dec. 1970), Box IS:1, WHSF, Nixon Papers; (quote) "Health Options, 1971" (13 July 1970), Box IS:1, WHSF, Nixon Papers; Ehrlichman to Richardson (15 July 1970), Box IS:3, WHSF, Nixon Papers; Cole to Price (18 Mar. 1971), Box IS:2, WHSF, Nixon Papers.

[48] (Quote) Medical Committee for Human Rights, "A Radical Alternative to National Health Insurance" (July 1971), Box 23, John Wiley Papers, SHSW; Moore to Cole (3 Feb. 1972), Box IS:1, WHSF, Nixon Papers; House Committee on Ways and Means, *Analysis of Health Insurance Proposals* 92:1 (Aug. 1971), 1–74; [National Assembly], *Report from Washington* (24 Feb. 1971), Box 4, Altmeyer add.

[49] House Committee on Ways and Means, *Hearings: National Health Insurance Proposals: Parts 1–13* 92:1 (Nov. 1971); Weinberger to Nixon (7 Dec. 1973), Box IS:3, WHCF, Nixon Papers; (quote) Willcox to Stoiber (11 July 1972), Box 150:2178, Series III, Falk Papers.

payroll-based contributions and taxation. The administration, reasoning that "we can't beat something with nothing," responded with a Comprehensive Health Insurance Program (CHIP) that combined a weak employer mandate with the HIAA's 1971 plan for subsidized private insurance. "If this health plan is what Mr. Nixon means by the 'new federalism,' " observed the United Auto Workers' Leonard Woodcock, "it should be called the new feudalism since it would make us all serfs of the insurance industry." Others noted caustically that dictionary definitions for "CHIP" included "a small piece, a very thin slice, anything trivial or worthless or dried up or without flavor, to shape or produce by cutting away pieces, to disfigure by breaking off fragments, [and]—perhaps the most appropriate definition . . . : a piece of dried dung."[50] Again reform faltered. Although the alternatives were much closer than they had been in 1971–72, neither the administration (distracted by Watergate) nor reformers (expecting post-Watergate electoral gains) were eager to compromise. Reformers were torn between their original vision of single-payer national health insurance (a government-financed, locally administered system on the Canadian model) and the pragmatic compromises urged by congressional Democrats. By late 1973 the CNHI conceded that it had lost momentum and lamented that "Health Security as a standard had reached the end of the road."[51]

Although efforts to expand coverage collapsed, efforts to control costs made greater progress: the health maintenance organization (HMO) emerged as a surrogate for reform in the early 1970s and would persist at the core of federal health policy. Determined to find a supply-side solution, the administration was captivated by the promise of health delivery systems (pioneered by Alain Enthoven, Paul Ellwood, and others) that would replicate the administrative and medical benefits of prepaid group practice and compete for patient dollars. Enthoven extolled the HMO as "a many-faceted jewel" and claimed (ironically, considering their subsequent record) that HMOs "provide an opportunity for cost

[50] Cole to Nixon (23 Apr. 1974), Box IS:3, WHCF, Nixon Papers; (quote) Timmons to Cole (29 Jan. 1974), Box IS:3, WHCF, Nixon Papers; Cavanaugh to Nixon (14 Dec. 1973), Box IS:3, WHCF, Nixon Papers; "Game Plan on the Health Issue" (2 Mar. 1974), Box HE:3, WHSF, Nixon Papers; "National Health Insurance: Diagnosing the Alternatives," *American Federationist* 81:6 (1974): 7; Woodcock quoted in House Committee on Ways and Means, *Hearings: National Health Insurance: Part 3* 93:2 (Apr.–July 1974), 1144; (quote) Brindle to Glasser (15 Feb. 1974), Box 105, all in Part II, Series VI, UAW-SSD Records.

[51] "National Health Insurance: Diagnosing the Alternatives," 7; Loen to Timmons (24 Apr. 1974), Box IS:3, WHCF, Nixon Papers; Starr, *Transformation of American Medicine*, 404–5; (quote) CNHI Technical Committee Meeting (23 Oct. 1974), Box 105; Joint Executive Committees [CNHI-HSAC] Meeting (12 Mar. 1973), Box 110; Joint Meeting of the Executive Committees of the CNHI and HSAC (2 Aug. 1974), Box 110; Fine to Kennedy (21 Dec. 1973) Box 110; all in Part II, Series VI, UAW-SSD Records.

control by physician judgment rather than by bureaucratic regulation."
Critics ranged from most reformers, who saw HMOs as an effort by for-
profit insurers and providers to highjack the group practice movement,
to the AMA, which rode the HMO bandwagon until it became apparent
that private intrusions in the doctor-patient relationship were no better
than public ones. The administration spurred HMO development by offering loans for pilot programs, pressing states (using Medicaid and Hill-
Burton funds as leverage) to run pilot programs, and requiring employers to give covered workers the option of choosing an HMO-based plan.[52]

After 1974, reform faded amid the urgency of controlling costs and a
fascination with "competitive" solutions. Congressional liberals hoped
the election of Jimmy Carter in 1976 might re-open the debate and proposed a system built around universal enrollment in private prepaid
plans. In response, Carter could come up with nothing better than a pale
echo of the 1974 Nixon plan, a development that at least one reformer
found "more than a little disturbing." Many in the new administration
were captivated by HMOs and spurred experimentation by relaxing minimum benefit standards (although others were equally convinced that
HMOs would do little to benefit the uninsured). The administration argued fruitlessly that costs could not be brought under control without
radical reorganization of the delivery system while admitting that radical
reorganization would be difficult as long as inflation ran unchecked.[53]
By 1978 increased coverage was secondary to "the priority that cost-containment has in connection with any national health insurance proposal." The administration's only significant reform foray was a hospital

[52] John Price to Cole (27 Jan. 1971) and handwritten notes (11 Mar. 1971), both in Box
HE:1, WHCF, Nixon Papers; "Fee for Service HMOs," *JAMA* 241:6 (1979): 589; "Health
Care Cost Controls" (6 Feb. 1974), WHSF, Nixon Papers; handwritten notation to "Proposed Health Game Plan" (12 Mar. 1971), Box IS:1, WHSF, Nixon Papers; "Report of the
Domestic Council Health Policy Review Group" (8 Dec. 1970), Box IS:1,WHSF, Nixon Papers; "Social Security Amendments of 1970 and 1971," Box 162, and Enthoven, "Overview
on HMOs" (18 June 1977), Box 489, both in Edgar Kaiser Papers, Bancroft Library, University of California, Berkeley; "Health Maintenance Organizations," *JAMA* 235:5 (1976): 537;
"Briefing Memo on HMOs" (1977), Box 489, Edgar Kaiser Papers; misc. HMO materials,
Box 48: 387–90, Series II, Caldwell Esselstyn Papers, Sterling Library; *BW* (30 May 1977),
104; *BW* (21 Apr. 1975), 31.

[53] "Outline of Possible Step-by-Step Development" (Apr. 1978), Box 228:2, Cohen Papers; "Publicly Guaranteed Health Protection," Box 228:2, Cohen Papers; (quote) Milton
Roemer, " 'Madison Avenue Elegance' Wrestles National Health Care Crisis," *APHA Newsre-
port* (Mar. 1979): 34; Starr, *Transformation of American Medicine*, 412–15; "Meeting with Califano" (22 June 1977), Box 489, Edgar Kaiser Papers; Mylon Winn, "Market Freedom/
Competition, Health Care, and the Black Community," *Urban League Review* 9:2 (1985–86):
59–60; "Retreat from National Health," *The Nation* 226 (11 Feb. 1978): 144–45; "The Battle
for Health Care," *The Nation* 229 (10 Nov. 1979): 455–56; Martin Halpern, "Jimmy Carter
and the UAW: Failure of an Alliance," *Presidential Studies Quarterly* 26:3 (1996): 764–66.

cost-containment measure—pursued less as a solution to the cost crisis, as one observer noted, than as a " 'shock' measure designed to scare the health industry into believing the administration is serious about holding down costs . . . to gain time for the administration to devise some concrete cost-containment methods." The AHA quickly and easily quashed the proposal in 1977 and again in 1979.[54]

Health care virtually disappeared from the political agenda in the 1980s. Democrats offered warmed-over versions of the mandates and Medicaid reforms proposed by Nixon in 1974 and Carter in 1978. The Reagan administration half-heartedly offered a combination of punitive tax incentives (counting "excessive" employer-paid health premiums as income) and its own version of managed competition. The latter, in keeping with the administration's broader ideological and political instincts, seemed the only viable way of meeting "the need to hold down the costs appearing on the federal budget, the need to allow private insurers to retain a major role in health care, and the need to limit the size and scope of government activity." Beyond the files of market enthusiasts, however, the proposals attracted little support. Business and labor dug in against any taxation of employee benefits. The AMA feared the professional implications of the market model. The Blues argued that competitive reforms would further encourage commercial insurers to "cherry pick" the best risks. Commercial insurers worried that they would bear the responsibility for containing medical and hospital costs. And while the AHA was generally supportive, hospitals that delivered a larger share of unbillable services (research or charity care) remained leery.[55]

Unable to drum up enthusiasm for market solutions, the administration cut spending. In its infamous 1981 budget, the administration

[54] Joseph Califano, *Governing America: An Insider's Report from the White House and the Cabinet* (New York, 1981), 129; Congressional Budget Office, *Controlling Rising Hospital Costs* (Washington, D.C., 1979); (quote) Bernstein to Cohen (22 Feb. 1978), Box 228:2, Cohen Papers; *BW* (7 Mar. 1977), 30; Weissman to Edgar Kaiser (23 May 1977), Box 489, Edgar Kaiser Papers; Daniel Greenberg, "Cost Containment: Another Crusade Begins," *NEJM* 296:12 (24 Mar. 1977): 700; "A Radical Prescription for Medical Care," *Fortune* 95:2 (Feb. 1977): 165–72.

[55] (Quote) Lorin Kerr, "Dear Colleagues" letter (n.d 1980), Box 3:38, Series I, Lorin Kerr Papers, Sterling Library; Vicente Navarro, *The Politics of Health Policy: The U.S. Reforms, 1980–1994* (Cambridge, Mass., 1994), 90–91; "Voodoo Medical Economics," *The Nation* 236 (19 Mar. 1983): 335–36; (quote) Alain Enthoven, *Health Plan* (Reading, Mass., 1980), 98; Thomas Oliver, "Health Care Market Reform in Congress: The Uncertain Path from Proposal to Policy," *Political Science Quarterly* 106:2 (1991): 453–57, 467–68; "Enthoven's Health Plan," *NEJM* 303:19 (6 Nov. 1980): 1116; Alain Enthoven, "How Interested Groups Have Responded to a Proposal for Economic Competition in Health Services," *American Economic Review* 70 (May 1980): 143, 146; John Iglehart, "The Administration's Assault on Domestic Spending and the Threat to Health Care Programs," *NEJM* 312:8 (21 Feb. 1985):

folded twenty-two separate health programs into four block grants (maternal and child health, drug abuse and mental health, primary care, and preventive health), slashed federal spending by nearly 25 percent, capped the federal share of Medicaid at an indexed increase over 1981 levels, and pared Medicaid's roles by squeezing eligibility for Aid to Families with Dependent Children (Congress later broadened Medicaid's base by severing its ties to AFDC). All of this marked the culmination of a long-standing determination to shift attention from means-tested programs for the poor to entitlements for the middle class. Perhaps most important, the administration's "singular belief" in paring federal spending led it to abandon interest in market solutions that promised no immediate savings. Both Congress and the Health Care Financing Administration leaned heavily on regulation of hospital and physicians' reimbursement under Medicaid and Medicare. And the administration (much to the AMA's dismay) dismantled Medicaid's "freedom of choice" provision, preferring the budgetary benefit of restricting patient and provider autonomy to the ideological benefit of protecting it. Through all of this, the Democrats offered few alternatives. Congressional Democrats generally agreed with the administration's program, especially as long as it focused attention on Medicaid and left Medicare and employment-based insurance alone. Democrats and liberal Republicans in state politics resented federal reforms that left them trying to keep public programs afloat, but could do little to stem the tide.[56]

Not surprisingly, health inflation continued unchecked. Between 1966 and 1990 per capita health spending (in 1990 dollars) ballooned from $700 to $2,500, and national health spending nearly doubled its share of net national product. By 1990 Medicare alone had outstripped its original spending projections fourfold. Observers trotted out a number of contributing causes (malpractice liability, technological sophistication, demographic change, demand induced by Medicare and Medicaid), but the central problem was the persistence of a fragmentary system that deferred health policy to private interests and squandered a quarter of

526–27; Sheila Sinler, "AHA Struggles to Reach Consensus," *Modern Healthcare* 14 (Mar. 1982): 28–29.

[56] Geraldine Dallek, "Frozen in Ice: Federal Health Policy during the Reagan Years," *Health/PAC Bulletin* (Summer 1988): 4–11; Thomas Bodenheimer, "The Fruits of Empire Rot on the Vine: United States Health Policy in the Austerity Era," *Social Science Medicine* 28:6 (1989): 531–39; "Changing Federal and State Relationships: A New Era in Health," *JAMA* 245:21 (1981): 2169–70; "Block Grants: New Federalism or Hot Potatoes?" *JAMA* 248:1 (1982): 53–54; Iglehart, "The Administration's Assault," 526–27; John Iglehart, "Medicaid Turns to Managed Care," *NEJM* 308:16 (21 Apr. 1983): 977; Helen Slessarev, "Racial Tensions and Institutional Support: Social Programs during a Period of Retrenchment," in *The Politics of Social Policy in the United States*, ed. Weir, Orloff, and Skocpol, 360–61.

its resources on the administrative task of sorting the insured from the uninsured. Although all industrial democracies faced increased health costs and expectations through these years, the U.S. experience diverged sharply. In 1965 the United States devoted just over 6 percent of its gross domestic product (GDP) to health care, a share that placed it on a par with Canada (shortly before the passage of the Canada Health Act) and just ahead of its European peers. By 1990 the U.S. share approached 13 percent (no other OECD nation spent more than 9 percent) and its per capita spending was nearly double that of its nearest OECD peers.[57]

At the same time, private and public insurance coverage began to slip. Rates of coverage remained closely tied to income and, by the early 1990s, nearly 30 percent of those with incomes below 150 percent of the federal poverty level went without basic coverage. Employer-sponsored coverage peaked at about 65 percent of the workforce in the early 1970s, after which jobs and job growth were confined to those corners of the economy—the service sector, small firms, part-time work—where such benefits were rare. By 1990 fully 85 percent of the thirty-eight million Americans without health insurance were workers and their families. The rate of uninsurance nearly doubled from around 10 percent in the wake of the 1965 reforms to almost 18 percent by 1990 and the likelihood of being uninsured increased dramatically for those who were poorer, younger, female, African American, or Latino. Again, the international comparison is striking: between the middle 1960s and the late 1990s, the percentage of Americans covered by public hospital insurance grew modestly from 20 to 40 percent and the percentage covered by public medical insurance grew from 6 to 25 percent. On both counts, no other OECD country covered fewer than 87 percent of its citizens under public programs.[58]

[57] *Economic Report of the President, 1985* (Washington, D.C., 1986), 129; Henry Aaron, *Serious and Unstable Condition: Financing America's Health Care* (Washington, D.C., 1989), 39–43, 58; Robert Evans, "Finding the Levers, Finding the Courage: Lessons from Cost Containment in North America," *JHPPL* 11 (1986): 589, 596; Gerard Anderson and Jean-Pierre Poullier, "Health Spending, Access, and Outcomes: Trends in Industrialized Countries," *HA* 18:3 (1999): 178–86; Henry Aaron and Robert Reischauer, "The Medicare Reform Debate: What Is the Next Step?" *HA* 14:4 (1995): 10.

[58] "Medicaid in Georgia," *The Nation* 221 (22 Nov. 1975): 529–30; Allen Whitfield Statement before the House Committee on Ways and Means (15 Nov. 1971), Box, II:11, Chamber of Commerce Papers; U.S. Department of Labor, *Health Benefits and the Workforce* (Washington, D.C., 1992), 3–5; U.S. Institute of Medicine, *Employment and Health Benefits: A Connection at Risk* (Washington, D.C., 1993), 28–29; Katherine Swartz, "Research Note on the Characteristics of Workers without Employer-Group Health Insurance," in *Health Benefits and the Workforce*, 13; Marc Berk et al., "The Growth in the U.S. Uninsured Population: Trends in Hispanic Subgroups, 1977–1992," *AJPH* 86:4 (1996): 573; Pamela Farley, "Who Are the Underinsured?" *MMFQ* 63:3 (1985): 494–95; OECD, *Measuring Health Care, 1960–*

Health interests followed the federal lead and tried to escape their share of spiraling costs. For insurers, this meant even more exclusionary underwriting practices for individuals and small groups, and increased pressure on employers to engage in their own risk management. Through the 1960s and 1970s, competition among insurers for group contracts had generally broadened benefits and coverage; from the late 1970s, the emphasis shifted to managed care and the cherry picking of good risks. Employers pared back work-based coverage by abandoning "first-dollar" (no deductible) coverage for higher premiums, coinsurance, and deductibles. Between 1979 and 1984 alone, the number of large firms requiring deductibles grew fourfold (from 14 to 52 percent), and from the late 1970s on, growth in the average employee share of premiums and services ran well ahead of health care inflation. In turn, large firms increasingly bypassed conventional insurance and chose to underwrite their own health plans. Self-insurance, which encompassed nearly 80 percent of large firms and over half of all covered workers by 1990, was essentially welfare capitalism: firms could change the terms of their health plans (for current or retired employees) at their whim.[59]

At the intersection of all of this sat the HMO. Increasingly, liberal reformers (following the logic of prepaid, group health coverage) and conservative opponents (reasoning from a free-market model) agreed that the solution rested on managed care within HMOs and competition among them. HMO membership grew from under two million in 1970 to almost forty million (about 27 percent of the health care market) twenty years later. And commercial insurers adopted many HMO practices, including limits on the choice of provider and close utilization review. The results, however, were mixed. Even champions of managed care conceded that its logic unraveled in settings without decent health care resources, cooperation from providers, and a population base sufficient to support two or three competing networks.[60] Often the savings

1983: Expenditures, Costs, and Performance, Social Policy Studies no. 2 (1985), 68–69; Joseph Simanis, "National Expenditures on Social Security and Health in Selected Countries," *Social Security Bulletin* 53:1 (Jan. 1990): 12–16.

[59] Deborah Stone, "The Struggle for the Soul of Health Insurance," *JHPPL* 18 (1993): 295–307; Robert Frumkin, "Health Insurance Trends in Cost Control and Coverage," in U.S. Department of Labor, *Employee Benefits Survey: An MLR Reader* (Washington, D.C., 1990), 79; U.S. Institute of Medicine, *Employment and Health Benefits,* 82–84, 101–103, 112–13; Regina Herzlinger, "Can We Control Medical Costs?" *HBR* 56:2 (Mar.–Apr. 1978): 108; Jacob Hacker, "National Health Care Reform: An Idea Whose Time Came and Went," *JHPPL* 21:4 (1996): 54–55; Margaret Farrell, "ERISA Preemption and Regulation of Managed Care: The Case for Managed Federalism," *American Journal of Law and Medicine* 23:2/3 (1997): 251–52, 265–76.

[60] "Strong Medicine for Health Bills," *Fortune* 115:8 (13 Apr. 1987), 70; Thomas Burke and Rita Jain, "Trends in Employer-Provided Health Care Benefits," *MLR* (Feb. 1991): 28;

claimed by individual firms under managed care reflected not the ability of HMOs to deliver care more efficiently, but their ability to shuffle costs to workers and patients. Measured against past performance or the experience of other countries, the rapid growth of HMOs since the late 1970s has done little to check health care costs and has inflated the administrative costs of "managing" and "competing" that are largely responsible for the exceptional American cost crisis.[61]

Dead on Arrival: The Rise and Fall of the Clinton Health Plan, 1992–1998

Shortly after the 1992 election, *The Economist* offered president-elect Clinton a facetious memorandum on health care. Its recommendations— frighten the insured, shift attention from increased coverage to cost control, and begin herding Americans into HMOs—echoed through the administration's initial plan and through the evaporation of reform in 1993 and 1994.[62] The Clinton health plan (CHP), which tried vainly to satisfy an array of often-contradictory goals and interests, serves as an appropriate postscript to nearly a century of frustrated reform. In its appeals to universal coverage, the CHP borrowed heavily on the liberal reform legacy that ran from the AALL through the national health insurance campaigns of the early 1970s. In its deference to medical interests and employment-based provision of care, the CHP underscored the privileged status of private interests in both the health system and in the broader logic of American politics.

The administration proceeded from a set of basic, if also contradictory, assumptions. First, health costs needed to be brought under control,

---

U.S. Institute of Medicine, *Employment and Health Benefits*, 100–101; "Industry Sponsored Health Programs," *NEJM* 296:23 (9 June 1977): 1351; Jeffrey Merrill et al., "Competition vs. Regulation: Some Empirical Evidence," *JHPPL* 11:4 (1986); David Himmelstein et al., "Mangled Competition: Clinton's Health Reform," *PNHP Newsletter* (Mar. 1993): 7.

[61] William Schwartz and Daniel Mendelson, "Why Managed Care Cannot Contain Hospital Costs without Rationing," *HA* 11 (1992): 100–107; William Glaser, "The Competition Vogue and Its Outcomes," *The Lancet* 341 (27 Mar. 1993): 805–812; Madelon Lubin Finkel, "Managed Care Is Not the Answer," *JHPPL* 18 (Spring 1993): 105–112; James Hadley and Kathryn Langwell, "Managed Care in the United States: Promises, Evidence to Date, and Future Directions," *Health Policy* 19 (1991): 91–118; Steffie Woolhander and David Himmelstein, "The Deteriorating Administrative Efficiency of the U.S. Health Care System," *NEJM* (2 May 1991): 1253–58.

[62] *Economist* (28 Nov. 1929): 24; "Clinton's Health Plan: A Push to Sell Peace of Mind," *NYT* (7 Apr. 1993): A1; Mark Peterson, "The Politics of Health Policy: Overreaching in an Age of Polarization," in *The Social Divide: Political Parties and the Future of Activist Government*, ed. by Margaret Weir (New York, 1998), 183–84; Theda Skocpol, *Boomerang: Clinton's Health Security Effort and the Turn against Government in U.S. Politics* (New York, 1996).

and reform could not involve any new federal spending. As one business group put it, pursuing "health care reform without cost control is like moving furniture into a burning house."[63] Second, some form of "managed competition" was both a means of cost control and an end in itself. The administration argued tirelessly that managed competition was "not the property of conservatives who distrust government and have little interest in dramatically expanding access" but a "compromise between competitive and regulatory reform approaches . . . [which combined] the means associated with conservatives (competition) and the ends associated with liberals (universal access)."[64] Third, private provision and private interests would not be displaced—a concession that reflected both budgetary anxieties and the political clout of health interests.[65] Finally, and not surprisingly given its other convictions, the administration dismissed the option of single-payer (governmental-financed), national health insurance. A single-payer bill cosponsored by Representative Jim McDermott (D-Wash.) and Senator Paul Wellstone (D-Minn.) was regarded less as an option than as a sort of legislative conscience; even its backers admitted the best they could hope for was that the administration not cozy up to the conservatives too quickly.[66]

The CHP developed fitfully as the task of drafting a workable bill became entangled with the task of accommodating health interests and political critics. Through a complex process of "tollgate" committees and working groups, the administration struggled with a parade of petty and profound questions involving the costs and scope of the employer mandate, the place of employment plans in the public insurance pools, the level and administration of global budgets, the pace and timing of expanded coverage, and the definition of a "standard" plan. The CHP was a tangle of contradictions and compromises, marked by rhetorical

[63] Cathie Jo Martin, "Together Again: Business, Government, and the Quest for Cost Control," *JHPPL* 18:2 (1993): 378; Enthoven to Starr (15 Feb. 1993), Box 1173, Clinton Health Care Task Force [CHTF] Records, National Archives; Uwe Reinhardt, "Health Insurance for All—Now," *NYT* (14 Dec. 1992): A11; Max Sawicki, "Deficit Delirium," *Dollars and Sense* (Sept. 1992): 16–18; Skocpol, *Boomerang*, 20–30.

[64] Navarro, *Politics of Health Policy*, 207–8; Magaziner to Zelman (16 Jan. 1993), Box 3308, CHTF Records; Paul Starr and Walter Zelman, "A Bridge to Compromise: Competition under Budget," *HA* (Supp. 1993): 7–23; Starr, "Design of Health Insurance Purchasing Cooperatives," *HA* (Supp. 1993): 58–64.

[65] Zelman to Senator Riegle (5 Nov. 1992), Box 3279; handwritten notes on "Principles Guiding the Attached Outline" (n.d.), Box 4001; "Insurance for Middle and Upper Income Persons" (n.d.), Box 600, all in CHTF Records.

[66] Laura McClure, "Labor and Health Care Reform," *Z Magazine* (Jan. 1994): 52–55; Navarro, *Politics of Health Policy*, 195, 207–8; "Briefing Book for the President and First Lady from the Informal Single Payer Group" (28 May 1993), Box 1183, CHTF Records.

concessions to single-payer advocates, substantial concessions to competition fetishists, cost-anxious employers, and large insurers, and whistle-in-the-dark fiscal premises. The CHP (like the health system it purported to reform) was unwieldy, expensive, and inaccessible. At 1,342 pages it was 1,340 pages longer than the Canada Health Act. This, of course, reflected the CHP's underlying purpose: like an aircraft carrier, most of its attention was occupied not in attacking the central problem, but in defending itself from incoming shells. Indeed, the records of the Task Force on National Health Care Reform suggest a drafting process much more attuned to potential political problems than to the health care crisis itself.[67]

The CHP's central elements included an employer mandate, a system of regional insurance purchasing cooperatives, a standardized health plan, income tax reform, and global spending caps. Little attention was paid to the problem of financing, save the hope for immediate or eventual savings through increased coverage, increased competition, simplified administration, and the old saw of cutting fraud and abuse. As one member of the administration confided, "the proposed savings are illusory because the assumptions are crazy." Chased in circles by the phantoms of taxes, deficits, and business displeasure, the CHP avoided new public burdens through the employer mandate—and then assumed much of the burden anyway for those willing to claim "job loss" or "competitive disadvantage."[68] The CHP unraveled almost as soon as it was unveiled. Although the plan portrayed itself as a variation on managed competition, the gurus of that approach (seeing spending caps and employer mandates as incompatible with market reform) washed their hands of the plan. But the CHP's fatal flaw was its insistence on combining employer mandates (which attracted health interests and repelled many employers) and cost control (which attracted employers and repelled health interests) without any effort to sort out the contradiction.[69] This set the tune for a slow dance to the right—reflected in the claims of

[67] "Work Plan for Health Care Task Force" (Jan. 1993), Box 3305, CHTF Records; Skocpol, *Boomerang*, 40–44, 63–67; "Ethical Foundations Briefing Book," Box 3294, CHTF Records.

[68] *NYT* (8 Sept. 1994): A11; *NYT* (12 Sept. 1993): A1, A18; *NYT* (19 Apr. 1993): A1, C12; *NYT* (23 August 1993): A12; *BW* (20 Sept. 93): 31; Carolyn Clancy, David Himmelstein, and Steffie Woolhander, "Questions and Answers about Managed Competition," *IJHS* 23:2 (1993): 215–16; *Fortune* (1 July 1991): 58; *BW* (7 Oct. 1991): 60; "Health Care Planners Urge Tax on Workers' Benefits," *NYT* (14 Dec. 1992): A1, C2.

[69] Robert Dreyfuss, "The Big Idea," *Mother Jones* (May/June 1993): 21; Paul Ellwood to Magaziner (14 Feb. 1993), Box 3305, CHTF Records; "Restructuring Health Care in the United States," *JAMA* 265:19 (1991): 2516–24.

congressional conservatives that there was "no health care crisis" after all, in various "mainstream" alternatives, and in the final and inevitable admission by congressional leaders that there was nothing left to pass.[70]

After the Clinton debacle, health politics collapsed into a pattern of piecemeal reform and persistent anxiety. This reflected the popular (if unfounded) conviction that "the public" had turned against the administration's "big government" solution and that market solutions were beginning to work. The business and health press leapt at any evidence that health inflation was abating, even though such savings proved short-lived. Both mainstream reformers and their opponents embraced "managed competition"—if only because such efforts confined attention to those already covered and avoided the budgetary politics of new programs. In turn, the persistence of cost inflation in Medicare and Medicaid put those programs in the spotlight. Echoing the debates of the 1940s, Republicans pressed to dismantle Medicaid (or at least push more of it onto the backs of the states) and to subject Medicare to a means test. The administration offered little dissent, save its effort to play up the sacred entitlement of Medicare by floating ideas like a prescription drug benefit. Behind these often theatrical battles, the task of making federal programs work fell to the states—where health politics was complicated by the fact that Medicaid was both an onerous fiscal burden and a means of leveraging federal matching funds. Most states responded, in some combination, by cutting spending, rolling state programs into Medicaid, and leaning increasingly on managed care.[71]

Efforts to actually increase coverage were lukewarm at best, and often recycled older piecemeal ideas. The State Children's Health Insurance Plan (SCHIP) of 1997 set aside $20 billion for state-level efforts to insure children. But enrollment was (and remains) spotty, and eligibility varies wildly from state to state. Similarly, the Health Insurance Portability and Accountability Act (HIPAA) of 1996 offered nothing to the uninsured, and "guaranteed" continued access to private insurance without making

[70] "Surprise! Health Care's Fever May Have Finally Broken," *BW* (26 Apr. 1993); "Radical Surgery for Medicine: Hold That Scalpel," *BW* (12 July 1993); Alain Enthoven and Sara Singer, "Health Care Is Healing Itself," *NYT* (17 Aug. 1993): A11.

[71] Thomas Rice, "Can Markets Give Us the Health Care System We Want?" *JHPPL* 22:2 (1997): 383–400; John Iglehart, "Republicans and the New Politics of Health Care," *NEJM* (6 Apr. 1995): 972–75; Henry Aaron and Robert Reischauser, "The Medicare Reform Debate: What Is the Next Step?' *HA* 14:4 (1995): 9–11; John Iglehart, "Health Issues, the President, and the 105th Congress," *NEJM* 366:9 (27 Feb. 1997): 671–75; "How to Heal Medicare," *BW* (2 Oct. 1995): 122–26; "Rewriting the Social Contract," *BW* (20 Nov. 1995): 120–34; Peterson, "The Politics of Health Policy," 197–208; Jacob Hacker and Theda Skocpol, "The New Politics of U.S. Health Policy," *JHPPL* 22:2 (1997): 322–29; Teresa Coughlin et al., "The Medicaid Spending Crisis, 1988–1992," *JHPPL* 19:4 (1994): 837–58.

any effort to regulate the costs of continuing a policy (routinely between 150 and 600 percent of the basic group rate). Not surprisingly, few participated in a program in which the right to continued coverage was compromised by the cost of exercising it.[72] Politicians increasingly focused on the regulation of managed care plans while ignoring their responsibility for herding patients and doctors into them in the first place. Patients' rights laws (over one hundred of which were proposed in 1996 alone) identified an array of HMO practices, including truncated hospital stays and various provider rewards for limiting coverage—in essence the very threats to patient choice and provider autonomy that private alternatives claimed to be saving patients from in 1992–94. Insurers, for their part, countered that new regulations would do little more than raise costs and shrink coverage.[73] The larger issue, of course, was that skirmishes over the rights of covered patients meant precious little to the growing ranks of the uninsured. "This Administration got into great political difficulty because it tried to achieve universal health coverage with a very complex regulatory approach," admitted one senior HEW official. "Now, ironically, we're getting all this regulation, and not very much of the coverage."[74]

---

[72] National Conference of State Legislatures, "State Children's Health Insurance Program: What the States Are Doing" (http://www.ncsl.org/programs/health/chiphome.htm); Peterson, "The Politics of Health Policy," 216; Katherine Eban Finkelstein, "Insuring Children: Health Care Reform Writ Small," *The Nation* 264 (3 Mar. 1997): 18–21; Robert Kuttner, "The Kennedy-Kassebaum Bill: The Limits of Incrementalism," *NEJM* 337:1 (1997): 64; "New Car, No Keys," *Lancet* 352: 9128 (22 Aug. 1998): 589; Senate Committee on Labor and Human Resources, *Health Insurance Portability and Accountability Act of 1996: First Year Implementation Concerns* 105:2 (Mar. 1998), 1–6.

[73] "Managing Managed Care's Tarnished Image," *NEJM* 337:5 (31 July 1997): 338–39; Iglehart, "Health Issues, the President, and the 105th Congress," 674–75; George Annas, "Women and Children First," *NEJM* 333:24 (14 Dec. 1995): 1647–51; Thomas Bodenheimer, "The HMO Backlash—Righteous or Reactionary?" *NEJM* 335:21 (21 Nov. 1996): 1601–4; Wendy Mariner, "State Regulation of Managed Care and the Employee Retirement Income Security Act," *NEJM* 335:26 (26 Dec. 1996): 1986–89.

[74] HEW official quoted in Kuttner, "The Kennedy-Kassebaum Bill," 67.

2

Bargaining for Health: Private Health Insurance and Public Policy

As a political alternative to national health insurance, private insurance had enormous appeal to a wide range of interests. As a practical alternative, it was a dismal failure—leaving public policy to subsidize private plans, mop up around their edges, and (in the process) stigmatize those they left behind. In turn, private coverage proved inherently fragmentary and discriminatory: it magnified the impact of job segregation by race and gender, perpetuated the ideal of family-wage male employment, and widened disparities in the social wage created by regional wage competition, uneven unionization, and a changing labor market. And private benefits, creating a tangle of private interests with substantial stakes in private and public provision, distracted or fragmented reform.

Employment-based health insurance has always been most commonly enjoyed by the upper tiers of the labor market: by the middle of the twentieth century, managerial and professional workers routinely received health coverage alongside private pensions, life insurance, paid vacations, and stock ownership plans. Employers viewed such fringe benefits as a source of employee loyalty and a defense against turnover. Managerial employees, in turn, viewed (and were encouraged to view) such benefits as important markers of class status, racial hierarchy, and masculinity. The provision and expectation of health benefits, in this respect, was intertwined with the emergence of a corporate culture and structure that privileged the occupational mobility and status of the company man. Fringe benefits not only flowed disproportionately into the white-collar ranks but, over time, also swelled those ranks as the task of administering the private welfare state fell to the same managerial class who benefited most from it.[1]

Although white-collar provision formed the foundation of the emerging private welfare state, I focus here on the extension of health benefits through collective bargaining to workers of more ordinary means. This was the frontier on which the parameters of private insurance were contested and defined. This was the frontier, through both the expansion

[1] Clark Davis, *Company Men: White-Collar Life and Corporate Cultures in Los Angeles, 1892–1941* (Baltimore, 2000), 124–25, 132–33; Gosta Esping-Anderson, *The Three Worlds of Welfare Capitalism* (Princeton, N.J., 1990).

of private coverage after the 1940s and its stagnation after the 1970s, on which health interests debated the merits of private coverage as a surrogate for public policy. And this was the frontier on which the limits of private provision—especially its relationship to a labor market and labor movement riven by race, region, and gender—were most starkly apparent. The labor movement, in its efforts to extend a benefit commonly claimed by managerial workers to the rank and file, contested the scope of the private welfare state without challenging its premises. The *need* for health coverage, as we shall see in this chapter and the next, was persistently confused with an *entitlement* to coverage flowing from occupational status or bargaining strength.

The Limits of Welfare Capitalism: Private Health Insurance before the New Deal

In its heyday between the wars, welfare capitalism encompassed a range of private, firm-level social policies—including innovations in personnel management, recreation, stock ownership, and cash benefits for retirement, unemployment, and sickness. Again, such benefits were most common and most expansive for white-collar employees whose occupational status rested on loyalty to the corporation and mobility within it. In a limited fashion, such benefits spread to small family-owned firms and company towns, and then to large industrial concerns facing new challenges in labor and community relations. At the core of both the benefits provided and the often onerous service provisions attached to them was the urgency of creating or re-creating workers' dependence upon and loyalty to the firm. "It is more important than installing cafeterias, medical service, or basketball games, etc.," one employer noted, "to engender in the minds of employees that they, themselves, have an interest in the plant they have invested themselves in." Although many employers balked at the concession of responsibility implied by some of the more expansive plans, most agreed that innovations in welfare capitalism were necessary to keep the alternatives—the state or organized labor—at bay.[2]

Beyond the managerial ranks, it is easy to exaggerate the scope and impact of welfare capitalism. Employers dispensed platitudes about "industrial democracy" or "employee loyalty" quite liberally, but few devoted

[2] Davis, *Company Men*, 143–69; (quote) Thomson in Roundtable on Industrial Relations, Chamber Proceedings (Apr. 1936), p. 352, Box I:8, Chamber of Commerce Papers, Hagley Museum and Library, Wilmington, Del.; P. Tecumseh Sherman in Roundtable on Social Insurance, Chamber Proceedings (Apr. 1931), p. 479, Box I:7, Chamber of Commerce Papers.

substantial resources to such programs and most abandoned them when employee contributions could not meet their costs. This was especially true of "sickness insurance." Employers maintained health and safety programs and viewed on-site care as a means of cutting occupational accidents and claims, dampening turnover and absenteeism, and lowering workers' compensation premiums. But even relatively expansive programs, as Gerald Zahavi notes of Endicott Johnson, were at the outset "limited, highly arbitrary, and designed more to deal with the threat of lawsuits than with the health of workers." Although employers responded to Progressive Era interest in social insurance with a range of private programs, they usually drew the line at health coverage. During the AALL debate of 1915–20, many went so far as to argue that only national health insurance could both accomplish public health goals and overcome the actuarial dilemmas faced by state-level or firm-level plans.[3]

Some employers did experiment with health coverage, often as a way of dealing with the parade of individual cases faced by personnel or relief departments or the peculiar challenges of workers' health in certain firms and industries. The most common innovation was the mutual benefit association (MBA), which peaked in popularity in the 1920s. MBAs were managerial initiatives motivated by anxieties about organized labor and, unlike most other welfare capitalist programs, required employee contributions. Employers often picked up the administrative costs or matched employee contributions, but by one 1931 survey, nearly half of all MBAs rested solely or substantially on workers' dues. MBAs most commonly offered death and permanent disability benefits; those offering sickness benefits varied widely, although cash benefits of between $7.00 and $12.00 a week (about half the wage rate) payable for ten to thirteen weeks were typical. Employers insisted that such plans were voluntary and supplemental to private responsibility. They believed that generous benefits would encourage malingering.[4]

[3] NAM, *Industrial Health Practices* (New York, 1941), 14–39; Andrea Tone, *The Business of Benevolence: Industrial Paternalism in Progressive America* (Ithaca, N.Y., 1997), 78–81; John Commons, "Social Insurance and the Medical Profession" (1914), American Association for Labor Association Papers [AALL], reel 62; CCMC, *Medical Care for the American People* (Chicago, 1932), 110–11; Beth Stevens, "Complementing the Welfare State: The Development of Private Pension, Health Insurance, and Other Employee Benefits in the United States," International Labour Office, Labour-Management Relation Series No. 65 (Geneva, 1986), 13–15; (quote) Gerald Zahavi, *Workers, Managers, and Welfare Capitalism: The Shoeworkers and Tanners of Endicott Johnson, 1890–1950* (Urbana, Ill., 1988), 22; "Recent American Opinion in Favor of Health Insurance," *ALLR* 6 (1916): 345; untitled testimony (March 1919), Box V:9; Seventh Meeting of the National Industrial Conference Board [NICB] (21 Dec. 1916), NICB Papers, Hagley Museum; Margaret Hobbs, "History of the Health Insurance Movement in America" (1919), reel 63, AALL Papers.

[4] Dean Brundage, "A Survey of the Work of Employees' Mutual Benefit Associations," *Public Health Reports* 46:36 (Sept. 1931): 2102–11; Relief Dept. Files, Box 267:14–26; A. J.

A few firms offered more expansive coverage. Montgomery Ward and Sears-Roebuck offered rudimentary group coverage (weekly benefits at one-half salary) as early as 1910. Kodak introduced a sickness insurance plan in the early 1920s and a hospital plan in 1935. DuPont offered occupational disability coverage before 1925 and added a limited range of non-occupational benefits (payable after the first sixty days to those with fifteen years service) after 1925. International Harvester covered 80 percent of its employees with wage-replacement sickness benefits. And Endicott Johnson offered full medical coverage to all its workers and any dependents not otherwise employed. At its peak in 1928, the Endicott Johnson Medical Service maintained a medical staff of over a hundred and spent just under $1 million (about $25.00 per employee) a year. Even at their most generous, however, sickness plans were subject to the absolute discretion of the employer: DuPont, for example, was careful to specify that its plan was "purely voluntary," that "no contractual obligation is assumed by the company," and that "in all instances and respects the Company reserves the right to terminate or alter Plans."[5]

The most extensive industrial health programs were found in remote and hazardous industries such as mining and lumbering. Resource-industry health programs, particularly in the Northwest and Appalachia, combined rudimentary hospital care with a company doctor. Because

---

County to Rea (26 Sept. 1924), Box 165:10; Insurance Fund Reports (1926–1960), Boxes 202:5, 238:4; misc. MBA material, Box 803:14; Relief Dept. Minutes (1933–1943), Box 267:14; "Obligations of Membership" (1952), Box 267:16; Address of Millard Loughner (20 Apr. 1926), Box 803:14, all in Pennsylvania Railroad [PRR] Papers, Hagley Museum; E. B. Hunt, "The PRR Voluntary Relief Department," in U.S. Department of Labor, *Proceedings of the Conference on Social Insurance*, Bureau of Labor Statistics Bulletin 212 (Washington, D.C., 1917), 491; "Mutual Benefit Associations" (15 Mar. 1923), Box V:8, NICB Papers; Constitution and By-Laws of Derby Relief Society (rev. 1 Nov. 1941), Box 540, Series II, Westmoreland Coal Papers, Hagley Museum; Alan Derickson, "The United Steelworkers of America [USWA] and Health Insurance, 1937–1962," in *American Labor in the Era of World War I*, ed. Daniel Cornford and Sally Miller (Westport, Conn., 1995), 73–74.

[5] Frank Dobbin, "The Origins of Private Social Insurance: Public Policy and Fringe Benefits in America, 1920–1950," *American Journal of Sociology* 97:5 (1992): 1425–26; Susan Porter Benson, *Counter Cultures: Saleswomen, Managers, and Customers in American Department Stores, 1890–1940* (Urbana, Ill., 1986), 146, 194; Bulletin of Bureau of Labor Statistics, *Health and Recreation Activities in Industrial Establishments, 1926*, Bulletin 488 (1928); NICB, *What Employers Are Doing* (New York, 1936); Laura Scofea, "The Development and Growth of Employer-Provided Health Insurance," *MLR* (Mar. 1994): 3–4; Sanford Jacoby, *Modern Manors: Welfare Capitalism since the New Deal* (Princeton, N.J., 1997), 98; Niles Carpenter, *Medical Care for 15,000 Workers and Their Families: A Survey of the Endicott Johnson Workers Medical Service* (Chicago, 1930), 9–32; Zahavi, *Workers, Managers, and Welfare Capitalism*, 48; (quote) "DuPont Welfare Plans" (1921), (quote) "DuPont Benefit and Pension Plans" (1925), Box 26, E. I. DuPont de Nemours [EIDPDN] Administrative Papers, Hagley Museum; George Ranney, "Employees' Benefit Association of the International Harvester Companies," in *Proceedings of the Conference on Social Insurance*, 484.

company doctors, in mining and elsewhere, were routinely used by management to minimize compensation claims, report malingering, and weed out employees and applicants on physical, behavioral, and political grounds, the most developed industrial plans were also the most widely despised.[6] Welfare-capitalist health programs were haphazard, meager, and deeply resented. By one 1917 estimate, only about 10 percent of industrial establishments maintained MBAs that covered wage loss or medical care, and the latter was provided almost exclusively by company doctors. "The wage earner who is insured at high cost in existing agencies," noted one observer, "is enabled to secure no more than a small pittance during illness and enough to give him a decent burial."[7]

Welfare capitalism also drew distinctions according to the gender or race of its beneficiaries. This was especially pronounced in white-collar work, in which the managerial ranks remained a white (even Anglo-Saxon) enclave and in which fringe benefits distinguished manly careers from the pink-collar rank and file.[8] In the industrial economy, programs for male workers focused on masculine diversions (sports) or breadwinner benefits. Programs for women, by contrast, were concerned largely with ameliorating the burden of work in such a way as to address the political assumption that women needed to be protected from wage labor. Although working women faced both a greater need for health coverage and a lower wage base from which to meet its costs, they were segregated, if not shunned entirely, by welfare capitalism. Of fourteen fraternal plans surveyed in New York in 1914, eight excluded women outright and the rest restricted coverage to partial benefits for wives and unmarried daughters. MBA and welfare-capitalist plans routinely ex-

[6] Robert Cunningham III and Robert M. Cunningham, Jr., *The Blues: A History of the Blue Cross and Blue Shield System* (De Kalb, Ill., 1997), 9; Raymond Munts, *Bargaining for Health: Labor Unions, Health Insurance, and Medical Care* (Madison, Wis., 1967), 7–9; Richard Mulcahy, "In the Union's Service: The Political Economy of the UMWA Welfare and Retirement Fund," *Maryland Historian* 23 (1992): 20–21; Stonega Hospital: Rules Governing the Admittance of Patients (1919), Box 538, Series II, Westmoreland Papers; Bureau of Cooperative Medicine Press Release (13 Mar. 1939), Director of Research Health Files, Box 8E:2, American Federation of Labor [AFL] Papers, State Historical Society of Wisconsin [SHSW], Madison, Wis.; Ranney, "Employees' Benefit Association of the International Harvester Companies," 488; Ivana Krajcinovic, *From Company Doctors to Managed Care: The United Mine Workers' Noble Experiment* (Ithaca, N.Y., 1997), 8–9; Alan Derickson, "Part of the Yellow Dog: U.S. Coal Miners' Opposition to the Company Doctor System, 1936–1946," *IJHS* 19:4 (1989): 709–17.

[7] Rick Halpern, "The Iron Fist and the Velvet Glove: Welfare Capitalism in Chicago's Packinghouses, 1921–1933," *Journal of American Studies* 26 (1992): 180–81; Edgar Sydenstriker, "Existing Agencies for Health Insurance in the United States," in *Proceedings of the Conference on Social Insurance*, 453, 472 (quote).

[8] Margery Davies, *Woman's Place Is at the Typewriter: Office Work and Office Workers, 1870–1930* (Philadelphia, 1982); Davis, *Company Men*, 68–69, 143–69.

cluded sex-specific conditions. Under the aegis of the family wage, women (whether they worked or not) were considered covered by benefits paid to husbands or fathers. "Most married women are here afforded ample support by their husbands," one observer noted, "and therefore no crying need exists for insurance of this type."[9] Black workers also had little claim on welfare capitalism. Such programs were rare in the agricultural and industrial labor markets in which black labor was concentrated, and employers excluded or segregated black employees. Industrial medical and hospital plans in the South echoed the region's broader pattern of Jim Crow medicine. Northern firms often maintained segregated MBAs: at the Pennsylvania Railroad, for example, the MBA was open to "white employees from every rank" (a restriction that lasted into the late 1940s) while black employees were relegated to a separate Colored Employees' Mutual Welfare Association.[10]

Given welfare capitalism's motives and methods, workers experimented with a range of alternatives. One such alternative was the fraternal lodge organized along ethnic, religious, or occupational lines (nearly one-third of men over the age of twenty belonged to such lodges in the 1920s). Major urban-industrial centers such as New York or Chicago boasted dozens of fraternal or benevolent societies, ranging from local lodges with membership in the hundreds to sprawling multichapter lodges, such as the Fraternal Order of Eagles, with membership approaching half a million. Such organizations were also popular among urban southern blacks, for whom fraternals offered a means of both paying for medical services and maintaining local hospitals. Most fraternals offered basic death and burial plans, but many also experimented with group medical plans: for a $2.00 annual fee, typically, members could receive basic medical care from a salaried doctor retained by the lodge. As a stable means of provision or an alternative to work-based coverage, however, fraternals made little headway. Fraternal medical care struggled with both the actuarial nightmare of open enrollment and the persistent opposition of medical societies. A 1914 survey counted almost two hundred fraternal lodges boasting seven million members and $100 million in annual benefit outlays, but barely 1 percent of this went to medical care.[11]

[9] Tone, *Business of Benevolence*, 11–13, 41–43, 140–81; Mary Van Kleeck, "Problems of Sickness Insurance for Women," in *Proceedings of the Conference on Social Insurance*, 589–92 (quote at 589); "Sickness Insurance in New York City" (1914), reel 62, AALL Papers; Sydenstriker, "Existing Agencies for Health Insurance," 471.

[10] Constance Kent, "The Wage Earner's Stake in Health," *American Federationist* 46:7 (1939): 750–51; Address of Millard Loughner (20 Apr. 1926), Box 803:14; F. Stone Report, "Personnel Practices of the PRR" (1947), Box 808:8; "Negro Welfare Work, 1923–1925," Box 1029:13, all in PRR Papers.

[11] David Beito, "The 'Lodge Practice Evil' Reconsidered: Medical Care through Fraternal Societies, 1900–1930," *Journal of Urban History* 23:5 (July 1997): 569–70, 572–73, 593;

Organized labor also competed with employers for the loyalty of workers by offering its own work-based plans. Through the 1920s, the American Federation of Labor scored MBAs as "calculated to benefit the employer and to work against trade union affiliation and loyalty" and encouraged workers to "provid[e] their own insurance rather than depending upon the humanitarian impulse of employers." Unions discouraged membership in company-run benefits: at the Pennsylvania Railroad, for example, barely 1 percent of unionized employees joined the MBA—which one union official dubbed "a menace to this Brotherhood and detrimental to the interests of our members."[12] While the AFL preferred high wages to benefits, many locals appreciated the union-building benefits and actuarial advantages of group practice or group payment. Again resource industries were important sites of innovation. Through the late nineteenth and early twentieth century, as Alan Derickson has shown, the Western Federation of Miners (WFM) established a remarkable network of union hospitals. Although the WFM hospital system would not survive the 1920s, it foreshadowed the landmark Health and Welfare Fund won by the United Mine Workers (UMW) in postwar bargaining.[13] In the garment industry, union health clinics offered routine care and performed exams for local sickness funds before World War I. These grew into more elaborate health plans in the late 1930s and early 1940s, as the International Ladies Garment Workers' Union (ILGWU) and the Amalgamated Clothing Workers (ACW) toyed with ways of pooling contributions across the industry in order to sustain some sort of an actuarial foundation for group insurance.[14] Others, following

---

Beito, "Black Fraternal Hospitals in the Mississippi Delta, 1942–1967," *Journal of Southern History* 65:1 (Feb. 1999): 109–11; Medical Advisory Board Minutes (29 Jan. 1935), p. 152, Box 67, Edwin Witte Papers, SHSW; Sydenstriker, "Existing Agencies for Health Insurance," 433–34; *JAMA* (1916): 1973; David Rosner and Gerald Markowitz, "Hospitals, Insurance, and the American Labor Movement: The Case of New York in the Postwar Decades," *Journal of Policy History* 9:1 (1997): 78–79; Jerome Schwartz, "Early History of Prepaid Medical Care Plans," *BHM* 39 (1965): 452.

[12] Dobbin, "Origins of Private Social Insurance," 1428–31; Stevens, "Complementing the Welfare State," 16–17; (quote) AFL, *Report of Proceedings, 44th Congress* (1924): 47–48; (quote) Grant Hamilton, "Proposed Legislation for Health Insurance," in *Proceedings of the Conference on Social Insurance*, 564; Special Circular (14 Mar. 1928) and membership calculations (1926–27), Box 1029:8, both in PRR Papers; AFL, *Report of Proceedings, 48th Congress* (1928): 38–41; Lawrence Root, "Employee Benefits and Social Welfare: Complement and Conflict," *AAAPSS* 479 (May 1985): 103–4.

[13] Alan Derickson, *Workers' Health, Workers' Democracy: The Western Miners' Struggle, 1891–1925* (Ithaca, N.Y., 1988): 57–124, 150–54; Derickson, "Part of the Yellow Dog," 709–17; Schwartz, "Early History of Prepaid Medical Care Plans," 453–55; Pierce Williams, *The Purchase of Medical Care through Fixed Periodic Payment* (New York, 1932): 109–10.

[14] Leo Price, "Health Program of the International Ladies Garment Workers' Union," *MLR* 49:4 (1939): 811–15, 826–27; Adolph Held, "Health and Welfare Funds in the Needle

the ILGWU-ACW lead, experimented with community-based group practice in the late 1930s. International Harvester employees, for example, established a medical center in Milwaukee in 1936 and offered coverage to other employee groups or individuals willing to pay the premiums. But such experiments were few and far between, and were eclipsed by collectively bargained group insurance.[15]

Welfare capitalism was widely resented by workers and poorly understood by employers. Although some firms persisted through the New Deal years and after, most retreated from welfare-capitalist programs in the mid- to late 1920s. The onset of the Great Depression further discouraged such experiments, as the chasm between demands for relief and management's willingness to fund them widened and public programs emerged to take their place.[16] The experience at Endicott Johnson was telling. In 1928, business conditions pressed the firm to deny medical benefits to new workers; to begin the practice (as company president George Johnson put it) of "differentiating between old and valued workers, and those younger and less responsive to kindness, and also less needing the help." In 1931 the firm retreated further, reducing wages 5 percent and shifting the burden of funding the Medical Services Department to the workers. While Endicott Johnson reestablished employer funding as conditions improved in 1934–35, cuts in benefits and another round of payroll deductions followed in 1938 and 1940. Efforts to maintain the program under difficult conditions, in this sense, only underscored its discretionary and tenuous coverage.[17]

Union and fraternal health plans also faltered through the 1920s and largely collapsed in the face of the Depression. Experiments in mining and the needle trades aside, union health provision was never widespread. By one estimate, there were thirty substantial union-based plans in 1900, thirteen in 1923, thirty in 1933, and nineteen in 1943. Unions

---

Trades," *ILRR* 1:2 (Jan. 1948): 248–49; "Union Health Center," *NYT* (10 Apr. 1949); Leo Price, "Guarding the Health of Garment Workers" (1940), Box 208, Witte Papers; Proceedings, NICB Conference on Union Health and Welfare Funds (Jan. 1947), pp. 35–38, Box I:29, NICB Papers; Helen Baker and Dorothy Dahl, *Group Health Insurance and Sickness Benefit Plans in Collective Bargaining* (Princeton, N.J., 1945), 68; *BW* (11 Mar. 1944), 102; Dorothy Sue Cobble, *Dishing It Out: Waitresses and Their Unions in the Twentieth Century* (Urbana, Ill., 1991), 425–26; Jennifer Klein, "Managing Security: The Business of American Social Policy, 1910s–1960" (unpublished ms., 2000), 292ff.

[15] "Milwaukee Labor Leads Fight for Medical Center" (1939), Box 208, Witte Papers; Andrew and Hannah Biemiller, "Medical Rift in Milwaukee," *Survey Graphic* (Aug. 1938).

[16] Jacoby, *Modern Manors*, 32, 36; Colin Gordon, *New Deals: Business, Labor, and Politics, 1920–1935* (New York, 1994), 253–79; Zahavi, *Workers, Managers, and Welfare Capitalism*, 99–104; Krajcinovic, *Company Doctors to Managed Care*, 10–11.

[17] Carpenter, *Medical Care for 15,000 Workers*, 14, 74–75; Zahavi, *Workers, Managers, and Welfare Capitalism*, 127–52, 178–79 (Johnson quoted at 127).

that did toy with health coverage often found that uncertain costs and actuarial dilemmas forced them to slash benefits, raise premiums, and retreat from direct investment in clinics—a combination that undermined efforts to offer an alternative to welfare capitalism and yielded more discontent than loyalty.[18] For unions and fraternals, medical society opposition remained the biggest obstacle. Local, state, and national medical societies, for example, met the multiunion Milwaukee plan of the late 1930s with "blank and uncompromising hostility." The county medical society expelled participating doctors, and the AMA instructed local hospitals to bar them as well. Union health programs generally survived only in remote settings in which local health provision was dominated by an employment-based plan, or when the union plan bent over backward to accommodate professional anxieties.[19]

In the early years of the Depression, private health provision seemed at a standstill as medical societies stifled experiments in group payment, employers retreated from welfare capitalism, and unions and fraternals faced the actuarial challenge of local provision in hard times. The Social Security debate of the mid-1930s, animated by both general economic stress and the failure of private provision, changed all of this. Social Security both socialized the burden of welfare capitalism (offering some employers and some workers an alternative to its uneven costs and tenuous benefits) and encouraged employers to weave public programs and private supplements into a seamless safety net of employment-based benefits. Some saw health care as intrinsic to any system of work-based social insurance; others (on both sides of the debate) questioned the wisdom of including a benefit that confounded the logic of contributory, family-wage, occupational coverage.[20]

Fringe benefits were not a major issue for labor through 1935–37 as the fledgling Congress of Industrial Organizations (CIO) focused on

[18] Krajcinovic, *Company Doctors to Managed Care*, 7; Lizabeth Cohen, *Making a New Deal: Industrial Workers in Chicago, 1919–1939* (New York, 1990), 193–95; Sydenstriker, "Existing Agencies for Health Insurance," 466–68; Held, "Health and Welfare Funds in the Needle Trades," 248; Baker and Dahl, *Group Health Insurance*, 11–16; Stevens, "Complementing the Welfare State," 7–10; Derickson, *Workers' Health, Workers' Democracy*, 130–31, 189–219.

[19] Biemiller, "Medical Rift in Milwaukee"; Schwartz, "Early History of Prepaid Medical Care Plans,"112–20; Beito,"The 'Lodge Practice Evil' Reconsidered," 579–80, 591–93; Joseph Garbarino, *Health Plans and Collective Bargaining* (Berkeley, Calif., 1960), 154–55; "Milwaukee Labor Leads Fight for Medical Center" (1939), Box 208, Witte Papers; Mulcahy, "In the Union's Service," 25–27; Mulcahy, "A New Deal for Coal Miners: The UMWA Welfare and Retirement Fund and the Reorganization of Health Care in Appalachia," *Journal of Appalachian Studies* 2:1 (1997): 40–41; Munts, *Bargaining for Health*, 44–45.

[20] Jacoby, *Modern Manors*, 2–8; Jennifer Klein, "The Business of Welfare: The Growth of Commercial Health Insurance, 1940–1955" (unpublished ms., 1995), 6–8; Root, "Employee Benefits and Social Welfare," 104–5; CES Minutes (15 Mar. 1935), pp. 21–23, Box

basic recognition and on the constitutionality of the new (1935) National Labor Relations Act (NLRA). Indeed the NLRA was unclear as to whether such benefits were even subject to collective bargaining. Both the AFL and the CIO supported national health insurance, but also recognized the union-building benefits of collectively bargained benefits. Leading CIO unions established social security departments to facilitate compliance with the federal Social Security program and work for its expansion. Unions in welfare-capitalist settings began exploring ways to incorporate health care as a contractual benefit. And established union health plans began pressing for more substantial employer contributions.[21] For most employers, health care remained incompatible with either welfare capitalism or payroll-based social security. Although a few mavericks argued that business interests should "regard an adequate public health service as a subsidy to industry, not as a burden," employers were leery of accepting responsibility for non-occupational or dependent coverage. Employers wanted to retain control, arguing that coverage should be "organized by 'industry' and varied to suit each industry [not] . . . communistically, with one stereotyped plan for all employments."[22] In the absence of any compulsion to pay for public health coverage under the Social Security Act or bargain over private coverage under the National Labor Relations Act, employers did what they could in the late 1930s to evade the issue entirely.

As business and labor faced off over the future of public and private health benefits, a flurry of innovation in group health coverage changed the terms of the debate and, by the end of the 1930s, made employment-based group coverage an attractive and pragmatic alternative. The Depression encouraged many experiments in group practice, including the Roos-Loos Clinic in Los Angeles, a cooperative hospital in Elk City, Oklahoma, the Kaiser health plan, and various group health initiatives. Although medical societies reacted predictably to such threats, they could not contain them—especially after losing a landmark antitrust case (brought by the Washington Group Health Association) in 1938.

65, and "Abstract of a Program for Social Insurance against Illness" (1935), p. 23, Box 67, both in Witte Papers.

[21] ICHWA, Proceedings of the National Health Conference (July 1938), 13–14; "Notes on Health Insurance" (1942); "National Health Program" (1939), all in Files of the Director of Research, Box 4, Series 8E, AFL Papers, SHSW; Derickson, "The USWA and Health Insurance," 70; Official Report of Proceedings before the Interdepartmental Committee (18 July 1938), 391–92, Box 29, ICHWA Records, Franklin D. Roosevelt Presidential Library [FDRPL], Hyde Park, N.Y.; Klein, "Managing Security," 227–28.

[22] (Quote) Draft copy: "The Nation's Health" (1938), Box 10, ICHWA Records; (quote) P. Tecumseh Sherman in Roundtable on Social Insurance, Chamber Proceedings (April 1931), p. 479, Box I:7, Chamber of Commerce Papers.

Through the late 1930s, hospital associations and medical societies concluded that the best course of action was to capture the group practice movement with Blue Cross and Blue Shield.[23] These plans depended not only on provider cooperation but also on enabling legislation exempting the Blues from conventional insurance regulation (the first such law passed in New York in 1934; Blue Cross ranged across thirteen states by 1935 and twenty-seven states by 1939). Local Blues were often organized around employee groups, and the labor movement allied itself closely with Blue Cross, which it viewed as a nonprofit alternative to commercial insurance.[24] Employers too were drawn to the prospect of group coverage, especially as full-blown political solutions entered national debate. "The constantly increasing and already high costs of medical care are such that unless an alternative is found to our present method of individual procedure, we are bound, eventually to find ourselves face to face with State medicine," argued one manufacturer. "If group hospitalization is not widespread within a relatively short time, additions will be made to the Social Security Act to provide for it, in which case the greatest burden will fall on the shoulders of industry."[25]

The late 1930s was a watershed in private health provision—especially for employers facing the failures of welfare capitalism, the demands of labor, the encroachment of the New Deal, and the emergence of new forms of medical payment. Important industrial health plans of this era included those at Kodak, DuPont, American Cast-Iron Pipe, Endicott Johnson, Heinz, American Tobacco, Goodyear, Youngstown Sheet and Tube, General Motors, Sun Ship, and Bethlehem Steel—for the most part mass production firms anxious to stave off the CIO.[26] In other cases (Endicott Johnson), these were carryovers from older welfare capitalist plans. In other cases (Sun Ship and GM), these were commercially insured hospitalization plans. In still other cases, industrial plans sponsored and relied upon communitywide hospital service plans (Rochester and Cleveland). And in some instances (Kaiser), these plans offered not

[23] Schwartz, "Early History of Prepaid Medical Care Plans," 450; Rickey Hendricks, *A Model for National Health Care: The History of Kaiser Permanente* (New Brunswick, N.J., 1993), 25–35.

[24] Rosner and Markowitz, "Hospitals, Insurance, and the American Labor Movement," 81–84; Cunningham and Cunningham, *The Blues*, 47–48.

[25] E. Morrel in *Manufacturers' Record* (clipping), Box 211, Witte Papers.

[26] Antiunion motives were often quite explicit. At DuPont, one manager reported (after delivering a health and accident check to a hospitalized employee) that "he was pleased with the visit and remarked that he and two CIO patients were in the same room in the hospital. The CIO patients were outspoken in their dissatisfaction of the treatment given them by the union . . . [the DuPont employee] remarked that you didn't have to belong to the CIO to get fair treatment from the employer." Evans to Harrington (11 Nov. 1937), Box 24, Willis F. Harrington Papers, Hagley Museum.

only an expansive range of prepaid care but the hospitals and clinics in which it was provided.[27] Although most relied on employee contributions, management retained substantial discretion and control. Employers preferred both a level of contribution that would help meet plan costs but not (as at DuPont) lead to demands that employees "be represented in the [plan] management" and a commercial insurance contract that would give employers the credit for providing coverage but relieve them of the headache of dealing with individual claims.[28]

Health Care in Wartime Bargaining, 1941–1945

Wartime mobilization and its regulation transformed private coverage. Federal health programs, especially those relating to military service, expanded dramatically. Existing group, industrial, and union plans swelled with the surge in war employment. And most important, a combination of labor demands, managerial strategy, and political regulation put fringe benefits on the bargaining table. Although few at the time appreciated the long-term implications, the war established the foundation for a private welfare state in which collectively bargained benefits both met some of the need for health coverage and displaced the urgency and feasibility of public alternatives.[29]

The war boom enhanced and restrained labor's bargaining power. Following the template cut in the Little Steel arbitration of 1941, the National War Labor Board (NWLB) protected union gains in exchange for regulated wage demands and a de facto no-strike pledge. For the NWLB,

[27] "Industrial Prepayment Medical Care" (1945), Box 54:3, Wilbur Cohen Papers, SHSW; AHA Round Table on Group Hospitalization (30 Sept. 1935), Box 212, Witte Papers; Sun Ship, "Announcement of Contributory Plan of Group Hospitalization Insurance" (1939); Minutes of the 14th Annual Meeting of the Board of Trustees [Bethlehem Relief Plan] (Feb. 1940), both in imprints collection, Hagley Museum; Hendricks, *A Model for National Health Care*, 36–37.

[28] "Employes' Cooperative Sickness and Non-Occupational Accident Insurance Plan" (1929), "Questions Your Men Will Ask . . ." (1929), Box 26; Lammot DuPont to W. B. Foster (25 Feb. 1930), Lammot DuPont to Group Hospital Service (22 Oct. 1935), Group Hospital to Lammot DuPont (25 Oct. 1935), Box 27, EIDPDN Administrative Papers; Summary of Benefits (1933), "Cost of Present vs. Proposed Industrial Relations Plans" (1932), Box 15, and "Comments on Recommendations" (16 Aug. 1938), Box 26, Harrington Papers.

[29] On the wartime developments, see correspondence in President's Official File [POF] 981–2, Franklin D. Roosevelt Papers, FDRPL; Clifford Staples, "The Politics of Employment-Based Insurance in the United States," *IJHS* 19:3 (1989): 419–20; Baker and Dahl, *Group Health Insurance*, 17–19, 31–54; Stevens, "Complementing the Welfare State," 17–20; Alan Siegel, *Caring for New Jersey: A History of Blue Shield of New Jersey, 1942–1986* (Montclair, N.J., 1986), 45–47; Dobbin, "Origins of Private Social Insurance," 1428–31; Hendricks, *Model for National Health Care*, 6–9, 41–76.

the problem lay in the demands labor was now in a position to make but also in the fact that "management under present war conditions will not perform its normal function of pressing to hold down wages [and] . . . are not adverse now to granting wage increases if thereby they can draw labor from other employers." With conventional bargaining suspended, one alternative was fringe benefits such as health insurance. Although the NWLB proceeded cautiously and did not often sanction labor demands for new group insurance plans, it did hold that employers could initiate such nonwage benefits.[30] In turn, the Revenue Act of 1942 encouraged private coverage by allowing employers (but not employees or individuals) to deduct their health insurance costs.[31]

For labor, NWLB policy was an opportunity to skirt Little Steel and ensure that employers shared in health plan costs and administration. Although unions such as the ACW or the UAW continued to experiment with union-based provision, most focused on the task of securing employer-paid group insurance.[32] For employers, health coverage was an important tool for recruiting and retaining employees. In turn, labor and management pointed to the tax benefits of employer contributions. "A dollar contributed by the employer will buy more in the way of benefits than a dollar given to the worker and then checked off," one unionist noted, "because the worker pays an income tax on his dollar while the employer receives a tax deduction for his." For defense contractors, the tax break was supplemented by a "cost-plus" contracting system that guaranteed a profit margin beyond the costs of production. Wartime employers, by one estimate, paid only about 20 percent of their health premiums. Health insurance was an inexpensive means of "persuad[ing] workers to stay on the job," one employer argued, since "it was a case of paying the money for insurance for their employees or to Uncle Sam in taxes."[33]

[30] (Quote) Leiserson to FDR (28 July 1942), POF 98:1, FDR Papers; Leon Henderson to FDR (4 Feb. 1942), William Davis to FDR (31 Mar. 1942), FDR to Davis (n.d. not sent), POF 98:1, FDR Papers; Lauchlin Currie, Re: Conversation with Philip Murray on Wage Rate Policy (16 Apr. 1942), POF 98:1, FDR Papers; misc. correspondence, POF 98:1, FDR Papers; *BW* (10 July 1943), 116; Klein, "Managing Security," 342–50.

[31] Christopher Howard, "The Hidden Side of the American Welfare State," *Political Science Quarterly* 108 (1993): 414, 422; misc. correspondence in POF 981–2, FDR Papers.

[32] Klein, "Managing Security," 355–61; correspondence in POF 142:2, FDR Papers; Murray memo (17 Jan. 1945), POF 98:2, FDR Papers; A. F. Whitney to Wagner (20 Dec. 1944), Box 60:528, Series II, Isidore Falk Papers, Sterling Library, Yale University, New Haven, Conn.

[33] (Quote) Harry Becker, "What Labor Wants in a Disability Benefit Program" (Dec. 1949), Box 201, Witte Papers; (quote) Baker and Dahl, *Group Health Insurance*, 25; Brief Submitted by the United Steel Workers In Re: United Steel Workers of America and United States Steel Corporation et al., NWLB 111–6230-D, Box 124, Alexander Sachs Papers,

While encouraging the spread of group insurance, the war left many issues unresolved. The NWLB was willing to accept benefits in lieu of wage increases, but refused to clarify whether such benefits were subject to collective bargaining. Many felt that wages would displace benefits in the postwar economy and that health insurance would revert to its welfare-capitalist status. At the same time employers were eager to demonstrate that private coverage made public intervention unnecessary, and workers continued to look for ways to democratize welfare capitalism. For its part, the Roosevelt administration was torn between the prospect of rounding out Social Security with a health insurance title and collapsing health coverage into the "full employment" logic of the postwar economy.[34]

Sporadic war-era provision, in turn, further widened the compensation gap between organized white male industrial workers and everyone else. As a consequence of job segregation, organizing strategy, and legal restrictions (including occupational exemptions and the separation of production and clerical workers in mass production bargaining), the CIO's gains were concentrated in bastions of white male employment. Although female union membership nearly tripled between 1935 and 1945, the labor movement still reached only one in fifteen female workers (compared with one in four male workers). Health provision, not surprisingly, followed union density and bargaining clout. Health plans often reflected that larger assumption (seen in Rosie the Riveter recruitment campaigns) that women's wartime work was exceptional and temporary. Just as firms and unions erected temporary job classifications or sex-segregated seniority lists, many health plans refused enrollment to new female employees on the assumption that their presence in the labor force was a wartime anomaly. Tellingly, war-era bargaining and policy viewed health insurance as an increasingly important component of employment-based family provision while rebuffing similar arguments surrounding child care.[35]

FDRPL; Siegel, *Caring for New Jersey*, 45; Derickson, "The USWA and Health Insurance, 1937–1962," 72.

[34] NICB Proceedings,"The Insurance Drive: What's Ahead at the Bargaining Table" (May 1950), pp. 18–19, Box I:33, NICB Papers; Clarence Hicks, *My Life in Industrial Relations* (New York, 1941), 107; Derickson, "The USWA and Health Insurance," 74–76; "Health and Income" (1941), Files of the Director of Research, Box 2, Series 8E, AFL Papers; Baruch to Byrnes (20 Nov. 1944), POF 98:2, FDR Papers; Harry Becker, "Organized Labor and the Problem of Medical Care," *AAAPSS* 273 (1951): 123–24.

[35] Sharon Hartman Strom, " 'We're No Kitty Foyles': Organizing Office Workers for the Congress of Industrial Organizations," in *Women Work and Protest: A Century of Women's Labor History*, ed. Ruth Milkman (New York, 1985), 213–15; Gladys Dickason, "Women in Labor Unions," *AAAPSS* 251 (1947): 70–71; Helen Baker, "Women in War Industries," *Princeton Industrial Relations Series* 86 (1942), 56; Heidi Hartman, "Changes in Women's Economic

Building a Private Welfare State: Bargaining and Politics, 1945–1950

In the aftermath of the war, private and public interests tried to decide whether a much-anticipated postwar boom meant new opportunities or new obstacles for New Deal social policy. Although the emerging politics of growth embraced established social insurance programs, the prospects for public health provision faded. War-era tax and wage policies assumed new importance as employers, insurers, and others viewed private benefits as a surrogate for public intervention. Many employers embraced (or conceded to) the political logic of employment-based benefits, and the Chamber of Commerce urged its members to patronize private insurers. Leading nonunion firms reinvented welfare capitalism as a bulwark against labor gains. Many unionists accepted (and defended) the emerging private welfare state. And private insurers aggressively promoted the virtues of group insurance on both welfare capitalist and political grounds. The result was not only the rapid expansion of private health insurance (from under five hundred thousand workers in 1946 to almost thirty million workers and dependents by 1954), but also an important shift in the focus and scope of postwar labor relations. Employment-based benefits were simultaneously an alternative to public policy, a means of identifying "deserving" citizens, and a contest for the loyalty of workers.[36]

Employers faced the rise of the private welfare state with considerable ambivalence. Those who supported any continuation of wartime benefits justified them on welfare-capitalist grounds—as discretionary programs designed to promote efficiency, stability, occupational health, and an open shop. And many saw the promise of full employment as sufficient social insurance: "Business through cooperation and regulation could then provide its answer to this Social Security problem . . . [by] employ[ing] every ABLE BODIED MAN in America at a wage sufficient to rea-

and Family Roles in post–World War II United States," in *Women, Households, and the Economy,* ed. Lourdes Beneria and Catharine Stimpson (New Brunswick, N.J., 1987), 58.

[36] Marie Gottschalk, *The Shadow Welfare State: Labor, Business, and the Politics of Health Care in the United States* (Ithaca, N.Y., 2000), 7–48; Altmeyer memo (29 Dec. 1942), President's Secretary's File 165, FDR Papers; Chamber of Commerce, "Business Support of Private Enterprise" (1950), Box, II:18, Chamber of Commerce Papers; Jacoby, *Modern Manors,* 44–45; Nelson Lichtenstein, "From Corporatism to Collective Bargaining: Organized Labor and the Eclipse of Social Democracy in the Postwar Era," in *The Rise and Fall of the New Deal Order, 1930–1980,* ed. Steve Fraser and Gary Gerstle (Princeton, N.J., 1989), 122–52; Michael Brown, *Race, Money, and the American Welfare State* (Ithaca, N.Y., 1999), 140–55; Klein, "The Business of Welfare," 39–40.

sonably support him and his dependents."[37] But employers had to juggle their faith in private employment with their fear that labor or the state might trespass on their "right to manage" if private plans did not meet social needs. For many, the postwar entrenchment of health bargaining came as a rude shock. Since labor, as the National Industrial Conference Board (NICB) reasoned, had "fallen back on the idea" of health coverage as an alternative to higher wages, workers should have allowed such plans to be displaced by wages in postwar bargaining. Some, such as the National Association of Manufacturers (NAM), went even further, arguing that wartime concessions were inadvertently "responsible for a major alteration in the theory and practice of collective bargaining [that] . . . placed new interpretations upon the concepts of employer responsibility for the welfare of employees and upon areas of management discretion which could be invaded by organized labor." More broadly, many feared the implication of unsettlingly open-ended commitments. Why should we "assume the cost of insurance for these various programs for the dependents?" asked one employer. "Where do you stop? Why shouldn't the employer pay the employee's taxes, or his water bill, or his telephone bill?" Others feared that employment-based care would ultimately assume much of the nation's health care burden. As one steel executive put it: "Is it up to the Sheet and Tube to prevent this community from having smallpox?"[38]

For many employers, the issue was not the existence of health plans but who controlled them. In 1947 the Chamber of Commerce defended the principle of private provision but worried about the drift toward contributory, collectively bargained plans in which employees claimed a vested interest and unions an administrative role: "The first thing you know the union contracts will whip it into some such shape that it is a fixed cost on you." For these reasons, NAM and others defended the welfare-capitalist model of cost-sharing and managerial discretion. Collective bargaining over benefits was not only an intrusion on managerial rights, in this view, but also put "'so-called welfare funds' in the hands

[37] NICB Conference on Union Health and Welfare Funds (Jan. 1947), 46–47, Box I:29, NICB Papers; "Health of Employees" (1946), clipping, Box 206, Witte Papers; Jacoby, *Modern Manors*, 81–82; "Highlights of the Health, Medical, and Safety Activities of the NAM, 1937–1951" (1951), Box 21, National Association of Manufacturers [NAM] Industrial Relations Department [IRD] Papers, Hagley Museum; (quote) "American Beveridge Plan and American Business" (1943), POF 1710:3, FDR Papers.

[38] (Quote) NICB Conference on Union Health and Welfare Funds (Jan. 1947), p. 2, Box I:29, NICB Papers; (quote) Control of Employee Benefit Plans During World War II, Box IV:109, NAM Papers; NICB Proceedings, (quote) "The Insurance Drive: What's Ahead at the Bargaining Table" (May 1950), p. 81, Box I:33, NICB Papers; (quote) Mahoning Valley Industrial Council, "Clinic on Health in Industry" (1940), Box 21, NAM-IRD Papers.

of labor leaders who could use them for the payment of strike benefits, for the support of sympathetic strikes, and for political activities." Such anxieties were captured in the bitterness surrounding the coal settlements of 1946 and 1950, in which management generally complained of the government's willingness to "step into the place of the owners of an industry and negotiate in their stead and then turn over the industry with new burdens to the owners" and argued that "the main issue of this agreement was not the wage issue but certain corporate union funds, the process amounts to a selective transfer of wealth and income out of owners and the consumers to the corporate entity of labor."[39]

But these concerns were complicated by simultaneous anxieties about political intervention. Although employers preferred the managerial discretion afforded by welfare capitalism, they also felt that only the rapid spread of private provision could stem the greater evil of national health insurance. In 1947 the Chamber of Commerce cautioned its members to "have in mind that if these benefits are provided by employers voluntarily it will have the effect of preventing the adoption of the Murray-Wagner-Dingell Bill" and resolved that "no compulsory legislation should be enacted at the state or federal level unless it should become clear that efforts to provide voluntary protection . . . have left substantial gaps in coverage." "As long as we can keep a fluid advancing front on our medical plans," agreed GE's director of employee benefits, "we can keep government intervention as only a threat."[40] Even NAM applauded each failure of health reform in these terms: health care "is management's job, and if management doesn't take the responsibility, somebody else will." "American industry has come off with just a warning this time," another NAM member noted in 1949, "[h]ad it not been for conscientious legislators in Congress, private employee benefit programs, one of the shining lights of the free enterprise system, might well have been locked in the vise of federal bureaucratic control." These fears were culti-

---

[39] (Quote) Resolutions, Chamber Proceedings (Apr. 1947), 132–35, Box I:10, Chamber of Commerce Papers; *BW* (22 Sept. 1945), 107–10; Minutes of the NAM Industrial Relations Program Committee (7 Feb. 1947) and Statement of Position . . . Health and Welfare Programs (1947), Box 3, NAM-IRD Papers; (quote) clipping from *Factory Management and Maintenance (1947)*, Box 3, NAM-IRD Papers; "NAM Position with Regard to Employee Benefit Programs" (Feb. 1947), Box I:103, NAM Papers; Proceedings, NICB Conference on Union Health and Welfare Funds (Jan. 1947), pp. 40–42, Box I:29, NICB Papers; (quote) Sachs, "Notes on the Coal Agreement," (7 June 1946), Box 123, Sachs Papers.

[40] (Quote) Resolutions, Chamber Proceedings (Apr. 1947), p. 131, and (April 1948), pp. 66–67; *Business Action* (13 May 1949), reprinted in Chamber Proceedings (April 1949), pp. 90–91, Box I:10, Chamber of Commerce Papers; (quote) E. S. Willis (GE) in NICB Proceedings, "Getting the Most for Your Insurance Dollar" (Jan. 1953), p. 130, Box I:43, NICB Papers.

vated by doctors and insurers, whose stake in private health care was more pressing and who persistently reminded employers of the larger implications of state intervention.[41]

For labor, private benefits were a necessary, if frustrating, alternative to national health insurance. Given its fragmented bargaining power and weak ties to national politics, labor's instinct was to win local benefits wherever possible. "We are willing to make any reasonable steps toward experimentation of voluntary programs of health and medical care," argued Kenneth Kramer of the Textile Workers, "prior to the eventual— and I say this advisedly—installation of a Federal Health Insurance Program." In 1949 the UAW demanded health coverage on the grounds that "workers cannot now look forward to an improvement in public social insurance programs." At the same time, labor also saw bargained benefits as a source of rank-and-file loyalty and union security and would have pursued them (at least as supplemental benefits) even if the push for national health insurance had succeeded in the late 1940s. In any case, health benefits spread quickly through unionized industry. Many unionists and health reformers hoped that this would "result in rendering many employers favorably disposed towards the alternative of governmental health insurance," although this was less a coherent strategy than a means of justifying bargaining gains as the momentum for national reform slowed. Instead, employers and unions and politicians viewed the private welfare state less as a precursor to the expansion of Social Security and more as a permanent alternative.[42]

Labor's options also reflected the legacy of welfare capitalism and changes in the organization of medical care. Contractual benefits marked the culmination of a long-standing drive to replace company paternalism with collective bargaining. This was especially true in coal and steel, where efforts to escape employer-dominated benefit societies

---

[41] (Quote) "Health of Employees" (1946), clipping, Box 206, Witte Papers; (quote) NAM Employee Health and Benefits Committee, "Industry Looks at the Welfare and Pension Plans Disclosure Act" (Feb. 1959), Hagley Museum Imprints; "To Members of Health and Benefits Committee" (2 Mar. 1962), Box I:23, NAM Papers.

[42] Kramer quoted in "The Insurance Drive: What's Ahead at the Bargaining Table" (May 1950), p. 35, Box I:33, NICB Papers; (quote) "Chrysler-UAW-CIO Workers Security Program" (1949), Box 78:851, Series II, Falk Papers; Michael Brown, "Bargaining for Social Rights: Unions and the Re-emergence of Welfare Capitalism," *Political Science Quarterly* 112:4 (1997–98), 657–59; Davis, "Subjects for Meeting" (15 Apr. 1948), Reel 1, Michael Davis Papers (microfilm), Harry S. Truman Presidential Library [HSTPL], Independence, Mo.; Baker and Dahl, *Group Health Insurance*, 21; Lichtenstein, "Corporatism to Collective Bargaining," 143; Reuther in *Proceedings of 8th CIO Convention* (Nov. 1946), 185; Alan Derickson, "Health Security for All? Social Unionism and Universal Health Insurance, 1935–1958," *JAH* 80 (Mar. 1994): 1350–56.

and company doctors predated the debate over national health insurance.[43] The postwar scramble by insurers and medical societies also opened some options and closed others. For commercial and nonprofit insurers, collectively bargained health care opened a vast new market by creating the large employee pools that made commercial insurance viable. Commercial insurers courted unions and employers, promising the former lower rates for those able to bring more employees and dependents into the pool and reminding the latter that "in offering our program to industry, we hope to assist in preventing regimentation in this country by an inroad through the medical profession which we are convinced would be but a stepping stone to more complete regimentation and control of private enterprise." In turn, state and local medical societies routinely prohibited group health organizations that were not controlled by doctors, and encouraged unions to forsake community plans for an employer contribution to commercial insurance. "Some of the international unions are beginning to think they have the bear by the tail," as one reformer noted. "They approach the limits of buying available health services, yet are forced towards greater coverage by pressure from their membership. Shall they fill in deficiencies by building their own hospitals and health centers. Where will they get the needed doctors, nurses, etc.? Shall they finance the training of future doctors? . . . Where does this end?"[44]

Of all the agreements reached between 1945 and 1950, the most important occurred in the coal industry. As the war drew to a close, UMW leaders wanted to protect members against mechanization, and the leading mines continued, as they had through the 1930s and early 1940s, to lean on union-enforced wage agreements to regulate competition. The solution, patched together by Interior secretary Julius Krug in 1946, was an industrywide Health and Welfare Fund financed by a royalty on tonnage. In signing this deal, the UMW's John Lewis explicitly placed his faith in the union as an alternative to state administration of benefits and in the industry as an alternative to state finance. While some in the

---

[43] Derickson, "Health Security for All?" 1349; Derickson, *Workers' Health, Workers' Democracy*, 189–219; Munts, *Bargaining for Health*, 8–9, 48–50; "Health and Income" (1941), Files of the Director of Research, Box 2, Series 8E, AFL Papers.

[44] "Notes for Use by Mr. Watt . . . September Radio Forum" (1944), Files of the Director of Research, Box 3, Series 8E, AFL Papers; The Travelers to Guy Wright (2 Mar. 1956), Box 850:1; draft memo (n.d. 1956), and Dulaney to Oram (25 May 1956), Box 850:2, PRR Papers; (quote) Siegel, *Caring for New Jersey*, 43; Brief Submitted by the United Steel Workers In Re: United Steel Workers of America and United States Steel Corporation et al., NWLB 111–6230-D, Box 124, Sachs Papers; preliminary draft of Proceedings, Association of Labor Health Administrators (28 Mar. 1957), and "History of Local 119 Health Fund of the Male Apparel Industry of Allentown" (1957), both in Box 37:212, Series II, Lorin Kerr Papers, Sterling Library; Robin Memo (2 July 1952), reel 4, Davis Papers.

labor movement viewed Lewis's break with the New Deal as a political betrayal, his bargaining strategy was hardly unique. The Health and Welfare Fund was part of a complex and ongoing effort to ensure the survival of the UMW in a volatile industry. Like his peers in other industries, Lewis weighed the prospect of national health insurance against the presence or promise of private benefits in his corner of the economy. And like most of his peers, Lewis found private provision—which promised stable benefits, union security, and substantial commitments from employers—the most compelling and realistic alternative.[45] The UMW Fund (paid for by the mine operators and controlled by the union) turned the logic of welfare capitalism inside out. Coal operators keenly resented this, and the larger business community routinely cited it as an example of union power run amok. In 1950 a compromise was struck in the form of a tripartite commission (one member representing the UMW, one the operators' association, and one the public). "The union asked for a cooperative administration of the Welfare Fund and we are giving it to them," noted one operator bitterly, adding that "the responsibility is [now] squarely on the shoulders of the union and if it fails, the public and ourselves will look directly at the union."[46]

It was scarcely surprising that workers would pursue private solutions. In the debate over state-level health insurance in California, labor support evaporated as workers "concluded that they could obtain all the benefits of [Governor Earl] Warren's bill as fringe benefits in their labor contracts and impose the entire cost of the system on employers." The AFL and CIO objected to the suggestion that payroll taxes as high as 6 percent might be needed to finance a national plan and remained unconvinced that a system financed out of general revenues would prove any more progressive. The AFL was torn between its traditional voluntarism and its recognition that bargained benefits would be confined largely to the CIO industries. The CIO, by contrast, had a firmer commitment to "social unionism," but also stood to satisfy those demands largely

[45] Brown, "Bargaining for Social Rights," 661–62; Lichtenstein, "Corporatism to Collective Bargaining," 143; Derickson, "Health Security for All?" 1345–47; Green to Wagner (20 Dec. 1944), Murray to Wagner (19 Dec. 1944), Whitney to Wagner (20 Dec. 1944), Murray to Wagner (19 Dec. 1944), all in Box 60:528, Series II, Falk Papers.

[46] Munts, *Bargaining for Health,* 31–35; George Goldstein, "The Rise and Decline of the UMWA Health and Retirement Funds Program, 1946–1995," in *The United Mine Workers of America: A Model of Industrial Solidarity?* ed. by John H. M. Laslett (University Park, Md., 1996), 243–50; Derickson, "Health Security for All?" 1347; Sachs, "Lights on Coal Crisis" (May 1946), Box 123, Sachs Papers; "National Bituminous Coal Wage Agreement of 1948," "Statement by UMW" (6 Dec. 1949), (quote) National Coal Association, "To All Members" (5 March 1950), "National Bituminous Coal Agreement" (1 Oct. 1952), all in Box 428, Series II, Westmoreland Papers; Krajcinovic, *Company Doctors to Managed Care,* 14–17; Mulcahy, "In the Union's Service," 28–29; J.P.N. to Symes (9 Sept. 1954), Box 849:1, PRR Papers.

in private bargaining. Labor leaders began to view health bargaining as a way of recouping some of the organizational and political ground lost during postwar reconversion. Such sentiments were especially prevalent in fragmented industries like construction or the garment trades, in which unions hoped industrywide benefits would provide a security and loyalty otherwise threatened by Taft-Hartley and state-level right-to-work laws.[47] As the prospect for reform evaporated, the alternative of private provision became an important source of organizational strength. Workers looked to unions not only to win basic coverage from employers but to bargain with insurers and providers over its scope and administration. At the same time, the complexities of health bargaining and the actuarial demands of group insurance further encouraged the labor movement's retreat to a narrowly contractual brand of "business unionism." Labor's postwar health policies, in this respect, marked a reprise of sorts of the pre-Depression pattern of voluntarism: faith in private solutions evoked a profound distrust of the state, the material and political uncertainty of labor's position, and the persistent conviction that organized male workers could and should provide for dependent women and children.

Through the early postwar era, the legal status of private benefits and the contentious issue of administrative control remained in the air. Employers wanted to administer and control fringe benefits; labor wanted to bargain over their terms and share in their administration; and both saw private benefits as an important source of rank-and-file loyalty. But aside from the NWLB's opinion that such plans did not constitute wages, labor law remained silent on the issue. This confusion figured prominently in the debate over Taft-Hartley in 1947. Alongside the "tyranny" of majority rule, employers and congressional conservatives identified union control over fringe benefits as a significant threat to managerial rights. And against the threat posed by Taft-Hartley, labor saw negotiated health benefits as an increasingly important source of union security. Taft-Hartley established close regulatory supervision of any plans to which management contributed and a framework (following the example in coal) for jointly managed multiemployer plans. But, just as important, its proponents did not succeed in excluding health coverage as a "condition of employment" and, in accepting the principle of regulatory oversight or joint management, made it harder to keep the terms of health provision off the bargaining table.[48]

---

[47] (Quote) Byrl Salsman OH in *Earl Warren and Health Insurance, 1943–1949* (Berkeley, Calif., 1971), 12; Stevens, "Complementing the Welfare State," 19–20; Cruikshank Memorandum (16 Apr. 1945) and Bittner Memorandum (12 Apr. 1945), both in Box 60:533, Series II, Falk Papers; Lichtenstein, "Corporatism to Collective Bargaining," 152 n63; Gottschalk, *The Shadow Welfare State,* 42–43, 51–52; Brown, "Bargaining for Social Rights," 662–72.

[48] Brown, "Bargaining for Social Rights," 662–72; Brown, *Race, Money, and the American Welfare State,* 154–55; Munts, *Bargaining for Health,* 10–11, 101.

Over the next two years, insurers and employers pressed private coverage as an alternative to the Truman health proposals. As the prospects for reform dimmed, core CIO unions also made the case for private coverage. In 1949 the Supreme Court (in the *Inland Steel* and *W. R. Cross* cases) held that health benefits were indeed a condition of employment subject to collective bargaining. Later the same year, the labor-management Steel Industry Board concluded "that all industry, in the absence of adequate government programs, owes an obligation to the workers to provide for maintenance of the human body in the form of medical and similar benefits and full depreciation in the form of old age retirement—in the same way as it does now for plant and machinery." Its legal status resolved, health coverage became a key feature of collective bargaining in 1949 and 1950. In some settings, such as steel, the scope and operation of existing managerial plans were put on the bargaining table for the first time. In other settings, such as automobiles, labor and management had put off health provision while the legal and political options played out. Across the industrial economy, labor and management turned to the complex task of determining the scope and the organization of coverage.[49]

A Reluctant Compromise: Consolidating the Private Welfare State, 1950–1965

In the late 1940s the interests of labor, business, and insurers converged around private health provision. Insurers, enthusiastic at the prospect of an exponential growth in health coverage, encouraged labor and management to pull together insurable groups of employees. "[W]hether or not we have a compulsory plan in the long run depends more on us than it does on the people who are advocating it so strongly," one insurer urged. "I think if we can make good we can protect people through these voluntary plans . . . and the people will prefer that to compulsion." Unions were eager to make basic coverage available and to gain a voice in older welfare-capitalist schemes. "[T]here is no choice for responsible unions," the ACW's Harry Becker argued, "but to take the position that, to the extent congressional action does not meet the need for workers' security, such provisions must be sought through collective bargaining." And employers offering health coverage cited a variety of reasons for doing so. Some maintained the logic of welfare capitalism that such programs would (as a GE executive put it) "pay a return to the owners of the business on the money invested in the program by improving produc-

---

[49] Becker, "Organized Labor and the Problem of Medical Care," 124–25 (Steel Board quoted at 124); Krajcinovic, *Company Doctors to Managed Care*, 12; Derickson, "The USWA and Health Insurance," 74–76.

tivity, raising morale, reducing turnover and increasingly loyalty." Others echoed the insurers' argument that voluntary coverage offered the best defense against state coverage. And still others noted the ability of health benefits, alongside industrywide wage agreements, to regulate competitive conditions.[50]

Private insurance, not surprisingly given its divergent motives, encompassed a bewildering array of benefits and financing arrangements. The initial round of substantive bargaining over health in 1949–50 preceded any real actuarial experience and proceeded with the uneasy recognition that local insurance terms and medical facilities varied wildly. Labor and management faced a choice between commercial indemnity insurance and nonprofit (Blue Cross/Blue Shield) service benefits, although other arrangements (including self-insurance and group practice) were common as well.[51] These issues were initially hammered out in the CIO industries. In steel, labor's efforts to retain wartime benefits and to eliminate the company doctor system led to both the *Inland* decision and, in its wake, a landmark deal with Bethlehem Steel that established joint (50/50) contributions to a Blue Cross–based health plan. In the automobile industry, Ford established a company-controlled plan in 1946 and some minor auto firms established collectively bargained plans as early as 1948, but the UAW did not show a sustained interest until 1949–50. After the 1950 bargaining round, all the major auto firms had contributory and collectively-bargained health plans in place.[52]

As private coverage spread, labor maintained few illusions about its scope or security. Simple tallies of subscribers or policies rarely considered overlapping coverage or the paucity of covered services. Although nearly half the population claimed some insurance by the end of the 1940s, most had only limited hospitalization coverage (barely 3 percent claimed comprehensive coverage). Of the nearly $10 billion expended on health care in 1949, patients' out-of-pocket share had fallen only

[50] Insurer quoted in "The Insurance Drive: What's Ahead at the Bargaining Table" (May 1950), p. 61, Box I:33, NICB Papers; (quote) Becker, "Organized Labor and the Problem of Medical Care," 129–30; Willis quoted in NICB Proceedings, "Getting the Most for Your Insurance Dollar" (Jan. 1953), p. 129, Box I:43, NICB Papers; D. A. Rhoades, "What Management Expects from the Industrial Relations Department" (Apr. 1956), Box 352, Edgar Kaiser Papers, Bancroft Library, University of California, Berkeley, Calif.; Brown, *Race, Money, and the American Welfare State,* 143–44; W. A. Sawyer in American Management Association, *Personnel Series* 39 (1939), Box 208, Witte Papers; J.P.N. to Symes (9 Sept. 1954), Box 849:1, PRR Papers.

[51] Stevens, "Complementing the Welfare State," 41–43; Munts, *Bargaining for Health,* 101–104; Garbarino, *Health Plans and Collective Bargaining,* 140–48.

[52] Derickson, "Health Security for All?" 1349–50; Sachs, "Emerging Labor Difficulties" (1947), Box 123, Sachs Papers; Munts, *Bargaining for Health,* 50–52; "Health and Welfare Plans in the Automobile Industry," *MLR* (Sept. 1951): 277.

slightly since 1929 (from 80 percent to 70 percent) and private insurance met barely 8 percent.[53] In turn, the poverty of health facilities left a yawning gap between contracted benefits and the ability to deliver them. In some settings (Milwaukee, Philadelphia, San Francisco), central labor councils established multiunion health plans that maintained both neighborhood clinics and central union hospitals (at its peak, the San Francisco Labor Health Center encompassed 141 locals and nearly 200,000 members and their families). In some instances (the Hotel Trades in New York City, the ILGWU in St. Louis and Philadelphia, the UMW through Appalachia) single unions established health centers that offered their services to the wider community as well.[54] And in some cases, prominent local unions invested in local facilities out of frustration with the limits and the costs of Blue Cross plans.[55]

Business, labor, and insurers agreed on the basic premises of the private provision, but they disagreed over fundamental details of organization, finance, and administration: How should costs be distributed? How should benefits be paid out? What was the appropriate scope of benefits? Who should act as the intermediary between payers and providers, and whose interests should that intermediary protect? Paying for health care was a complex issue, involving not only the share borne by workers or employers but also the uneasy relationship between contributory social insurance and employment provision. Employers and insurers argued that employment-based plans should rest on contributions from employees. "Employees appreciate the insurance more," Met Life's Gilbert Fitzhugh argued in 1949, "if they feel they are sharing in its cost." Increasingly, this perspective also reflected employers' anxieties about the costs of health care. Employee contributions, in this view, ensured responsible consumption: "where the employer pays the check, the union invariably displays an endless appetite and orders the best and the most." And this reliance on employee contributions reflected the difficulty of ensuring

[53] "Roundtable Session on National Health Insurance," pp. 166–67 (Madison, Wisc., Nov. 1949), Box 206, Witte Papers, SHSW; Senate Committee on Labor and Public Welfare, *Health Insurance Plans in the United States*, Report 359:1, 82d/1 (Washington, D.C., 1951), 1–2, 8.

[54] Albert Deutsch, "A New Union Health Plan," *The Nation* 175 (20 Sept. 1952): 232–33; "Philadelphia Shows the Way," *American Federationist* 64:4 (1957): 30; Garbarino, *Health Plans and Collective Bargaining*, 149–54; HEW, *Management and Union Health and Medical Programs*, Public Health Service Pub. 329 (1954); Barbara Berney, "The Rise and Fall of the UMW Fund," *Southern Exposure* 6:2 (1978): 97–98.

[55] "Report of Meeting Regarding the CHA" (Jan. 1957) and "Program and Development" (1957), both in Box 3, Community Health Association Papers, Records of the United Auto Workers Social Security Department [UAW-SSD], Archives of Labor History and Urban Affairs, Wayne State University, Detroit, Mich.; Munts, *Bargaining for Health*, 59–64, 75–78.

stable employer contributions in fragmented or seasonal industries. As leading employers and labor appreciated, contributory benefits in such industries were less dependent on the employer and were (ideally) portable within the industry.[56]

Generally, labor pressed for full employer financing, a point many employers conceded. Commercial insurers typically required a subscription rate of 75 or 80 percent before they would extend group coverage, and such thresholds were easier to meet in plans paid for by employers. In turn, employers' contributions were tax deductible and employee contributions were not—encouraging employers and unions to treat wages deferred to health premiums as business costs rather than as payroll deductions. Employer financing sustained the benefits of welfare capitalism by identifying the company as the source of the benefit. And employer financing seemed the only means of maintaining employer control over health plans—although this goal was often frustrated in scattered industries (like coal) in which "the labor organizations almost always dominate, since there is generally a single union but a large number of participating employers."[57] Indeed the specter of union control over employers' contributions animated much of the backlash against "union corruption" in the 1950s.[58]

Through the 1950s, full employer financing (what auto executive Benson Ford dubbed "private, industrialized, socialized medicine") became increasingly common. A 1951 NAM survey found employers bearing the full cost in about a quarter of all health plans, and over half of the costs in another quarter. CIO unions typically contracted a 50/50 share in their first Blue Cross and Blue Shield offerings, but by the early 1960s

[56] Fitzhugh quoted in Hoey Hennesy to Industrial Relations Group (5 Dec. 1949), I:75 NAM Papers; (quote) A. A. Imberman, "Racketeering in Health and Welfare Funds," *HBR* 32 (Nov.–Dec. 1954): 72–80; "Company Group Insurance Programs" (Aug. 1953), Box I:75, NAM Papers; Proceedings, NICB Conference on Union Health and Welfare Funds (Jan. 1947), pp. 38–39, Box I:29, NICB Papers.

[57] (Quote) Towers, Perrin, Forster, and Crosby, "Report on Hospital, Medical, and Surgical Benefits" (July 1954), Box 849:1, PRR Papers; Harry Becker, "Trends in Bargaining on Health Benefit Plans," *American Management Association Personnel Series* (Sept.–Oct. 1960): 60–61.

[58] Jennifer Klein, "Welfare Capitalism in the Era of the Welfare State: The 1958 Welfare and Pension Disclosure Act and the Privatization of New Deal Liberalism" (paper presented at a conference of the Social Science History Association, Chicago, Nov. 2001); Bureau of National Affairs, "Administration of Health and Welfare Plans" (1954), Box 849:1, PRR Papers; NAM Employee Health and Benefits Committee, "Industry Looks at the Welfare and Pension Plans Disclosure Act" (Feb. 1959), imprints collection, Hagley Museum; Imberman, "Racketeering in Health and Welfare Funds," 72–80; Bituminous Coal Institute, "What Did the Coal Miners Offer John L. Lewis?" (Apr. 1946), Box 428, and Harlan County Coal Operator's Association to All Members (17 May 1962), Box 429, Series II, both in Westmoreland Papers.

had won full employer financing. By 1963 over a third of all health plans were employer financed, about half were jointly financed, and less than 10 percent still rested solely on employee contributions.[59] As benefits became more expansive and costs rose, however, employers introduced copayments or deductibles in order to provide "a sounder base upon which to develop future extensions, such as the provision of dependent coverage." And many (at the urging of commercial underwriters) sought to rein in the moral hazard of routine care, arguing, as a Sears executive put it, that the "hospital plan should not endeavor to do any more than simply help take the sting out of the employee's medical expenses."[60]

Employers and workers and insurers also confronted each other over the form of the benefit. Traditionally, sickness insurance was paid as a wage-based indemnity (by which workers compensated for lost wages rather than for the costs of health care), reflecting both the family-wage premise of such benefits and the fact that, into the late 1940s, lost wages posed a more substantial burden than the costs of care. In turn, employers and insurers viewed wage-based benefits as an important safeguard against malingering. "Employees will not stay at home for minor reasons while wages and hours are favorably high," argued an Equitable Life executive, "especially when benefits are nominal." Into the early 1950s, health plans routinely offered benefits at between 40 and 60 percent of regular wages, payable for anywhere from thirteen to fifty-two weeks. For their part, unions preferred service benefits of the kind pioneered by Blue Cross, especially as the costs of health care began to overshadow the cost of lost wages.[61] Service-based coverage, however, was complicated by the necessity of ensuring the cooperation of hospitals and doctors and intermediaries. Beyond prepaid service plans such as Blue Cross,

[59] (Quote) Benson Ford, "A Businessman Looks at Health" (1955), Box 208, Witte Papers; NAM, "Industrial, Medical, and Safety Practices" (1951), Box 21, NAM-IRD Papers; Arno Mayer, "Union Welfare Programs" (1948), Box 206, Witte Papers; Munts, *Bargaining for Health*, 54–88; "Employees Benefit Plan" (1952), Box 348, J. E. Rhoades Company Papers, Hagley Museum; Falk, "The Situation in the Steel Industry," Box 115:1387, Series II, Falk Papers.

[60] (Quote) Towers, Perrin, Forster, and Crosby, "Report on Hospital, Medical, and Surgical Benefits" (July 1954), Box 849:1, PRR Papers; Sears executive quoted in NICB, "Getting the Most for Your Insurance Dollar" (Jan. 1953), p. 164, Box I:43, NICB Papers; "Group Practice Prepayment Plans" (10 Nov. 1964), Box 111:1325, Series II, Falk Papers.

[61] (Quote) NICB Conference on Union Health and Welfare Funds (Jan. 1947), p. 28, Box I:29; "The Insurance Drive: What's Ahead at the Bargaining Table" (May 1950), p. 23, Box I:33, NICB Papers; William Rafsky to Andrew Janaskie (5 May 1950), Series 3, Box 11, American Federation of Hosiery Workers [AFHW] Papers, SHSW; J. Oram to B.O.W. (2 Apr. 1957), Box 855:1, PRR Papers; Baker and Dahl, *Group Health Insurance*, 61–62; Klein, "The Business of Welfare," 20; "Comments on Employee Sick Benefits" (1955), Box 21, NAM-IRD Papers.

providers were not obligated to accept negotiated benefits as full payment for services, and health inflation often rendered fee or benefit schedules obsolete almost the moment they were drafted. Many large employers and unions clung to indemnity coverage, because it was the only way to offer workers in diverse local settings equitable coverage. Indeed, as unions such as the UAW discovered, Blue Cross plans varied so much that, as of the early 1960s, over half the union membership did not have local access to the benefits won in national contracts.[62]

Debates over contributions and services reflected the increasingly expansive scope of private health coverage. Into the early 1950s commercial group health insurance typically included hospitalization, surgical reimbursement based on a negotiated fee schedule, and a range of flat allowances for maternal care and outpatient medical services. Often basic hospitalization was covered by Blue Cross while other services were commercially insured.[63] Expanding coverage to nonhospital services proved quite difficult: private physicians dug in against contracted coverage or fee schedules, employers were reluctant to accept responsibility for dependents or retirees, and commercial insurers continued to hold that coverage of routine care posed an unacceptable risk. Bargaining, however, yielded gradual expansion. Many plans added major or catastrophic medical coverage in the early 1950s, an innovation that accommodated labor's demands and insurers' anxieties. Many introduced limited dependent coverage. And many added retirees (either allowing them to continue group coverage at their own expense or including them in the current workers' plan), especially as coverage for the elderly entered national debate in the late 1950s.[64]

[62] Report and Recommendations to the Negotiating Committee (Oct. 1951), Series 14, Box 1, AFHW Papers; Bureau of National Affairs, "Administration of Health and Welfare Plans" (1954), Box 849:1, PRR Papers; "Union-Management Welfare Plans" (10 Nov. 1949), Box 69:708, Series II, Falk Papers; Munts, *Bargaining for Health*, 67–70; NICB Conference on Union Health and Welfare Funds (Jan. 1947), pp. 7–8, Box I:29, NICB Papers.

[63] Towers, Perrin, Forster, and Crosby, "Report on Hospital, Medical, and Surgical Benefits" (July 1954), Box 849:1, PRR Papers; S. Gwyn Dulaney, "Can Employers Afford Comprehensive Medical Plans?" *American Management Association Personnel Series* (Jan.–Feb. 1959), 52–59; Texas Company, "Description of Accident and Sick Benefit Plan" (1951); "Standard Oil Plan" (1950); Worth Steel, "Benefit Plan" (1950); International Harvester, "Group Hospital and Surgical Benefit Plan" (1946), all in imprints collection, Hagley Museum; "Schedule of Benefits and Standards (26 July 1954), "Hospital-Medical-Surgical Benefits for Non-Operating Employees" (12 July 1954), Box 849:1; R.N.C. to J.B.P. (4 Nov. 1954), Box 849:4; "Copy of Group Policy Contract" (Jan. 1955), Box 849:7; Relief Department file, 1960–1964, Box 884:18, all in PRR Papers; *General Electric Commentator* (15 Aug. 1952), Box 170, Witte Papers; NAM, "Industrial, Medical, and Safety Practices" (1951), Box 21, NAM-IRD Papers; Comments on Employee Sick Benefits" (1955): Box 21, NAM-IRD Papers.

[64] Stevens, "Complementing the Welfare State," 34–38, 44–45; *BW* (3 Sept. 1955): 89; *BW* (15 Oct. 1955): 46; Munts, *Bargaining for Health*, 54–55, 96–97; *BW* (27 Sept. 1941): 68–

Perhaps the most vexing issue facing labor and management was the choice of the insurer, a role that involved both the actuarial task of administering group coverage and the practical task of ensuring the availability and cooperation of providers. By and large, the choice lay between the Blues, commercial insurance, and prepayment plans (such as Kaiser). The nonprofit Blues offered group-based service benefits at locally determined community rates. As organizations of providers, the Blues were able to offer full service coverage without (at least through their early history) copayments or deductibles. Open enrollment periods and continuation allowances allowed individuals access to group rates and retirees to maintain coverage.[65] While the Blues began as systems of group coverage and struggled to accommodate individual subscribers, commercial insurance was designed to deal with individual risks and accommodated employee groups only when the Blues showed it could be done. The commercials offered experience-rated (different rates for different industries and firms) indemnity coverage and viewed only major expenses such as hospitalization or catastrophic care as truly insurable. And increasingly the commercials used experience-rating to guard against adverse selection and to cherry pick good risks. Indemnity-based payment reflected the absence of any stable relationship between providers and insurers, and the conviction (shared by many employers) that cash payment served to check malingering and maintain the status of health care as a consumer good.[66] Prepayment plans (forerunners of the modern HMO) incorporated the service benefits of the Blues and the cost-consciousness of commercial insurance by offering full coverage in settings that closely monitored utilization.[67]

For practical and philosophical reasons, labor preferred the Blues. Service benefits were an obvious attraction, especially as the costs of health care began to rise (in 1949 Blue Cross met nearly 80 percent of subscrib-

---

69; "Medical Care for Retired Workers," *Fortune* 62:1 (July 1960): 211; Derickson, "The USWA and Health Insurance," 80; Lane Kirkland to California State Chamber of Commerce (29 Nov. 1956), Box 207, Witte Papers; "Interim Report of the HRRC" (20 Jan. 1962), and "Notes Re 'Mutual Problems' for HRRC" (14 Jan. 1962), Box 110:1316, Series II, Falk Papers.

[65] George Heitler, "The Blue Cross in Cost Control" (3 May 1960), Box 884:25, PRR Papers; "UAW Experience with Retiree Health Insurance" (Apr. 1964), Box 1, Part I, Series I, UAW-SSD Records; Health Information Foundation, "Voluntary Health Insurance for the Individual Subscriber" (Mar. 1953), Box 208, Witte Papers.

[66] Klein, "The Business of Welfare," 47–50; Lane Kirkland to California Chamber of Commerce (29 Nov. 1956), Box 207, Witte Papers; Report to NAIC on Definition of "Noncancelable Insurance" (11/30/59), Box 21, Orville Grahame Papers, University of Iowa Special Collections, Iowa City, Iowa.

[67] Elliott memo: Permanante-Auto Workers (Mar. 1952), Box 68, Henry Kaiser Papers, Bancroft Library.

ers' bills while commercial insurance met barely 50 percent). Blue Cross outpaced the commercials in the provision of dependent and retiree coverage and, in some settings, offered group coverage that was portable among participating firms. Unions routinely blasted commercials for their meager coverage (disguised by "sham additional benefits") and objected bitterly when employers moved groups from Blue to commercial coverage. Labor nurtured a close political alliance with Blue Cross and expected that it would champion the worker at both the operating table and the bargaining table. And the Blues pitched their services to labor on the basis of both their community-rated service coverage and their "organic relationship" with doctors and hospitals.[68] For the same reasons, management favored commercial coverage. Commercials offered most employee groups experience rates that undercut the local community rate. Commercial plans could be tailored to fit individual firms and offered a variety of cost-sharing mechanisms (copayments, deductibles). Firms could negotiate health coverage as part of a larger insurance and pension package, and national firms could negotiate standard benefits rather than a variety of deals with local Blues. Just as the Blues sold their services to labor, commercials aggressively promoted group insurance and offered firms a variety of ancillary services to manage and monitor claims. Commercials also paid dividends when claim experience outshone expectations, a kickback that could approach the cost of the premiums themselves.[69]

The choice between commercials and the Blues was rarely simple. Although the Blues invented the practice of group health coverage in the 1930s and claimed a substantial head start in the race to sign up employee groups, the commercials gained ground steadily. Blue Cross and Blue Shield were strong in northern industrial states but made much slower progress elsewhere. The experience rates offered by the commercials undermined the Blues and ultimately pressed them to experiment with "merit rates" for major corporate clients as well. Commercial coverage surpassed the Blues in the early 1950s, and by the early 1960s most

[68] Health Information Foundation, "Voluntary Health Insurance for the Individual Subscriber" (Mar. 1953), Box 208, Witte Papers; NICB, "The Insurance Drive: What's Ahead at the Bargaining Table" (May 1950), p. 35, Box I:33, NICB Papers; Louis Goldblatt, "Workers Health: The ILGWU Program," *The Nation* 179 (18 Dec. 1954): 530; (quote) "To Reps Serving Ford Plants and Ford Local Unions" (7 Sept. 1955), Box 8, Part I, Series II, UAW-SSD Records; John Carney to Travelers (24 Feb. 1955), Box 849:9, PRR Papers; "The Case for Blue Cross" (1952), Series 14, Box 1, AFHW Papers; workers' letters in Box 849:9 and 850:4, PRR Papers.

[69] Stevens, "Complementing the Welfare State," 43–49; Bureau of National Affairs, "Administration of Health and Welfare Plans" (1954), Box 849:1, PRR Papers; Baruch to Humphrey (9 July 1942), Box 374, Series II, Westmoreland Papers; Klein, "The Business of Welfare," 8–10, 24–35; J.P.N. to J. W. Oram (13 Nov. 1958), Box 855:1, PRR Papers.

local Blues had dropped the practice of community rating.[70] Contracted benefits also hinged on the services offered by commercials and local Blue Cross or Blue Shield plans, and routinely combined them. In some settings, labor and management used Blue Cross hospitalization insurance to supplement established commercial indemnity plans. In some settings, commercial insurance was employed to fill in benefits not offered by the Blues. Some unions, such as the UAW, boasted success in displacing commercial insurance and ensuring that members' health benefits flowed through largely community-based nonprofit channels. Others, such as the electrical workers, found it difficult to loosen the cozy ties between management and commercial insurance. And in many cases, national contracts had to accommodate an array of local arrangements according to the availability of local providers.[71]

Labor's allegiance to the Blues weakened over time. Labor worked closely with Blue Cross in the late 1940s and early 1950s, sometimes even cooperating (as the UAW did in its 1948 negotiations with the Michigan Plan) on a rate increase in order to buttress a nonprofit alternative to commercial insurance. But as commercials picked off the good risks and health costs rose, rate increases became an annual event. Labor increasingly resented premium inflation and the unwillingness of Blue Cross to press providers to control costs. Opposition to Blue Cross, however, was muted by the paucity of alternatives, by concerns that labor might abet "hit and run attacks" on the principle of nonprofit insurance, and by the dismal state of labor relations in the hospitals themselves. The record of Blue Shield, whose coverage had always been spottier and whose relationship with the labor movement had always been weaker, was even worse. As early as 1954, labor leaders noted a "chronic grievance against Blue Shield—the continuing decline in the value of the benefits in relation to doctors' charges."[72] Equally troubling was the persistently uneven nature of Blue Cross and Blue Shield coverage. The UAW, for example,

[70] CFNH Bulletin 11 (8 June 1950), Box 60, Caroline Ware Papers, FDRPL; Harvey Sapolsky, "Empire and the Business of Health Insurance," *JHPPL* 16:4 (1991): 753; NAM, "Industrial, Medical, and Safety Practices" (1951), Box 21, NAM-IRD Papers; Glasser to Cruikshank (17 Apr. 1964), Box 1, Part I, Series I, UAW-SSD Records; "New Blue Cross Rates" (1959), Box 855:1, PRR Papers.

[71] Harry Becker Address (25 June 1950), Box 212, Witte Papers; "Ford" (13 July 1955), Box 8, Part I, Series II, UAW-SSD Records; "Chrysler-UAW-CIO Workers Security Program" (1949), Box 78:851, Series II, Falk Papers; Klein, "The Business of Welfare," 40–46; Falk, "Situation in the Steel Industry," Box 115:1387, Series II, Falk Papers.

[72] Harry Becker, "Recent Blue Cross Increase" (6 July 1948), Box 5; McNary to Gettlinger (16 Sept. 1958), Box 4; UAW Press Release (18 Apr. 1963), Box 1; (quote) Statement by Emanuel Mann before the Insurance Department of the Commonwealth of Pennsylvania (13 Nov. 1958), Box 1; (quote) Harry Becker to Jerome Pollack (5 Mar. 1954), Box 5, all in Part I, Series II, UAW-SSD Records.

won uniform national health benefits in its 1955 contract, but found that many local Blues could not deliver them. Frustration with foot-dragging by local Blues prompted the UAW and others to look to alternative community arrangements, subscribe to Kaiser-like plans where available, and later reluctantly support the development of HMOs.[73] For labor and management, it became increasingly apparent that the Blues represented providers rather than patients. Unions, which had relied on cooperation with Blue Cross in order to bargain effectively, increasingly accused it of "running interference for the hospitals" in the setting of rates or benefits.[74]

Political Costs, Practical Limits: Dilemmas of the Private Welfare State

In their collective fascination with private coverage, labor and management and insurers paid little attention to either the political consequences of relying on employment-based provision or the fate of those left behind. Labor was an ambivalent champion of private coverage: bargaining for health benefits was a logical strategy, even if such benefits undermined the efforts of reformers and girded the arguments of their opponents. Employers and insurers, in turn, argued that innovations in private coverage made public programs unnecessary, even in areas (such as care for the elderly) where such coverage remained rare. "Private employee benefit plans with their inherent flexibility to adapt to the almost infinite requirements of employees and employers," NAM argued in 1965, "should be encouraged to grow and prosper within a favorable government policy and climate."[75]

[73] "Ford" (13 July 1955), Box 8; "Ford Motor Company Health Insurance Problems" (17 Aug. 1956), Box 8; "Hospitalization and Surgical Operation Plans" (27 Jan. 1956), Box 8, all in Part I, Series II, UAW-SSD Records; [UAW] *Social Security Reporter* (Nov. 1955); Derickson, "The USWA and Health Insurance," 77–79; Munts, *Bargaining for Health*, 75–78; Falk to I. Grossberg (7 June 1964) and "Group Practice Prepayment Plans for Steelworkers and Their Families" (May 1964), Box 111:1322, Series II, Falk Papers.

[74] "Labor Council Orders Inquiry" clipping (Nov. 1958), Box 1; telegram to Indiana Blue Cross (21 Jan. 1958), Box 1; (quote) *Washington Evening Star* clipping (17 July 1959), Box 1; Michigan Hospital Service to Walter Reuther (19 Mar. 1948), Box 5; Superintendent of Insurance to Jacob Hurwitz [UAW] (28 Aug. 1962), Box 1; Becker to Pollack (5 Mar. 1954), Box 5; Glasser to Dunlop (27 Oct. 1965), Box 5, all in Part I, Series II, UAW-SSD Records; Rosner and Markowitz, "Hospitals, Insurance, and the American Labor Movement," 86–89.

[75] NAM, "Medical Care for the Aged: An Information Kit" (Jan. 1960), Box I:23; "Proposed Position on Public Policy on Private Welfare and Pension Plans" (Oct. 1965), Box I:103, both in NAM Papers.

Generally speaking, public policy followed suit by sanctioning and subsidizing the private welfare state. Tax policy of the World War II era, refined and reinforced in 1961, encouraged private benefits and rewarded employers who provided them. In the shadow of the debate over the Truman health plan, Taft-Hartley quietly established the framework for private provision in fragmented multiemployer industries like construction ("Taft-Hartley plans" pooled employers and allowed workers to carry coverage from one employer to another within the pool).[76] As the Truman initiative collapsed, the Federal Security Agency turned to private provision as well, conceding that the best coverage would probably come from a "truly expanding economy" that afforded "the breadwinner" the opportunity to "continue producing as long as he wants to without being forced out of the labor market by sickness or disability." The Eisenhower reinsurance proposals were animated by the fear that "time is running against those who seek to keep health insurance on a voluntary basis" and the hope that reinsurance would "in the traditional American way of individual responsibility and private endeavor . . . compress the experimentation of the next 20 years into less than half that time through the simple mechanism of a broad sharing of risks." Medicare and Medicaid, which many feared might serve as a "first step towards socialized medicine," were crafted in such a way as to support the practice and principle of private coverage by shoring up its edges.[77]

There have always been stark limits to the scope of private coverage. Private insurance was slow to offer group coverage and slower still to offer anything approaching comprehensive coverage. In the eyes of insurers, not only those left behind by employee group coverage but a substantial percentage of the gainfully employed were always "uninsurable." Such risks were avoided by pricing individuals and small groups out of the market, dropping retirees from group coverage, and experience rating covered groups. Given employment patterns and insurance practices, private benefits magnified existing disparities in the social wage. Those with jobs got benefits and those with good jobs got better benefits. Most public spending, in turn, went into social insurance programs rather than into public assistance, and the middle and upper-income brackets garnered virtually all of the benefit of the tax expenditures that underwrote private benefits.[78] Although private coverage was

[76] Gottschalk, The Shadow Welfare State, 44–46.

[77] (Quote) FSA recommendations for 1950 State of the Union Address (2 Nov. 1949), POF 419F, Box 1264, Harry S Truman Papers, HSTPL; (quote) "Health Reinsurance" (Jan. 1955), Box I:275, NAM Papers; Nancy Jecker, "Can an Employer-Based Health Insurance System Be Just?" JHPPL 18:3 (1993): 658; (quote) Eugene Caldwell, "Industry's Viewpoint on Medical Care" (10 May 1962), Hagley Imprints.

[78] Proceedings, NICB Conference on Union Health and Welfare Funds (Jan. 1947), pp. 50–52, Box I:29, NICB Papers; "Health Insurance Is Next," Fortune 41:3 (Mar. 1950): 64–

widely justified as a contractual "right" flowing from employee contributions, such rights proved quite tenuous. Coverage rested on past contributions *and* continued employment; employees had no right to carry that coverage into retirement or from one firm to another. Under commercial insurance, the key contractual relationship was not between employee and employer but between employer and insurer, and the latter routinely pressed changes in coverage (or canceled policies outright) if claims experience did not prove profitable. As insurers gathered claims experience on standing group contracts and competed for new ones, employers routinely switched carriers—a business decision that exposed covered workers to new waiting periods, new opportunities for exclusion on the basis of preexisting conditions, and new care arrangements.[79]

Private benefits, in turn, were marked by an ongoing tension between unions, who saw covered employment as a conduit for dependent and retiree care, and employers and insurers, who saw it as a means of avoiding such liabilities. Into the early 1960s, most firms made no provision for retiree care. Those with retiree plans required fifteen or twenty years of service for eligibility and offered substantially lower benefits. Over time, labor too grew leery of retiree coverage—in part because there was "no assurance that any given group of retirees will, throughout their lifetime, continue to be backed by an active working group," and in part because the inclusion of retirees threatened preferential experience rates.[80] Dependent care was widely offered by the early 1960s, though usually on a contributory basis. Such coverage marked an important advance for workers, especially as the costs of care outpaced lost wages. At the same time, dependent coverage also reinforced the family-wage premises of job-based coverage and left many children (especially children of the working poor) without access to private or public insurance.[81]

The private welfare state clearly conceived of women as "dependents" rather than as workers and replicated and magnified the family-wage assumptions of managerial employment, collective bargaining, and social insurance. Insurers marketed group and individual policies as guar-

---

65; Howard, "Hidden Side of the American Welfare State," 416–17; Martin Rein, "The Social Policy of the Firm," *Policy Sciences* 14 (1982): 132.

[79] Staples, "Politics of Employment-Based Insurance," 418; Allen Atkinson to Travelers (17 May 1955), Box 850:4, PRR Papers; NICB Conference on Union Health and Welfare Funds (Jan. 1947), p. 9, Box I:29, NICB Papers; Janaski to McKeown (10 Aug. 1949), Series 3, Box 11, AFHW Papers: Smith to Murkovich (4 Nov. 1954), Series 14, Box 1, AFHW Papers; Poland to Becker (17 Aug. 1950), Box 5, Part I, Series II, UAW-SSD Records.

[80] Merriam to Cohen (20 July 1961), Box 126:10, Cohen Papers; (quote) Brindle to Becker (20 Nov. 1961), Box 1, Part I Series II, UAW-SSD Records; Garbarino, *Health Plans and Collective Bargaining*, 224–32.

[81] HEW, "Self-Insured Health Plans" (May 1955), Box 208, Witte Papers.

antees of family provision, a viewed routinely echoed by employers. As Benson Ford argued in 1955, "every American has a definite and primary responsibility to meet his own and his family's health needs to the full extent of his ability." Organized labor viewed health plans in similarly masculine terms, arguing typically that "every free man has the right to a chance to build up a good home, to give his children education, to get ahead himself and equip his family for a good life." And even health reformers proceeded with the understanding "that a wage-earning man and a housewife can well be recognized as a normal family, particularly when either sickness or unemployment create added strains . . . until the continuation of masculine employment."[82] This reasoning rested on a pair of increasingly untenable assumptions: that the population was neatly organized into familial units headed by male breadwinners; and that sustaining the incomes of those breadwinners would yield adequate health coverage for them and their dependents.[83]

As workers, women did not have the same access to health benefits. Persistent patterns of job segregation relegated women to those jobs least likely to offer health benefits: unorganized firms and industries, domestic and agricultural employment, seasonal or part-time employment, and (especially after 1970) the service sector. Labor market participation was also shaped by female responsibility for children (including the health care of children). As the labor market participation of single (excluding widowed and divorced) women progressed in fits and starts (from 48 percent in 1940, to 44 percent in 1960, to 62 percent in 1980) and the participation of married women grew more dramatically (17 percent in 1940, 32 percent in 1960, 51 percent in 1980), patterns of work still depended closely on the presence and age of dependent children.[84] Movement in and out of the labor force in order to meet familial responsibili-

[82] Jerome Miller, *Selling Accident and Health Insurance* (New York, 1940), 5; (quote) Ford, "A Businessman Looks at Health" (1955), Box 208, Witte Papers; (quote) *Labor's Monthly Survey* (Oct. 1942) in POF 142:1, FDR Papers; "American Beveridge Plan and American Business" (1943), POF 1710:3, FDR Papers; (quote) Williamson to Falk (8 Jan. 1943), Box 68:699, Series II, Falk Papers.

[83] Joni Hersch and Shelly White Means, "Employer Sponsored Health and Pension Benefits and the Gender/Race Wage Gap," *Social Science Quarterly* 74:4 (1993): 854; Jecker, "Can an Employer-Based Health Insurance System Be Just?" 662–65.

[84] Claudia Goldin, *Understanding the Gender Gap: An Economic History of Wage-Earning Women* (New York, 1990), 17; "Families with own children: Employment status of parents by age of youngest child and family type, 1998–99," at www.stats.bls.gov/news.release/famee.t04.htm; Howard Hayghe, "Development in Women's Labor Force Participation," *MLR* (Sept. 1997): 41–46; Lynn Weiner, *Working Girl to Working Mother: The Female Labor Force in the United States, 1820–1980* (Chapel Hill, N.C., 1985), 93; Ann Corinne Hill, "Protection of Women Workers and the Courts: A Legal Case History," *Feminist Studies* 5:2 (1979): 247–71.

ties made it difficult to establish vested rights in firm-level social insurance—a dilemma especially true of health insurance that exposed workers to preexisting condition restrictions whenever they changed jobs. And even working women were, in the calculus of social insurance, dependents of men. As late as 1967, for example, ILGWU officials argued that lesser benefits for its predominantly female membership were justified by the assumption that "many of these women are married, and the major health needs of their husbands and children may be financed from the husbands' wages or fringe benefits"—even as they acknowledged that "it is not known, however, to what extent this is true."[85]

The occupational and temporal patterns of women's work and the premises of social insurance were compounded by the deeply gendered nature of medical underwriting. Commercial insurers had always maintained higher group rates for industries and firms that employed mostly women and often declined to offer individual coverage to women at all.[86] Insurers, employers, and unions alike assumed that women posed a peculiar risk and crafted benefit plans accordingly. Insurance plans routinely disallowed claims (as at Bethlehem Steel) "in the case of female participants, from any sickness which is recurrent or peculiarly due to their sex" or (as at Westmoreland Coal) which involved "any sickness or condition to which both sexes are not subject." Riders usually excluded maternity, reproductive health ("claims involving the female organs") and other "female disorders."[87] In turn, women were often subject to the sort of attention and interference associated with charitable rather than contractual social policy. Consider the following account of maternity policy in the early 1940s at AC Spark Plug:

> There is such close observation of the women working in the plants that a pregnancy is known not later than the second month. The woman is invited in to the office of the social worker and urged to contact a good physician,

---

[85] Max Shain, "Survey of the Union Health Center and Hospital Benefit Program" (1967), 10:252, Series I, Caldwell Esselstyn Papers, Sterling Library.

[86] Hersch and Means, "Employer Sponsored Health and Pension Benefits," 851, 855; Beth Stevens and Lauri Perman, "Industrial Segregation and the Gender Distribution of Fringe Benefits," *Gender and Society* 3:3 (1989): 389–90, 395–96; Baker, "Women in War Industries," 56; Health Information Foundation, "Voluntary Health Insurance for the Individual Subscriber" (Mar. 1953), Box 208, Witte Papers; Tom Eilers, "The Case for Accident and Sickness Insurance" (1954), Box 208, Witte Papers.

[87] NICB Conference on Union Health and Welfare Funds (Jan. 1947), pp. 73–75, Box I:29, NICB Papers; (quote) Minutes of the 14th Annual Meeting of the Board of Trustees [Bethlehem Relief Plan] (Feb. 1940), Hagley Imprints; (quote) Casper to Rogers (10 Aug. 1942), Box 374, Series II, Westmoreland Papers; (quote) Andrew Janaskie to Locals (15 Oct. 1963), Series 14, Box 1, AFHW Papers; Naomi Naierman and Ruth Brannon, "Sex Discrimination in Insurance," in United States Commission on Civil Rights, *Discrimination against Minorities and Women in Pensions and Health, Life, and Disability Insurance* (1978), I:480–84.

and advised that she is to be reported to the health department as prenatal. We check our records to determine whether she shows up in any of our mothercraft classes. If she fails, we report back and the gal is prompted by both the public health nurse in the district of her residence and the social worker to "play ball". . . . Under the medical and hospitalization insurance plan, and under an agreement between management and labor women must discontinue work at the fifth month . . . but are followed by us to see that they get acceptable instruction and care. Under the plan, hospitalization and medical insurance takes over at delivery, and then unemployment compensation again takes over when the mother returns from the hospital.

Sex-specific exclusions not only allowed employers and insurers to avoid maternity coverage (until the passage of the 1978 Pregnancy Discrimination Act), but also figured prominently in constraints on reproductive and occupational freedom. The foremost obstacle to abortion rights would always be their exclusion from private and public insurance coverage. And reproductive "protections" were often used to camouflage efforts to ease women out of nontraditional jobs.[88]

Even as covered and contributing workers, women were often treated as undeserving recipients because their place in the labor force was always suspect and their claims on insurance plans were considered excessive. In 1947 national officials of the American Federation of Full-Fashioned Hosiery Workers (AFFFHW) faced escalating premiums and warned locals of "excessive" female claims. "One of the most discouraging things which cannot slip by unnoticed," union officials reasoned, "is the type of claims that is being made by our female membership. They are not the types which are definite and positive such as female operations or appendectomy or thyroid. They are principally claims which leave a broad avenue of doubt of total disability open, such as, anemia, neurosis, nervousness, extremely nervous exhaustion, tired eyes, neuritis, menopause, etc. etc."[89] The punch line, at least for the union, was that "this kind of ratio is bound to kill our splendid insurance coverage and if this happens, and we must turn to some other insurance company to write a much less favorable policy, the real sufferer is going to be the family of the breadwinner or the male member of our Union." Such sentiments also emerged in the classification of eligible dependents.

---

[88] AC Spark Plug account in Sappington to Eliot (5 May 1942), Box 148, Central File, 1941–1944, RG 102, Records of the Children's Bureau, National Archives, College Park, Md.; Lisa Hayden, "Gender Discrimination within the Reproductive Health Care System," *Journal of Law and Health* 13:2 (1998–99): 171–80; Wendy Chavkin, "Occupation Hazards to Reproduction," *Feminist Studies* 5:2 (1979): 310–20.

[89] William Smith to Branch Secretaries (26 July 1947) and Smith to Katz (27 June 1945), both in Series 3, Box 11, AFHW Papers.

Under most plans, wives were held to be dependents of employed husbands, but female employees could only claim children as dependents. "There is quite a difference in the interpretation of the dependent husband as compared to the dependent wife," acknowledged the AFFFHW. "The policy does not consider the husband as a dependent for that disability which caused the husband to be a dependent of the wife." By the same reasoning, elderly mothers were dependents, fathers were not.[90]

Private Benefits in Crisis, 1965–2000

Even during the most robust years of postwar growth, employment-based group insurance offered tenuous and uneven coverage. As postwar growth slowed in the late 1960s and stumbled into the 1970s, so too did the fate of the private health provision. Deindustrialization displaced high-wage, high-benefit industrial employment with low-wage, no-benefit service employment, and drove industrial unions into a pattern of concessionary bargaining in which fringe benefits were often the first casualty.[91] The new service economy attenuated the long-standing divide between the managerial strata and a white-collar working class. Indeed, the latter was increasingly defined by patterns and practices (subcontracting, part-time employment, high turnover) that undermined benefits.

To make matters worse, all of this was accompanied by health inflation that predated and outpaced the general inflationary crisis of the 1970s. Employers lamented the steady increase in costs and the incentives that fed it: doctors "told us frankly that they had had mill business for a long time and never made much money out of it," one noted, "and now that the insurance was in they were going to get the insurance plus whatever the person had in his pocket." Just as important, employers increasingly complained that labor got credit for winning health benefits but that management's contribution went "unnoticed until the cost of the plan has risen so far out of line that the company tries to revise and restrict the benefits." Insurers were "perfectly ready to write the most liberal plans any company insists upon . . . after all, if the price is right, it is the company's dollars we are going to be spending," but they increasingly

[90] International Harvester, "Group Hospital and Surgical Benefit Plan" (1946), in imprints collection, Hagley Museum; (quotes) Anne Murkovich to Branch Secretaries (21 May 1951), Series 14, Box 1, AFHW Papers; Alice Kessler-Harris, "Designing Women and Old Fools: The Construction of the Social Security Amendments of 1939," in *U.S. History as Women's History*, ed. Linda Kerber, Alice Kessler-Harris, and Kathryn Kish Sklar (Chapel Hill, N.C., 1995), 95–100; Ida Merriam to Wilbur Cohen (20 July 1961), Box 126:10, Cohen Papers.

[91] Kim Moody, *An Injury to All: The Decline of American Unionism* (London, 1988), 165–92.

questioned "the soundness of giving the doctor, the hospital, or the employee the blank check that many Comprehensive plans do." And having won the principle of employer-funded health care, labor found itself "on some sort of a treadmill . . . just as fast as they could negotiate money to provide more and better health services for their members, doctors raised their fees and hospitals boosted their charges."[92]

Business and labor began noting inflation in the early 1950s (by one estimate, health costs more than doubled through the 1950s) and blamed increased costs on "doctors and hospitals taking advantage of group plans." At the same time, labor continued to press for more comprehensive services—leaving most health plans, as Benson Ford noted, "squeezed between the pincers of fast rising medical costs on the one hand and a growing demand for broadened benefits and coverage on the other." "The premium has been growing so steadily as to remind one of the sorcerer's apprentice," added a union official in 1958, "even when cut in half, each half being shared by the employees and the industry . . . the half now costs more than the earlier whole, and there is nothing in sight that even suggests a change ahead."[93] In response, labor and management launched various initiatives, including the first efforts at utilization review and non-occupational health services, and closer attention to risk and benefit management.[94]

The cost of private health insurance rose through the late 1950s and early 1960s, and settled into a pattern of double-digit inflation by 1964—reflecting, in large part, the widespread adoption of the "usual, customary, and reasonable" system of billing. Doctors insisted on UCR billing in order to maintain some autonomy while participating in Medicare and Medicaid, and insurers and employers accepted the practice as a

[92] George Heitler, "The Blue Cross in Cost Control" (3 May 1960), Box 884:25, PRR Papers; (quote) NICB Proceedings, "The Insurance Drive: What's Ahead at the Bargaining Table" (May 1950), pp. 26–27, Box I:33, NICB Papers; (quote) Dulaney, "Can Employers Afford Comprehensive Medical Plans?" 56; (quote) George Meany in "The Nation's Health" (conference proceedings, Nov. 1969), Box 112:1336, Series II, Falk Papers.

[93] (Quote) "Administration of Health and Welfare Plans" (1954), Box 849:1, PRR Papers; *BW* (30 Oct. 1971), 104; HEW, *Medical Care Prices* (Feb. 1967), Box 21, Edgar Kaiser Papers; Walter Pollner, "Influence on the Rate of Growth of Expenditures for Voluntary Health Insurance" (1959), Box 208, Witte Papers; Anne R. Somers and Herman Somers, "Health Insurance: Are Cost and Quality Controls Necessary?" *ILRR* 13:4 (1960): 588; (quote) Ford, "A Businessman Looks at Health" (1955); (quote) Jerome Pollack, "Health Insurance Today and Tomorrow: A Labor View" (Feb. 1958), Box 206, Witte Papers.

[94] Cecil Sheps and Daniel Drosness, "Prepayment for Medical Care," *NEJM* 264:10 (9 Mar. 1961): 496; Robert Page, "Industry Calls in the Doctor," *HBR* 31:5 (Sept.–Oct. 1953): 108–17; Marilyn Field and Harold Shapiro, *Employment and Health Benefits: A Connection at Risk* (Washington, D.C., 1993), 73–77; Mulcahy, "New Deal for Coal Miners," 40–41; Brumm to the Executive Committee (29 June 1955), Box J49:4, Walton Hamilton Papers, Rare Books and Manuscripts, Tarlton Law Library, University of Texas, Austin, Tex.

compromise between rigid fee schedules and "blank check" service coverage. Unions, willing to "gamble on the risk of inflation in order to achieve service," conceded to UCR as an alternative to coinsurance or deductibles. Not surprisingly, UCR billing, as one UAW official noted in 1964, provided "the occasion for physicians to probe the outer limits of acceptable fees and to justify higher fees on the basis of those charged by other physicians." "You cannot control costs," as I. S. Falk observed in retrospect, "and give a signed check to doctors, hospitals, and insurance companies."[95] Private health spending ran steadily ahead of inflation, growing (on average) just over 10 percent each year between 1968 and 1998. Between 1965 and 1990, health costs swelled from 6 to nearly 15 percent of the gross domestic product while health spending by business alone ballooned from to 1 to 4 percent of GDP, and from 14 percent to over 100 percent of after-tax profits.[96]

Almost as soon as employer-financed service benefits became the norm, employers began looking for ways to escape them and looking for others to shoulder the burden. "Confronted by a staggering rise in employee health care costs over the past five years," as *Business Week* noted in the early 1970s, "employers have tried to staunch the flow of cash by switching to self-insurance, monitoring claims, participating in regional health planning agencies, and even appealing to employees to double-check their own medical bills. Mostly they have simply wrung their hands in frustration." Such anxieties prompted a variety of solutions but, most important, employers brought their concerns to the bargaining table and began to retreat from their commitment to the private welfare state. "I hope that none of us will abandon our employees," NAM's Richard Heckert testified in 1990, "but we are going to cut our losses."[97] Such losses, it should be noted, were not nearly as

[95] (Quotes) Hurwitz to Glasser (31 Mar. 1964) , Box 1, Part I, Series II, UAW-SSD Records; Russ to Tomayko (31 Mar. 1964), Box 111:1322, Series II, Falk Papers; Joint Subcommittee on Medical Care with Representatives of Blue Cross (6 Apr. 1961), Box 110:1314, Series II, Falk Papers; (Falk quote) Minutes, CNHI Technical Committee (5 July 1972), Box 3, Arthur Altmeyer add., SHSW.

[96] Cost figures from "Public and Private Expenditures for Health and Medical Care, 1950–1967" (1968), Box 109:4, Cohen Papers; John Iglehart, "The American Health Care System," *NEJM* 326:25 (18 June 1992): 1716; Robert Evans, "Finding the Levers, Finding the Courage: Lessons from Cost Containment in North America," *JHPPL* 11 (1986): 589, 596; Gail Jensen, "Cost Sharing and the Changing Pattern of Employer-Sponsored Health Benefits," *MMFQ* 65:4 (1987): 522; Regina Herzlinger, "Can We Control Medical Costs?" *HBR* 56:2 (Mar.–Apr. 1978): 102; Health Care Financing Administration, "National Health Expenditures, 1960–1998," archived at www.hcfa.gov.

[97] (Quote) *BW* (17 May 1971): 144; Stanley Jones, "What Is the Future of Private Health Insurance?" in *Social Insurance Issues for the Nineties* (proceedings of the Third Conference of the National Academy of Social Insurance), ed. Paul Van de Water (Dubuque, Iowa, 1992), 20–21; U.S. Department of Health, Education, and Welfare, *Trends Affecting the U.S. Health Care System* (Washington, D.C., 1976), pp. 211–21; U.S. Senate, Subcommittee on

frightening as they were often portrayed. Costs to business were over-drawn to the extent that they represented deferred wages or were offset by tax advantages. And for most of corporate America, increased health costs had little effect on the bottom line. As employers retreated from health coverage in the 1980s and 1990s, corporate profits also climbed steadily (the after-tax profit rate in the late 1990s of between 7 and 8 percent approached the postwar peak of the early 1960s). Business anxiety over health costs—and the cuts and cost sharing that followed from them—were part of the broader assault on labor standards and labor costs that accompanied the competitive anxieties of the postgrowth economy.[98]

Through the 1980s and early 1990s, the rate of employment provision for civilian workers slipped from 61 percent to 54 percent; for low-wage workers it fell from 30 percent to 14 percent. Deindustrialization undermined the very premises of the private welfare state. Employment-founded on health benefits had always been based on the assumption that commercial insurance or self-insurance could only be offered to large, actuarially sound employee groups. After 1980, job growth was concentrated in small and service firms with little record of health provision. By one estimate (for 1985–91), every 100 jobs lost in manufacturing represented a net loss (including dependents) of 224 covered persons, while every 100 new service jobs yielded only 40 covered workers or dependents. In turn, economic and demographic shifts reopened the race and gender gap. Employment opportunities for women in the burgeoning service sector were compromised by conditions that undermined the provision of benefits: small firms, low levels of unionization, increased utilization of part-time and contingent workers. By the late 1990s about three-quarters of white men but just over half of all other workers claimed health coverage. Although women and men made up roughly equal portions of the uninsured population (a reflection of spousal benefits), as single household heads men (at 80 percent) were far more likely than women (at 50 percent) to be covered.[99]

Health, Committee on Labor of Public Welfare, *Inflation of Health Care Costs, 1976* (Washington, D.C., 1976), 118–46, 829–38; U.S. Congress, House, Subcommittee on Health, Committee on Ways and Means, *National Health Insurance* (Washington, D.C., 1976), passim; Heckert testimony in U.S. House, Subcommittee on Labor Management Relations, Committee on Education and Labor, *The Growing Crisis in Health Care* (Washington, D.C., 1990), 60.

[98] Gottschalk, *The Shadow Welfare State*, 121, 123; profit rates from Dean Baker and Lawrence Mishel, "Profits Up, Wages Down," *Economic Policy Institute Briefing Paper* (Sept. 1995): 7–8.

[99] HIAA (1990) figures in Senate Committee on Labor and Human Resources, *Health Security Act of 1993: Part I* 103:1 (Oct.–Nov., 1993), 365; impact of deindustrialization in Deborah Chollet, "Employment-Based Health Insurance in a Changing Work Force," *HA* 13:1 (1994): 315–21; Hersch and Means, "Employer-Sponsored Health and Pension Bene-

Employers who could not escape coverage altogether began demanding concessions or cost sharing in contract negotiations—indeed, attempts to chisel away at health coverage provoked many of the major labor disputes (including the Baby Bell and Pittston strikes) of the 1970s and 1980s. Contracts introduced higher deductibles, caps on the employers' share of health care premiums, and copayment of plans previously funded entirely by employers. Such measures reflected both the ongoing cost crisis and the long-standing anxiety that "hospital-oriented first-dollar coverage" represented a dangerous moral hazard. As early as 1971 the Chamber of Commerce championed deductibles on the grounds that only "the personal involvement of the insured" could ensure responsible utilization. Although most firms continued to accept a role for employer contributions, most also felt that that contribution should not exceed half of the premium cost. Nearly three-quarters of providing firms paid the full costs of their respective health plans by the late 1970s; barely a third continued to do so in the mid-1990s. Only a handful (14 percent) of firms required deductibles by the late 1970s; a majority (55 percent) did so by the mid-1980s. Employers also began toying with "cafeteria plans" that allotted employees a dollar amount for benefits, and then left it to them to make hard choices with scarce resources from a menu of benefits.[100]

Many employers ducked their commitments to retiree care. In terms of both its direct costs and its impact on group-rated premiums, retiree coverage was relatively expensive. Equally important, a 1993 Financial Accounting Standards Board (FASB) ruling forced firms to record health

---

fits," 851, 855; James Tallon and Rachel Block, "Changing Patterns of Health Insurance Coverage: Special Concerns for Women," *Women and Health* 12:3 (1987): 119–22; Goldin, *Understanding the Gender Gap*, 179–83; Current Population Survey, "Work experience of the population during the year by sex and extent of employment, 1998–99," at http://stats.bls.gov/news.release/work.t01.htm; Sara Kuhn and Barry Bluestone, "Economic Restructuring and the Female Labor Market: The Impact of Industrial Change on Women," in *Women, Households, and the Economy,* ed. Beneria and Stimpson, 3–30.

[100] William M. Davis, "Collective Bargaining in 1990," *MLR* 113/1 (Jan. 1990): 3–18; "Companies Cut Medical Costs," *NYT* (7 Nov. 1989); "Developments in Industrial Relations," *MLR* 112/12 (Dec. 1989): 55; *MLR* 113/3 (Mar. 1990): 65; *MLR* 113/7 (July 1990): 52; "Health Care Vigilantes," *NYT* (24 Sept. 1989); "Are Companies Cutting Too Close to the Bone?" *BW* (30 Oct. 1989): 143–44; "Corporate Health Care Costs," *The Economist* (9 Mar. 1991): 70; NICB,"Issues in Health Insurance" (Jan. 1977), Box I:190, NICB Papers; (quote) Chamber of Commerce, "Improving Our Nation's Health Care System: Proposals for the 1970s" (1971), Box II:27, Chamber of Commerce Papers; "Who's Saying No to Uninsured Kids?" *Business and Health* 15:3 (1997): 33; Marilyn Werber Serafini, "Getting Stuck with the Tab," *National Journal* (19 Oct. 96): 2252; Jensen, "Changing Pattern of Employer-Sponsored Health Benefits," 528–42; NICB, "Employee Benefits: Promises and Realities" (Jan. 1977), Box I:190, NICB Papers; *BW* (8 Sept. 1986): 50; *BW* (16 Apr. 1984): 50.

care liabilities as they accrued rather than as they were paid. In 1988, for example, American firms paid out $9 billion in health care to retirees. However, retiree liabilities totaled almost $230 billion, or nearly 10 percent of the stock market value of the firms concerned. Had the FASB rule been in effect in 1988, corporate profits would have been cut by $21 billion (the year's increase in liability). This prospect left *Business Week* worrying that the FASB ruling might shorten the fuse of a "demographic time bomb" that "could virtually wipe out profit as we know it for the top 1,000 public companies." Slashing retiree coverage often depended on the type of insurance offered or even the wording of the policy. Self-insured firms and industries found it relatively easy to cut retiree coverage; those operating under collective bargaining and commercial insurance contracts found it harder to retreat.[101]

Another common strategy was self-insurance, an arrangement by which the employer underwrote the health plan and employed commercial insurers only to handle the administrative details. This was an attractive option, especially for large firms, because self-insured plans escaped the regulatory attention of both the 1974 Employment Retirement and Income Security Act (ERISA) and state insurance regulation. The drift to self-insurance began in the early 1960s and accelerated in the 1970s and 1980s as firms sought greater managerial control. By 1990 over half of covered workers were enrolled in self-insured health plans.[102] This retreat to a more discretionary welfare-capitalist model of provision was also reflected in the proliferation of in-house health programs. Firms increasingly hired their own doctors, instituted fitness or substance-abuse programs, and required employers to pass health exams in order to qualify for good-health rebates.[103]

The most important change in private health care was the spread of the health maintenance organization and other innovations in managed care. Competition among health plans and close utilization review within them, argued proponents, would allow "the market" to reform a health system "characterized by uninformed consumers, a lack of management

[101] "Corporate Health-Care Bills," *The Economist* (6 Jan. 1990): 62, 66; (quote) "Broken Promises or Broken Budgets," *BW* (10 Dec. 1990): 34; "Retiree Benefits," *BW* (27 Feb. 1989): 39; *BW* (16 Apr. 1984): 50; *BW* (17 Dec. 1984): 106.

[102] HIAA Annual Report of the General Manager (1964/1965), Box 20, Grahame Papers; Joe Peel to D. A. Paulman (2 July 1964), Box 23, Grahame Papers; Jensen, "Changing Pattern of Employer-Sponsored Health Benefits," 543–44.

[103] Employee Benefit Research Institute, *The Changing Health Care Market* (Washington, D.C., 1987), 1–30; "New Incentives to Take Care," *NYT* (21 Mar. 1989); Camille Colatosi, "Who Benefits from Flexible Health Care?" *Labor Notes* (Apr. 1990): 7; "Preventive Medicine," *Nation's Business* (Sep. 1995): 32–33; David Calkins and Regina Herzlinger, "How Companies Tackle Health Care Costs," *HBR* 64:1 (Jan.–Feb. 1986), 70–80.

skills, small and fragmented delivery units, noncompetitive cost-plus pricing features, and inefficient incentives for both buyers and sellers of
health services." By either employing providers directly or organizing
them into "preferred provider" networks, the HMO gave employers and
insurers greater control over health costs and patterns of utilization. At
least for employers, the strategy was a qualified success. As enrollment
in HMOs swelled (to 85 percent of covered employees in the late 1990s),
growth in employer spending on health slowed (the average annual increase fell from 12 percent in the 1980s to 5 percent in the 1990s). The
bigger picture, however, was somewhat muddier, as HMO enthusiasts
rarely distinguished among the savings realized by actually lowering the
costs of services, by rationing services, and by shuffling employers' costs
elsewhere (usually onto employees or public programs).[104]

Workers and their unions dug in against increased costs and decreased
benefits, but lost ground on both fronts. Unions proved necessarily shortsighted, battling to retain existing benefits but often joining employers in
efforts to rein in costs or utilization. Many defended experience rating,
encouraged self-insurance, or promoted HMOs for the same reasons as
their employers; they wanted to retain coverage by controlling its costs.
In turn, unions had little choice but to accept increased out-of-pocket
costs or HMO coverage when they were presented as essential to the
survival of private provision.[105] Consider the experience of the UMW
Fund, which began to falter in the 1960s as health costs rose and royalties
(based on declining tonnage) fell. As early as 1962 some mines tried to
break the fund by withdrawing their contributions and farming health
coverage out to Blue Cross and Blue Shield. After ERISA, the fund had to
manage its retirement and health plans as separate accounts, effectively
orphaning the latter. In 1978 the fund shuffled the responsibility for
medical care (with the exception of some retirees) back to the individual

[104] Paul Ellwood and Michael Herbert, "Health Care: Should Companies Buy It or Sell
It?" *HBR* 51:4 (July–Aug. 1973): 99–102 (quote at 99); Ernest Saward and Merwyn Greenlick,
"Health Policy and the HMO," *MMFQ* 50:2 (Apr. 1972): 166–68; NICB Proceedings, "Em-
ployee Benefits: Promises and Realities" (Jan. 1977), Box I:190, NICB Papers; Employment
Benefits Research Institute, "Employer Spending on Benefits in 1997" (Nov. 1999); EBRI,
"Employment-Based Health Care Benefits" (Sept. 1998); Lawrence Brown, *Politics and Health
Care Organization: HMOs as Federal Policy* (Washington, D.C., 1983): 172–91.

[105] "Health Insurance Legislative Update," *JNMA* 84:1 (1992): 17; Sparks to Glasser (14
June 1971), "Draft Memo Re: proposed Model Neighborhood/Blues Health Program" (4
Oct. 1971), Loren to Sparks (4 Oct. 1971), "UAW Role in MNCHP" (22 Nov. 1971), all in
Box 41, Part II, Series III, UAW-SSD Records; Marie Gottschalk, "The Missing Millions:
Organized Labor, Business, and the Defeat of Clinton's Health Security Act," *JHPPL* 24:3
(1999): 495–96; Lawrence Weil, "Organized Labor and Health Reform: Unions Interests
and the Clinton Plan," *Journal of Public Health Policy* 18:1 (1997): 36–38.

mines. This undermined the stability of the fund and invited companies (as underscored in the Pittston strike) to escape the accord altogether.[106]

Despite the inherent limits of private provision and the wavering commitment of employers from the early 1970s on, reformers and their opponents alike increasingly viewed private benefits as the cornerstone of national health policy. Prescriptions for the ongoing health care crisis, including the reform efforts of the early 1970s and early 1990s, generally concentrated on stabilizing employment-based provision, expanding its reach, or cleaning up around its perimeter. Debate narrowed to often arcane confrontations over how best to achieve these goals. By and large, liberal reformers leaned toward mandated employment-based provision, usually coupled with some mechanism for cost control and some provision for pooling small employers or individuals.[107] Conservatives put more faith in supply-side managed care or managed competition initiatives, usually coupled with income tax reform that would encourage or subsidize (through premium deductibility or medical savings accounts) "personal responsibility" for health provision.[108] But both—for a tangle of political, fiscal, and practical reasons—accepted the premises and the promises of the private welfare state.

[106] Mulcahy, "In the Union's Service," 30–41; Mulcahy, "Partitioning the Miners' Welfare State: The Destruction of the Medical Program of the UMWA Welfare and Retirement Fund," *Mid-America* 77:2 (1995): 182–95; Harlan County Coal Operator's Association to All Operators (11 Sept. 1962), Josephine Roche to "Coal Company" (5 Sept. 1962), Roche to "Employee" (29 Aug. 1962), all in Box 429, Series II, Westmoreland Papers; Goldstein, "Rise and Decline of the UMWA Funds," 239–41, 257–65; Berney, "The Rise and Fall of the UMW Fund," 99–102; Colin Gordon, "Miners' Health Bargain," *Z Magazine* (May–June 1992): 56–57; "Retired Coal Miners Rally," *Labor Notes* (Apr. 1992); "Fiercest Fight on Taxes: Health Care For Miners, *NYT* (15 Mar. 1992): 13.

[107] Draft of the Minutes of the Technical Advisory Group of CNHI" (16 Dec. 1969) and (10 Mar. 1970), Box 3 (Mss 400), Arthur J. Altmeyer Papers, SHSW; Marsh Berzon [AFL] to Karen Ignani (13 May 1993), Box 961; Zelman to Magaziner (11 Mar. 1993), Box 3308; "Short-term options to promote managed care" (n.d.), Box 1173, all in Records of the Clinton Health Task Force, National Archives.

[108] Enthoven to Califano, Memo on National Health Insurance (22 Sept. 1977), Box 228:2, Cohen Papers; *BW* (8 Feb. 1982): 58–60; "Taking the Taxes out of Health Care," *Nation's Business* (Dec. 1996): 29–30; NICB Proceedings, "Employee Benefits: Promises and Realities" (Jan. 1977), Box I: 190, NICB Papers.

3

Between Contract and Charity: Health Care and the Dilemmas of Social Insurance

THE United States has always had a notoriously weak sense of social citizenship. The confusion of citizenship and property rights, a characteristic of modern liberalism exaggerated in the American setting, has created a two-tracked welfare system in which contractual employment benefits or contributory public programs have always been more important and more legitimate than means-tested charitable assistance. From early in the twentieth century, fascination with contractual benefits imbued social provision with the family-wage premise of the private economy: women were viewed as either maternal conduits for charitable family assistance or dependents of contracted employment benefits, and health care was confined to either male breadwinners or especially deserving fragments of the population. And the focus on property rights had profound racial implications, not only because for much of American history African Americans *were* property, but also because the relationship between social provision and industrial employment segregated the emerging welfare state. Any sense of universal entitlement remained very weak: "For the poor and sick—well and good, reasoned a typical reaction to the health debate of the 1940s, "but plenty of us are neither poor nor sick—so what about us?"[1]

Against the broader emergence of social insurance in the United States, health care posed an enduring dilemma. Reformers leaned heavily on the political and administrative appeal of social insurance, and yet (as opponents tirelessly pointed out) health-care provision defied the logic of such programs. This confusion spilled over into the question of how to pay for health care, a persistent tug-of-war between the medical, actuarial, and administrative logic of universal provision, on the one hand, and the political appeal of contributory financing, on the other.

---

[1] Nancy Fraser and Linda Gordon, "Contract vs. Charity: Why Is There No Social Citizenship in the United States?" *Socialist Review* (1992): 5–47, 52–53, 62; William Forbath, *Law and the Shaping of the American Labor Movement* (Cambridge, Mass., 1991), 25–29; Gwendolyn Mink, "The Lady and the Tramp: Gender, Race, and the Origins of the American Welfare State," in *Women, the State, and Welfare,* ed. Linda Gordon (Madison, Wis., 1990), 92–93, 99; Olive Wheeler to HST (19 Nov. 1945), President's Personal File [PPF] 200, Box 257, Harry S. Truman Papers, Harry S. Truman Presidential Library [HSTPL], Independence, Mo.

Employment-based health care exemplified the political and fiscal logic of contributory social insurance but also underscored its limits. As a result, reformers sought out other deserving recipients—children, veterans, the indigent, the elderly—in such a way as to both supplement employment-based care and fragment any sense of universal provision.

The American Way: Social Insurance as Social Policy

The idea of workingmen's insurance or social insurance emerged in the late nineteenth and early twentieth century as American politicians and academics began take note of the welfare regimes emerging in western Europe. Although some pressed for European-style welfare systems, most approached the problem as one of adapting European ideas to American conditions—of reconciling the consequences of industrial society with the practical and cultural limits of American government. Indeed American social insurance advocates ascribed a wide range of meanings to the term. Some leaned on its "social" implications and pressed for compulsory state programs. Some leaned on the idea of voluntary "insurance" against the interruptions in employment. Some saw social insurance as a means of compensating workers for dismal industrial conditions. Some hoped that social insurance would force employers to improve those conditions. But most would agree, as the American Federation of Labor would put it, that social insurance was the "principle of making a series of small payments when you are well and earning money" against the risks of sickness, unemployment, or retirement.[2]

Although social insurance made little headway in the Progressive Era, its basic premises had enormous implications for the future of the American welfare state. Perhaps most important, it understood poverty as a consequence of industrialism and focused political attention on industrial workers. "Social insurances in the United States grew out of the employer experience," one observer stressed. "They extend to all the principles found effective by leading employers [and] . . . put a floor on competition by short-sighted employers who have avoided the true costs of an effective labor force." Although such views retreated from the excesses of Social Darwinism and accepted some responsibility for the conditions of modern employment, they also drew a clear boundary between

---

[2] Theda Skocpol, *Protecting Soldiers and Mothers: The Political Origins of American Social Policy* (Cambridge, Mass., 1992), 160–204; David Moss, *Socializing Security: Progressive-Era Economists and the Origins of American Social Policy* (Cambridge, Mass., 1996), 60–75; "New Directions in Health Benefits," *American Federationist* 72:9 (1965), 6–7.

the worthy poor (industrial workers) and others.[3] The needs of women and children were subsumed by the family-wage logic of "workingman's insurance." Social provision reflected and reinforced patterns of occupational and racial segregation. And farmers, farm laborers, domestics, and the self-employed would claim uneven access to a welfare state provided or paid for at the workplace.

Social insurance proponents hammered away at the political, moral, financial, and psychological connection between contributions and benefits. The term "insurance" rarely carried the full actuarial implications of pooled risk and was meant only to distinguish social insurance from charity. "The wage earner has a more real basis for feeling the benefits he receives are rights to which he as a citizen is entitled," one reformer argued, adding that a contributory system "removes all taint of charity which so often accompanies employers' welfare work."[4] This reasoning collapsed as state-level efforts stalled and employers experimented with firm-level plans. Between the Progressive Era and the New Deal, welfare capitalists designed discretionary and noncontributory programs precisely to avoid any implication of legal entitlement: such benefits were considered "a voluntary act of the employer who, in most cases, admits no contractual obligation on his own part nor any legal right there to on the part of the employee," as the National Industrial Conference Board stressed in 1925, allowing only that employers might "acknowledge a moral obligation and a corresponding moral claim."[5]

The Depression underscored the limits of welfare capitalism and the urgency of a more expansive system of relief. The New Deal drew heavily on social insurance ideas and accepted both the logic of contractual provision and its limits. For the architects of Social Security, contributory social insurance solved a tangle of political and fiscal and ideological problems. "We put those payroll contributions there so as to give the contributors a legal, moral, and political right to collect," recalled Roosevelt famously, ". . . with those taxes in there, no damn politician can ever scrap my Social Security program." Strategic and political considerations were buttressed by arguments about the psychology of contributory programs. "This approach starts from the premise that what workers really

---

[3] (Quote) J. Douglas Brown, "Management's Stake in the Survival of Contributory Social Insurance," Box 64:614, Series II, Isidore Falk Papers, Sterling Library, Yale University, New Haven, Conn.; Moss, *Socializing Security*, 40–43, 56–68.

[4] Statements before the Advisory Committee in Box 9, Decimal File 025, Records of the Social Security Board [SSB], Office of the Commissioner, RG 47, Social Security Administration [SSA], National Archives, College Park, Md.; "Report of the Committee on Social Insurance," *JAMA* (17 June 1916): 1975.

[5] NICB, *Industrial Pensions in the United States* (New York, 1924), 24.

want is continued employment rather than any benefit which gives them a part only of their former wages," argued the Committee on Economic Security, adding that "this is also assumed to be by far the best policy for society at large." Turning its attention to health insurance, the CES was even less equivocal: "The question of whether insurance should be contributory or non-contributory has almost ceased to be discussed . . . . In the eyes of the workers and of the public in general the contribution is the feature which distinguishes insurance from relief, [and] creates a right to benefits."[6]

This principle was repeated and reinforced in every refinement of Social Security after 1935 and in every effort to add health insurance to the Social Security system. In discussions leading up to the 1939 Social Security amendments, Social Security Advisory Council member J. Douglas Brown stressed that the council "had in mind that we in America were interested in a system that involved the paying of a larger benefit to a man who had contributed more . . . as a matter of paralleling the basic idea that runs through all our American culture, so to speak." Arthur Altmeyer of the Social Security Board urged his colleagues to pursue compulsory insurance rather than tax-supported programs because "under health insurance, medical service is received as a 'right;' under public medical service, until the stage is reached where free medical care is available to all, medical care is given as a form of charity and is available to people only in connection with a 'means test.' " Indeed the consensus at the board in the late 1930s was that health insurance "should be *Personal.* If not *Personal* will soon be just a gift, a charity, a political football to be used by the demagogue, the crack-pot, urging higher and higher 'benefits' on [the] theory that the beneficiary is getting something for nothing—that beneficiaries must organize into political pressure groups to get their just rights." While some saw compulsory insurance as the first step toward more universal provision, others argued the dangers of moving beyond the pool of contributors. "To be liberal to this group [the poor] is to penalize those who finance the system," reasoned one reformer. "If the program is self-supporting, then the contributors who are completely eligible will have to pay the cost for those . . . who are

<hr />

[6] FDR quoted in Arthur Schlesinger, *The Coming of the New Deal* (Boston, 1959), 308–9; Edwin Witte, "Possible General Approaches to the Problem of Economic Security" (16 Aug. 1934), Box 1, Committee on Economic Security [CES] Records, SSA Records; Round Table Conference on Medical Care (14 Nov. 1934), p. 214, Box 65, Edwin Witte Papers, State Historical Society of Wisconsin [SHSW], Madison, Wis.; "Compulsory Health Insurance: A Short Summary of Present Tendencies" (Dec. 1934), Box 21, CES Records; CES, Final Report on Risks to Economic Security Arising Out of Illness (1935), Box 67, Witte Papers.

brought in by liberal interpretations. If the system is not self-supporting, such extra cost must be met by the general taxpayers. In neither case does it seem hardly fair."[7]

The importance of this approach was not just the right that accompanied contributions, but also the distinction it drew between that right and charitable assistance. One reformer put it bluntly: "Denial of benefits to even a relatively few people would, by furnishing a convenient contrast, make those who are covered somewhat more aware of their benefits, and would thereby strengthen the concept of a purchased right." Indeed, there was little disagreement "that indigent medical care requires one set up and that the self-supporting group must be handled in an entirely different way," one state medical officer concluded in 1939. He continued: "It is essential that they be kept separate." Business leaders generally agreed, although they were less interested in federal programs than in ensuring that employers not pick up the whole tab for employment-based benefits. National Association of Manufacturers officials argued that "the contributory principle makes service a right and dissociates [sic] it from the onus of charity." In the wake of the bitter steel dispute of 1949, Colorado Fuel and Iron officials agreed that contributory benefits were "the only way that needed security can be provided without destroying the fabric of our society." And while labor generally supported proposals for national health insurance, it too hammered away at the distinction between charitable and contractual benefits. Workers were willing to "pay part of the tax for this sickness insurance," noted the *American Federationist* in 1940, in order to ensure that "a worker and his family would have the cash benefits as a right, not a charity." The New York Labor Federation went so far as to insist that the state agency be called the Department of Insurance and Pensions rather than the Department of Welfare because the latter invited "a particularly repugnant reaction among even our working people."[8]

---

[7] Altmeyer to Lape (27 Dec. 1938), Box 11, Decimal 025, SSB Records, Office of the Commissioner, SSA Records; "Social Security" (1939), Box 34, Decimal 056, General Classified Files [GCF] (1939–1944), Records of the Department of Health, Education, and Welfare [HEW], RG 235, National Archives; Myers to Williamson (17 Dec. 1941), Box 2, Decimal 11, Correspondence of the Executive Director, SSA Records; NRPB, *Security, Work, and Relief Policies* (Washington, D.C., 1942), 206.

[8] Advisory Council on Social Security, "Report to the Senate Committee on Finance" (May 1948), Box 16, Decimal 025, SSB Records, Records of the Executive Directory, SSA Records; Oregon medical officer quoted in "Abstract of Hearings," *JAMA* 112:24 (1939): 2521; handwritten comments (27 Sept. 1946), Box 63:579, Series II, Falk Papers; "Principles of a Nation-Wide Health Program" (1945), Box 4, National Association of Manufacturers [NAM] Industrial Relations Department [IRD] Papers, Hagley Museum and Library, Wilmington, Del.; Holtzmann quoted in Alan Derickson, "The United Steelworkers of America [USWA] and Health Insurance, 1937–1962," in *American Labor in the Era of World*

The propriety and necessity of contributory programs also underscored the persistent assumption that male breadwinners were responsible for their wives and children. "The population which a state law required to be covered would, for practical purposes, have to be defined in terms of employed persons," observed the CES typically, "although the social purpose of the plan involves medical service also to their families." Efforts to tinker with Social Security consistently tied "the dignity of men (defined as their capacity to provide)," as Alice Kessler-Harris argues, "to the virtue of women (their willingness to remain dependent on men and to rear children)." Postwar reformers echoed such assumptions and saw them as a key selling point. Indeed, accommodation of the family wage was one of the few exceptions to the logic of contributory benefits. "The man who has made a payment into the national health trust fund, whether it is called a 'contribution' or a 'health tax,' will presumably feel that he has . . . . his entitlement to services," argued one reformer, adding that "the inclusion of the contributor's dependents . . . is consistent with the 'contributory principle,' in spite of the fact that the dependents themselves have paid nothing." Women and children were covered by benefits provided to men, or relegated to the less legitimate stream of charitable means-tested assistance.[9]

Through the late 1940s, the contributory principle was employed freely by proponents and opponents of national health insurance alike. Opponents argued that compulsory health insurance was incompatible with social insurance and that the virtues of contractual benefits could only be achieved through private bargaining. Reformers, by contrast, viewed the contributory argument as a necessary political strategy, only to find that it hardened the distinction between vested rights and other claims for state attention. "The majority of Congress, and especially its leaders or key men, abhor 'free' benefits, but HAVE been sold on and accept the social insurance approach restricting benefits by formula to those paying," conceded the architects of the Wagner-Murray-Dingell

---

War II, ed. Daniel Cornford and Sally Miller (Westport, Conn., 1995), 76; "The National Health Bill," *American Federationist* 47:5 (1940): 528; NYFL to HST (11 Nov. 1949), Official File 670A, Box 1521, Truman Papers.

[9] CES, "Final Report on Risks to Economic Security Arising out of Illness" (1935), Box 67, Witte Papers; Alice Kessler-Harris, "Designing Women and Old Fools: The Construction of the Social Security Amendments of 1939," in *U.S. History as Women's History*, ed. Linda Kerber, Alice Kessler-Harris, and Kathryn Kish Sklar (Chapel Hill, N.C., 1995), 86–106 (quote at 95); Special Report on Proposed 1946 Social Security Expansion (rough draft), p. 17, Box 3, Arthur Altmeyer Papers, SHSW; 47; CES, Preliminary Report of the Staff of the Committee on Economic Security (Sept. 1934), Box 70, Witte Papers; "Health Insurance" (1935), Box 41; handwritten comments (27 Sept. 1946), Box 63:579; (quote) "National Health Bill—Coverage" (6 Nov. 1946), Box 63:579; Alanson Willcox to Harry Rosenfeld (25 Nov. 1946), Box 63:579, all in Series II, Falk Papers.

health bill. "The contributory plan, segregating THOSE WHO PAY and the needy for who Gov't pays is a less abrupt transition from present private purchase—and has a better chance of being enacted." Some felt it important to stress that WMD "rejects the charity principle, [and] is based on providing benefits as a right to all contributors and their dependents in return for a very small pay-roll deduction," and even those who held out for more universal programs were careful not "to belittle the political or psychological values inhering in the "contributory principle.' " When congressional Republicans countered with a means-tested program, reformers were quick to point out that the proposal "ditches completely the typically American insurance principle under which a person could obtain benefits as a matter of right because he had made his proportional contribution," and blasted the GOP for "adoption of the public assistance as against the social insurance approach."[10]

Although the Truman health initiative faltered, the contributory basis of Social Security was persistently reaffirmed. The 1950 Social Security Amendments underscored the principle that the Social Security Administration (SSA) be self-supporting and independent of general revenues, and efforts to expand the scope of "covered occupations" were animated by a widely shared conviction that means-tested programs would "melt away" as the contributory system expanded. For this reason, many congressional Republicans jumped aboard the Social Security bandwagon in the 1950s, many Democrats objected to means-tested alternatives such as the 1948 Taft bill or the 1960 Kerr-Mills program, and many reformers saw the Social Security pension pool as the only realistic frontier for health insurance. "Under a contributory social insurance system there is a direct relationship between wages, contributions and benefits," emphasized Altmeyer, "Accordingly, to the extent that an individual is able to develop his capacities, add to the productivity of the country, and achieve a higher wage, he receives higher social security benefits." Some were troubled by the fact that Social Security's means-tested old-age assistance program did cover medical care, while the contributory old-age insurance program did not. Reformers used this as an argument for adding a contributory health program for the elderly, while at the same time emphasizing that a medical benefit received under the assistance pro-

[10] (Quotes) Handwritten comments (27 Sept. 1946), and "National Health Bill—Coverage" (6 Nov. 1946), both in Box 63:579, Series II, Falk Papers; "Comparison of Three Major Health Bills," Box 211, Witte Papers; Summary of Hearings (23 May 1946), Box 3, Decimal 11.1, Division of Research and Statistics, SSA Records; W. L. Mitchell to Watson Miller (12 May 1947), Box 117, Commissioner's Correspondence (1936–1969), SSA Records; Robert Lieberman, *Shifting the Color Line: Race and the American Welfare State* (Cambridge, Mass., 1998), 70.

gram was "not a right, but only a payment on a needs basis, which subjects the beneficiaries to the stigma of relief."[11]

Not surprisingly, the contributory principle took center stage in the gestation of Medicare and Medicaid—though often in ways that confounded reformers. Medicare's architects leaned heavily on the popularity of Social Security. "President Johnson's proposed hospital insurance program," the administration argued, "is consistent with the underlying principles of our free enterprise system, since the protection is made available on terms which reinforce the interest of the individual in helping himself." Organizations of the elderly concurred that, as a spin-off of Social Security, Medicare would be seen as "a right arising from his prior contributions to the plan." Reformers pushed the Social Security model because "[it] avoids the necessity of a means test because benefits are available as a matter of earned right." "There can be no place in such a system for a means test or any similar device to make benefits available only as a matter of charity and not as a matter of right," as even *Business Week* argued, adding that contributory financing was the only way "of keeping old people from feeling that they are beggars living off society's handouts." Kaiser officials saw Medicare's principal virtue as the opportunity for the wage earner to "make a dignified contribution in advance for the medical care he will need when he becomes 65." And congressional debate echoed the assumption, as one senator put it, that "the social security approach—and only such an approach—provides assurance that practically everyone will have needed hospital insurance protection in old age as an earned right . . . benefits are paid to each as a consequence of contributions."[12]

The last-minute inclusion of Medicaid in the Medicare bill hardened the distinction between social insurance and "welfare medicine" and in-

[11] Alvin David, "Old-Age, Survivors, and Disability Insurance: Twenty-Five Years of Progress," *ILRR* 14:1 (Oct. 1960): 15; Gareth Davies, *From Opportunity to Entitlement: The Transformation and Decline of Great Society Liberalism* (Lawrence, Kans., 1996), 23–29; Marion Folsom, "How to Pay the Hospital," *Atlantic* (June 1963): 79–83; Altmeyer, "The American Approach to Social Security" (July 1950), Box 3, SSB Records, Office of the Commissioner, SSA Records; Edwin Witte, "Economic Aspects of the Health Problems of the Aging" (1952), Box 74, Witte Papers.

[12] (Quote) Moyers to Dr., Don Boston (8 Oct. 1964), WHCF IS 2, Lyndon B. Johnson Papers, Lyndon Baines Johnson Presidential Library [LBJPL], Austin, Tex.; (quote) National Committee on Health Care for the Aged, "A National Program for Financing Medical Care for the Aged" (1963), in HEW, *Background on Medicare, 1957–1962*, Box 10, Gaither Office Files, LBJPL; David, "Old-Age, Survivors, and Disability Insurance," 10; "Why Physicians Support Hospital Insurance for the Aged" (1962), Box 5, Physician Committee on Health Care for the Aged [PCHCA] Papers, SHSW; (quote) *BW* (16 Jan. 1965): 132; *BW* (16 Apr. 1960): 184; " 'Medicare,' the Cure That Could Cause a Setback," *Fortune* 67:5 (May 1963): 172; (quote) Weissman to Keene (10 Dec. 1964), Box 387, Edgar Kaiser Papers,

sulated the former from pressures for expansion. The argument that "no stigma would be attached" to Medicare benefits was also a way of pointing out that Medicaid recipients—who did not make "dignified contributions," whose eligibility was means-tested, and whose benefits were considered handouts—would be stigmatized. HEW opposed the use of sliding-scale deductibles for Medicare because it "would be contingent on an income test. The earned right idea under social security, without a needs or income test, means that a worker knows he will not lose his benefits if he saves his money." Characteristically, HEW labeled Medicare patients "beneficiaries," and Medicaid patients "clients" or "recipients." More broadly, reformers understood the relationship between Medicare and Medicaid as part of the larger tug-of-war between social insurance and welfare and warned that, in the absence of a Social Security–based program for the elderly, the only option would be to bring more and more of the population under the stigma of means-tested coverage.[13]

After 1965 the contributory logic persisted, although fiscal crises and episodic concern for the solvency of Social Security began to expose the actuarial uncertainty of the "purchased right." Health reformers in the early 1970s argued that "it would be suicide to move away from the [contributory] trust fund approach" and hammered away at the "simplicity, understandability, general acceptance" and "inherent virtues of a contributory social insurance system . . . [which maintains] "the feeling on the part of the worker and the public that he along with his employer is paying for the benefit he receives." But when the Nixon administration floated the idea of tying unemployment and pension benefits more closely to contributions, staffers at HEW worried that this would encourage "demands for vesting of interests by contributors in all such programs." In an era of fiscal restraint, it was harder to make the case for new social insurance programs and harder to defend the integrity of old ones. Social Security remained the untouchable "third rail" of American social policy, but health programs—whose spiraling costs were more urgent and whose logic as social insurance was more tenuous—were easy

---

Bancroft Library, University of California, Berkeley; (quote) *Congressional Record* 111:11 (1965), 15630.

[13] National Committee on Health Care for the Aged, "A National Program for Financing Medical Care for the Aged" (1963), in HEW, *Background on Medicare, 1957–1962*, Box 10, Gaither Office Files; (quote) Cohen to O'Brien (20 May 1964), Box 291, Secretary's Subject Files [SSF] (1955–1975), HEW Records; Ribicoff, "Health Insurance for the Aged under Social Security" (July 1961) in HEW, *Background on Medicare, 1957–1962*, Box 10, Gaither Office Files; Helen Slessarev, "Racial Tensions and Institutional Support: Social Programs during a Period of Retrenchment," in *The Politics of Social Policy in the United States*, ed. Margaret Weir, Ann Orloff, and Theda Skocpol (Princeton, N.J., 1988), 363–64; Rashi Fein, *Medical Care, Medical Costs: The Search for a Health Insurance Policy* (Cambridge, Mass., 1989), 115; Paul Starr, *The Social Transformation of American Medicine* (New York, 1982), 370.

targets. Indeed, Medicare was cut loose from the Social Security system (and its political and philosophical anchors) in 1977 with the creation of the Health Care Financing Administration, an agency animated more by fiscal restraint than by social insurance principles.[14]

Through the 1970s and after, concern for the "contributory" principle compelled Democrats and Republicans alike to train their fiscal sights on means-tested programs. When the Reagan administration singled out Medicaid in the early 1980s, for example, many (especially in state politics) worried less about Medicaid itself than about new pressures that such cuts might put on social insurance programs such as Medicare. In other respects, the assault on social spending also blurred the line between contributory and charitable programs (underscored by the ability of the Reagan administration to make "entitlement" a dirty word), and debates about the future of Social Security abandoned the assumption that past contributions ensured future benefits. The Reagan administration considered Medicare as closer to Medicaid than to Social Security, and proposals for means-testing Medicare dredged up the arguments (pressed by the AMA and others as early as the 1940s) that expansive care for the elderly would burden the young and provide benefits to many who could easily afford to purchase them privately.[15]

When national health insurance resurfaced in national debate in the early 1990s, the contributory principle persisted largely in the Clinton administration's deference to private plans and employer provision. In seeking to mandate employment-based coverage, the Clinton health plan (CHP) acknowledged the important political and fiscal distinction between insurance premiums and payroll taxes. "A premium is now and will continue to be the cost of their own personal health insurance policy," argued CHP architect Paul Starr, "and the money will go, not to the government, but from their employer to the health plan . . . a premium is a *price* paid for something in return."[16] But the older social insurance

<hr>

[14] (Quote) Minutes of the Meeting of the CNHI Technical Committee (5 July 1972), Box 3, Arthur J. Altmeyer Papers (add.), SHSW; (quote) Altmeyer to Falk (30 Apr. 1970), Box 144:2082, Series III, Falk Papers; House Committee on Ways and Means, *Hearings: National Health Insurance: Part 3* 93:2 (Apr.–July 1974), 1144; "Middle Class Economic Issues" (Feb. 1972), Box IS:1, White House Central File [WHCF], Richard M. Nixon Papers, National Archives; Falk to Harper (9 May 1972), Box IS:1,WHCF, Nixon Papers; Theodore Marmor, "Coping with a Creeping Crisis: Medicare at Twenty," in *Social Security: Beyond the Rhetoric of Crisis*, edited by Theodore Marmor and Jerry Mashaw (Princeton, N.J., 1988), 186–99.

[15] Slessarev, "Racial Tensions and Institutional Support," 376; Fred Block et al., *The Mean Season: The Attack on the Welfare State* (New York, 1987); Marmor, "Coping with a Creeping Crisis," 186–99.

[16] Starr to Magaziner (22 Apr. 1993), Box 3210, Clinton Health Care Task Force [CHTF] Records, National Archives.

approach was clearly in shambles: the link between contributions and benefits, as the administration saw it, could be maintained only in private, employment-based insurance plans. And that link (in the logic of "managed competition") was aimed less at establishing a right to benefits than at disciplining those who would exercise it.

The Square Peg: Health Care and Social Insurance

It was never entirely clear whether reformers saw contractual provision as a moral imperative, an administrative necessity, or a political concession. Certainly most believed in the virtue of distinguishing between contractual entitlements and charitable assistance, while some hoped that universal programs would ultimately erase that distinction. In any case, such assumptions perpetuated the "two-track" approach to social policy and made it increasingly difficult to accommodate health care on either track. Universal health care was a difficult sell because it did not ensure (or even pretend) any direct relationship between contributions and benefits. This not only forced reformers into all sorts of political and actuarial contortions, but also handed opponents some of their most potent arguments.

The first problem confronting health reformers was that sickness, unlike retirement or unemployment or occupational health, was not a consequence of industrial employment. The AALL struggled with this in 1914–1920—at times, as in the emphasis on compensation for lost wages, leaning heavily on the employment-based contributory logic; at others, as in its argument for employer, employee, and state contributions, acknowledging the broader basis of the risk. The wage-loss, employment-basis first floated by the AALL would remain the organizing principle for subsequent reform efforts, even as most reformers acknowledged its limits. "An analysis of European experience with workingmen's systems of insurance," admitted the CES in 1934, "shows that some of the most serious weaknesses—especially in regard to medical benefits—rest upon the fact that these are *workingmen's* systems," but the committee still recommended that the insured "be defined in terms of [the] employed person . . . and his dependents." Subsequent efforts—whether they sought to prolong employment-based coverage, supplement it, or subsidize it—persistently organized the coverage and financing of health care around industrial payrolls, even as they just as persistently admitted (as a HEW staffer put it in 1959) that "the principles of social insurance aimed at providing a base of income maintenance do not apply in the development of insurance to pay for personal health services."[17]

[17] Moss, *Socializing Security*, 72–75; (Quote) "Abstract of a Program for Social Insurance against Illness" (1935), pp. 26–28, Box 67, Witte Papers; Dr. Farran, "A Coordinated Plan

This confusion was not lost on those who were expected to foot the bill. Employers complained that the AALL plan would burden them with things ("alcoholism, feeble-mindedness, venereal disease") that were not their fault and argued that employment-based coverage would be too meager to accomplish any public health goals. Through the Social Security debate, employers showed no inclination (as they would with pensions and unemployment insurance) to use federal law to sort out disparities in private and state-level programs. And as employment-based service benefits grew in the 1940s, employers argued that they were assuming costs and risks that far outstripped their logical responsibilities. "[We recognize] the obligations which have always existed between employer and employee incident to the hazards of that employment," argued one employers' association, but health care was clearly "beyond that . . . an entirely different matter." It warned that "we have arrived at the point where we must decide whether we want to cross that line." This sentiment was exaggerated by the postwar trajectory of expanded coverage and spiraling costs. By the 1980s large unionized firms monotonously complained (as an American Airlines executive put it) that by raising premiums or hospital charges, "the providers of medical care are shifting these costs to people who have generous employer-provided programs."[18]

Just as reformers conceded and employers argued that health was not logically a risk of employment, many also recognized that health coverage scrambled the contractual premise of social insurance. "[I]n at least two important respects," one reformer admitted in 1946,

> health insurance differs markedly from the other social insurances. The risk insured against is not a function of earning capacity, either present or past; from which it follows, first, that there is no basic reason (as there is in other insurances) to exclude non-earners from the benefits; second, that the quantity of benefits available to eligible persons will not vary with earnings or contributions. The latter consideration seems to us to heighten the inequity of the dividing line between those contributors who get nothing because their contributions are too small and those who get everything the system has to offer.

---

to Achieve Health Security," in Medical Advisory Board Minutes (29 Jan. 1935), pp. 82, Box 67, Witte Papers; (quote) "Meeting with Consultant on Health Insurance" (20 Nov. 1959), Box 225, Decimal 900.1, Secretary's Subject Correspondence [SSC] (1956–1974), HEW Records.

[18] Margaret Strecker, "Critical Analysis of the Standard Bill for Compulsory Health Insurance" (1920?); and untitled testimony (Mar. 1919), Box V:9, Seventh Meeting of the National Industrial Conference Board [NICB] (21 Dec. 1916), all in NICB Papers, Hagley Museum; NAM, *Industrial Health Practices* (New York, 1941), 14–39; (quote) Martin Hilfinger in NICB, "Compulsory or Voluntary Health Insurance" (1946), Hagley Imprints; Hoey Hennesy to Industrial Relations Group (5 Dec. 1949), Box I:75, NAM Papers; McNamara quoted in "Calling for a Bigger U.S. Health Role," *NYT* (30 May 1989).

The dilemma was that health insurance promised service benefits according to need rather than cash benefits according to contribution. Reformers clung to the political and fiscal appeal of contributory financing, but they could not pretend that contributors would enjoy commensurate benefits: the healthy might see no return on their contributions and the sick, the elderly, and the malingerers could claim more than their share. This would "eliminate the old sense of personal responsibility and fraternal integrity," the AMA argued, continuing that patients would be interested only in "getting as much as possible out of the great financial bureaucracy to which they were forced to contribute," that compulsory insurance would only foster " 'greediness,' the feeling that enforced contributions have created a 'right' to cash and service . . . that the insurance funds belong to the contributors," and concluding that insurance would "implant the idea in the consciousness of a simple man: 'Now that I have paid so long, I will at last get something out of it!' " Proposals to extend OASI coverage to health were routinely characterized as "unfairly taxing working people throughout the nation to pay the bills for people to whom they owe no obligation whatever" or "burden[ing] the young people who are raising children so that old, retired people can misuse medical facilities." Medicare, as one opponent observed, "deviates from the previous position of Social Security in providing benefits instead of cash, thus *dictating* how each recipient must spend his benefits."[19]

The social insurance case for health coverage was further complicated by the confusion with which reformers approached the very concept of insurance. Social insurance was designed to spread the risks of industrial employment across the life span of an individual worker. Pensions, for example, underwrote a known risk with regular payments. Unemployment insurance was not so clear-cut, because the risk was less predictable and because there remained disagreement as to whether the goal was to bridge gaps in employment or encourage continuous employment. Health care posed an even greater riddle, especially as it graduated from compensation for wage loss to service benefits for workers and their dependents. Most reformers saw health insurance as a means of regularizing individual payments for individual care in a given year (as in the

[19] Milton Roemer, "Universal Coverage under a National Health Insurance System" (23 Sept. 1946), Box 131, Decimal 056.1, GCF (1944–1950), HEW Records; "Principles of a Nation-Wide Health Program" (1945), Box 4, NAM-IRD; "A Critical Analysis of Sickness Insurance," *JAMA* 29:4 (1934): 54, 64; Dr. Robert Cates to Wilbur Mills (22 May 1964), Box 32, and Dr. John Toth to Wilbur Mills (15 Sept. 1964), Box 1, both Medicare Correspondence, Records of the House Committee on Ways and Means, 88th Congress, RG 233, Records of the House of Representatives, National Archives; Bridget Mitchell and Willam Schwartz, "Strategies for Financing National Health Insurance: Who Wins and Who Loses," *NEJM* 295:16 (14 Oct. 1975): 867.

AALL proposals) or across a worker's lifetime (as in Medicare). Reformers hoped to reap the political advantages of contributory social insurance while acknowledging that health insurance was either incompatible with such a system or (more tortuously) that " 'insurance' refers to income, and not to some form of mathematical or actuarial relationship between money collected from and money disbursed to any individual." Reformers were persistently unsure whether health and hospitalization benefits were "a substitute for earnings" or "a substitute for individual budgeting of the costs of such care."[20]

Actuarial assumptions were even more uncertain. For some, the social insurance goal of budgeting individual health costs required some form of group-based, first-dollar coverage. But, as commercial insurers and others pointed out, such coverage ignored the moral hazard of providing benefits over which the insured exercised some control. "Sickness is an indefinable condition," argued the AMA in 1934, "frequently desired by the insured individual and therefore created in part by insurance itself." For this reason, insurers and many reformers turned their attention to catastrophic coverage—the only service benefit that conformed to conventional actuarial assumptions. By the same token, the social insurance goal of "regularizing payments" made little sense to commercial insurers, who viewed risk as something properly spread across a large population. But while health insurers sought an insurance pool large enough to bear the risk of individual injury or sickness, they also sought pools that were small enough to rule out bad risks altogether. "We encourage insurers to test where appropriate," as one state insurance commissioner put it, "because we don't want insurance companies to issue policies to people who are sick, likely to be sick, or likely to die." Private insurers, in this sense, liked the political implications of private contributory benefits but balked at any implication that contributions created a right to coverage. "Any insured buying an A & H [accident and health] policy with no age limit," HIAA officials noted in the early 1960s, "begins to feel that he has a property interest therein and that it is not fair for the insurer to refuse renewal of such a policy after a claim."[21]

[20] CES (Medical Advisory Board), Interim Report (Jan. 1935), Box 67, Witte Papers; Ball to the Secretary (20 June 1962), Box 166, Decimal 056.1, SSC (1956–1974), HEW Records; Witte, "Possible General Approaches to the Problem of Economic Security" (Aug. 1934), Box 48, Harry Hopkins Papers, Franklin D. Roosevelt Presidential Library [FDRPL], Hyde Park, N.Y.; Bureau of Research and Statistics, "Memorandum on Health Insurance" (1937), pp. 2–5, Box 34, Decimal 056, Chairman's File, Commissioners' Records, SSA Records; NRPB, Security, Work, and Relief Policies, 3; "Social Security by Any Other Name," Fortune 11:3 (March 1935): 86–87; Falk, "Comments on H.R. 7534" (12 Nov. 1942), Box 60:536, Series II, Falk Papers.

[21] Paul Starr, The Social Transformation of American Medicine (New York, 1982), 292–93; "A Critical Analysis of Sickness Insurance," JAMA 29:4 (1934): 49, 79–80; "The Insurance

On balance, neither commercial insurance nor social insurance could fully accommodate health-care provision. As organized labor won more expansive benefits, and employers and insurers scrambled to assemble actuarially viable employment groups, the end result was a social insurance benefit masquerading as an insurance risk. Labor's fight for the right to health care yielded a system of private insurance that assiduously denied such a right existed. The consequences—as insurers pursued good risks, and unions and employers pursued lower premiums—included the gradual fragmentation of the insured population into small and homogenous groups (each according to its own risks) and the relegation of bad risks to public responsibility. The politics of contractual benefits and the practice of private insurance combined to encourage private coverage while restricting its scope, to direct attention to those who needed it the least, and to stigmatize those who could not lay claim to the "purchased right" of employment-based coverage.[22] Private and political efforts to sustain the contributory principle ran parallel to the insurers' drive to fragment the actuarial pool. When faced with the prospect of reestablishing broader community pools in the early 1990s, Blue Cross officials underscored what they considered the inequity of "asking younger, healthier groups to do more to subsidize older, sicker groups."[23]

These riddles resisted easy answers and, as a result, provided hay for opponents. Having made the argument that compulsory health insurance could regularize and socialize one of the pervasive risks of industrial employment, the AALL was ill prepared for the strident opposition of employers and organized labor, the latter arguing that "so called compulsory health insurance is not health insurance at all, but only a thinly-veiled scheme for forcing charity on a portion of the community which neither requires nor desires charity." In the 1930s members of the CES labored to present health insurance as a contributory social insurance, only to have opponents spit the logic back at them. "It has been stated

Principle in the Practice of Medicine," *JAMA* 102:19 (1934): 1612–15; Cecil Sheps and Daniel Drossness, "Prepayment for Medical Care," *NEJM* 264:8 (23 Feb. 1961): 390; insurance commissioner quoted in Deborah Stone, "The Struggle for the Soul of Health Insurance," *JHPPL* 18 (1993): 308; memo to Mr. Grahame (28 Feb. 1964); and (quote) Minutes of Special Subcommittee to Review Regulatory Policy (25 Feb. 1964), both in Box 24, Orville Grahame Papers, University of Iowa Special Collections, Iowa City, Iowa.

[22] "Reforming the Health Insurance Market," *NEJM* 326:8 (1992), 565–69; Stone, "Struggle for the Soul of Health Insurance," 288–89, 290, 292–93, 308.

[23] Mary Nell Leonard (Blue Cross/Blue Shield) testimony in House Committee on Ways and Means, *Hearing: Private Health Insurance Reform Legislation* 102:2 (March 1992), 188; "Insurance: Starting Off on the Wrong Foot," *American Federationist* 78:11 (1971): 21; Donald Light, "Excluding More, Covering Less: The Health Insurance Industry in the U.S.," *Health/PAC Bulletin* (Spring 1992): 7–13; Thomas Bodenheimer, "Should We Abolish the Private Health Care Industry?" *IJHS* 20:2 (1990): 199–220.

that the funds that are to be used . . . . are to be *contributions* and not a tax," noted one medical conservative. "Anything that is compulsory is a tax and when people generally understand this it seems to me they will take a different attitude towards health insurance." Others noted both the tortured logic of contributory health programs and the discrepancy between contributions and benefits. For its part, the AMA envisioned a future in which "the waiting rooms of insurance practitioners are crowded with patients who wish cash benefits, or attempt 'to get something back' for their contributions, or come to obtain free drugs." However self-serving these protests, it was certainly true, as an insurance executive noted in 1937, that reformers were eager to "quote private insurance principles frequently when they do not apply and [to] discard them when they interfere."[24]

Opponents repeated these arguments in their battle against the health proposals of the 1940s. The Truman health plan could not possible fly as a "contributory" program, stated the AMA, because "money is to be taken from every income receiver and the benefits paid not according to amount paid but according to incidence of illness." Means-tested alternatives were animated by a conviction that "the benefit promised" by the Truman plan "has no relation or a very remote relation to the amount of the payments made." The only conclusion (for the AMA, Republicans, and others) was that "if similar families do not pay similar premiums for similar services, a means test, or the lack of it, does not obscure the fact that charity is being given and that a system of taxation rather than insurance is involved." This argument reflected, in part, a broader attack on the Social Security system itself in which "the villain," as Rulon Williamson of the Insurance Economic Society scoffed, "is the 'pretender' *contributory insurance* . . . at this cooperative dinner for the aged, the guest who brings a spoon acts as though he has paid for the full meal."[25] Although most conservatives gradually reconciled themselves to Social Security, social insurance logic continued to haunt the cause of health reform.

This was especially true in the wake of the 1960 Supreme Court decision in *Flemming v. Nestor,* which held that Social Security contributions did not amount to "an accrued property right" and that the interest of

[24] E. M. Stanton, "Some Fundamental Defects Inherent in Compulsory Health Insurance," *JAMA* (24 Jan. 1920): 272; clipping from Philadelphia County Medical Society (1935?) in Box 207, Witte Papers; Bureau of Medical Economics, Statement on Sickness Insurance (1935?), Box 67, Witte Papers; Williamson memo Re: Dr. Falk's Presentation (9 Dec. 1937), Box 10, Decimal 025, SSB Records, Office of the Commissioner, SSA Records.

[25] Frank Dickinson, "Analysis of the Ewing Report," *AMA Bulletin* 69 (1949): 12; Taft address (19 Feb. 1949), Box 43, Decimal 011.4, Federal Security Agency, Office of the Administrator, GCF (1944–1950), HEW Records; statement of Rulon Williamson (15 Apr. 1954), Box 28, Grahame Papers.

the contributor "cannot be soundly analogized to that of the holder of an annuity, whose right to benefits is bottomed on his contractual premium payments." In dissent, Justice Hugo Black could offer little more than the importance of maintaining the appearance of contracted benefits as an assurance that a retired worker might "receive his benefit in dignity and self-respect."[26] *Nestor* confirmed what many had suspected about the legal limits of the Social Security "contract," but did little to threaten its sanctity. Still, *Nestor* was widely cited by opponents of health reform, who seized on the Court's admission that contributions were really taxes and on its distinction between the legal and political status of social insurance. The AMA greeted the 1960 King-Anderson bill with the argument that it "would not be an insurance or prepayment program. Social Security is strictly a tax program with current taxes used to provide current benefits for those now retired." Weaving *Nestor* into its long-standing doubts about the contractual logic of service benefits, the AMA argued that "King-Anderson would compel, not permit. It would tax, not allow contributions. Taxpayers would pay for today's beneficiaries, not for themselves at retirement. . . . King-Anderson does not provide insurance or prepayment of any type, but compels one segment of our population to underwrite a socialized program of health care for another, regardless of need."[27]

Such arguments became increasingly prominent leading up to 1965 and, while not stemming the passage of Medicare, shaped the law and its administration. Again the problem lay in the uncertain relationship between contributions and benefits. "Introducing a flat benefit—the same amount of protection against health care costs to everyone—means that those with higher earnings will pay much more in Social Security taxes than others—expecting the *same health care protection* in old age," asked the Chamber of Commerce. "Will this be acceptable to Americans who have been accustomed to receive more when they have paid more?" The AMA agreed that workers' contributions "would not be set aside for their health care in their own later years [but] would pay taxes today for

[26] *Flemming v. Nestor,* 363 U.S. 603 (1960), at 622, 610, 623; Robert Cover, "Social Security and Constitutional Entitlement," in *Social Security: Beyond the Rhetoric of Crisis,* ed. Marmor and Mashaw, 73–77.

[27] (Quote) Blasingame to Appel (29 Jan. 1961), Box 244, Decimal 910, SSC (1956–1974), HEW Records; Chamber of Commerce, "Adding Health Benefits to Social Security: Are There Basic Conflicts? (June 1963), Hagley Imprints; "Comments on AMA Telecast" (1962), and "The Real Story about AMA Charges," both in Box 126:7, Wilbur Cohen Papers, SHSW; "Memo: From Your Doctor" (1962), Box 6, PCHCA Papers; AMA, "Health Care for the Aged" (1963), Box 6, PCHA Papers; (quote) Leonard Larson address (27 Nov. 1961), Box 244, SSC (1956–1974), HEW Records; Cohen, "Is OASDI Insurance?" (6/5/62), Box 14, Wilbur Cohen Papers, LBJPL.

today's beneficiaries," adding that almost twenty million elderly "would be immediately eligible, most of whom have paid nothing for the benefits." As the 1965 Advisory Council on Social Security reluctantly agreed, Medicare "differs profoundly from our system of paying cash benefits to beneficiaries under social security."[28]

For reformers, this meant that the passage and implementation of Medicare posed peculiar fiscal and political challenges. For opponents, it meant that health coverage, as the AMA complained, "would alter the basic philosophy of our Social Security system." Indeed the AMA took a new tack after 1964 and played up fears that Medicare might bankrupt Social Security. "The addition of the so-called medicare provision to the social security program represents a radical departure," agreed Senator John Williams (R-Del.), continuing that Medicare "taxes workers under the social security program for later benefits—if needed—of a specific type. . . . This would seem to violate the concept of social security which holds that the individual has a right to benefits under the program whether he needs those benefits or not, to do with as he pleases because he has paid for them." Because benefits would be determined by medical need rather than by past contribution, as congressional Republicans argued, it only made sense to tie those benefits to economic need instead— and to avoid the prospect of providing open-ended medical care to pensioners who could pay for it themselves.[29]

After 1965 the dilemmas of contributory social insurance persisted in both the debate over broader public coverage and the practice of private employment-based benefits. The Johnson administration identified the expansion of maternal and children's health programs as an important and politically viable program, but paying for it raised an intractable dilemma. Although there was a moral imperative to cover children who could neither provide for themselves nor be held responsible for their parents' inability to do so, children could not really participate (as contributors or beneficiaries) in social insurance. Some argued, through 1967 and 1968, that a marginal increase in Social Security taxes would mean that "benefits as an insured right under the social security system would be payable in the case of over 95 percent of births." But the relationship between contributions and benefits remained murky. The ad-

---

[28] Chamber of Commerce, "Adding Health Benefits to Social Security"; Edward Annis, "Government Health Care: First the Aged, Then Everyone," *Current History* (Aug. 1963): 106; draft report of the 1965 Advisory Committee, Box 298, Commissioner's Correspondence (1936–1969), SSA Records.

[29] "Facts about Fedicare" (1964), Box 2, Donovan Ward Papers, University of Iowa Special Collections; "The Final Push to Win Hospital Care," *American Federationist* 72:2 (1965): 3–4; Williams quoted in *Congressional Record* 111:12 (1965): 16147; Edward Berkowitz, *Mr. Social Security: The Life of Wilbur J. Cohen* (Lawrence, Kans., 1995), 227–29.

ministration insisted that contributions made by parents yield benefits for which only *their* children were eligible and hoped such an arrangement would still give "beneficiaries the psychological feeling that they have helped pay for *their* protection." In turn, the proposal dredged up the problem of providing categorical benefits from a relatively universal pool of contributors. For this reason, planners floated the option of a government contribution in order to dampen "the argument by those who are beyond childbearing years or who engage in family planning that they are being asked to make payments on behalf of those who do not plan, some of whom have illegitimate children." Finally, "kiddycare" underscored the tendency of existing contributory health programs to extend care to those who needed it the least or to those years in life when it was of the least benefit. "Medicare taxes are accepted because *everybody* now working expects to face the hazards of old age," noted a Bureau of the Budget analysis of the proposal, "but a 'Kiddicare' tax would be imposed on everyone over 45 years of age; it finances risks he (or she) are no longer facing."[30]

Employment-based benefits represented the most literal construction of the contributory principle but were also a clear departure. The "contributor" in employment-based plans was not the beneficiary but the employer—whose goal was not an equitable return on contributions but (especially as costs soared) an escape from that burden. Copayments, deductibles, and preferred providers recast the contributory principle: the employee's share was seen less as the root of dignity and entitlement than as an incentive to play the responsible consumer. As large firms turned to self-insurance through the 1980s and 1990s, health coverage resembled less a contractual right than a discretionary welfare-capitalist benefit. Reform efforts of the 1970s and 1990s also struggled with the logic of social insurance. Reformers leaned on the contractual logic of private provision and tried to build near-universal coverage around mandated employment benefits. This perpetuated a basic confusion, as a member of the Clinton Health Care Task Force (CHTF) put it, as to "whether the Administration wants to set social insurance or private insurance as the fundamental direction of public policy." By this time, the social insurance arguments of the 1930s and 1940s had lost much of their appeal. Most now saw the connection between "earmarked" contributions and benefits less as a moral imperative than as a source of market discipline or fiscal restraint. Senator Joseph Lieberman (D-Conn.) cap-

---

[30] Cohen to Califano (10 Jan. 1968), Box 191, Gaither Office Files; Cohen to Califano (17 Jan. 1968), Confidential File LE 64, LBJ Papers; Bureau of the Budget, "Insured Medical Care for Mothers and Children" (Jan. 1968), Box 191, Gaither Office Files.

tured the new prevailing wisdom during a 1999 debate over a proposal to add prescription drug benefits to Medicare, which he dismissed as "another big costly benefit that nobody pays for even though everybody wants it."[31]

Who Pays? Social Insurance and the Financing Riddle

Attempts by reformers to reconcile health coverage with social insurance were uneven, inconsistent, and ultimately counterproductive. This confusion was most pronounced in the shadow of any reform effort: the debate over how to pay for coverage. Time and time again, reform efforts stumbled over the question of who should (or could) be covered by new programs and who should (or could) pay for them. Though often obscured by arcane calculations of contribution percentages, income thresholds, or budget implications, the financing question underscored the ways in which devotion to social insurance imprisoned reform.

The core dilemma was clear. Reformers were reluctant to provide benefits to some (based on an income or means test, for example) from general revenues, or to finance general benefits from those willing or able to contribute via payrolls—and they endlessly debated whether the "economic advantage inherent in a system financed out of general revenues," as Altmeyer put it, "outweighed the inherent long range social, psychological, and political advantages of a contributory social insurance system."[32] In opting for the latter, reformers not only allowed the administrative detail of running contributions through payrolls determine the scope of coverage, but then turned around and defended the virtues of covering only (some) workers. This, as we have seen, weakened arguments for expanded coverage and stigmatized any residual benefits. Faced with the argument that contracts were binding but voluntary commitments, reformers were constantly distracted by the task of accommodating individuals or firms who might want to opt out of public programs. Finally, the task of financing public health programs was complicated after the mid-1960s by overlapping inflationary and budgetary anxieties. In this atmosphere, the appeal of reorganizing (and re-

[31] Colin Gordon, "Dead on Arrival: The American Health Care Debate," *Studies in Political Economy* 39 (1992): 141–58; Herman Somers and Anne Somers, "Major Issues in National Health Insurance," *MMFQ* 50 (Apr. 1972): 179–81; Marilyn Field and Harold Shapiro, *Employment and Health Benefits: A Connection at Risk* (Washington, D.C., 1993), 41; (quote) Gatz to Magaziner (8 Mar. 1993), Box 3305, CHTF Records; Lieberman quoted in *Daily Iowan* (28 June 1999): 6A.

[32] Arthur J. Altmeyer, *The Formative Years of Social Security* (Madison, Wis., 1966), 109.

straining) private expenditures through more universal programs collided with the political necessity that health programs either pay for themselves or hide their costs "off budget."

The schedule of contributions accompanying the AALL's 1914–15 proposal reflected its overlapping and conflicting purposes: employees, as a means of budgeting for the costs of medical care, would pay 40 percent; employers, as a token of their responsibility for workers' welfare, would pay 40 percent; and the state, as a redistributive commitment to its poorer citizens, would pay 20 percent.[33] As both a last gasp of Progressivism and a precedent for future efforts, the AALL financing proposal was remarkable in two respects. First, it made sense to no one but those who drafted it. Employers resented any implication of responsibility beyond the boundaries of workers' compensation, and organized labor objected to compulsory contributions, employer's contributions (assumed to come out of wages), and the stigma that accompanied the state's contribution. Second, and despite its failure, the AALL proposal firmly established the principle of both contributory financing and employment-based coverage. Subsequent efforts saw these, at worst, as the outer boundaries of reform and, at best, as the only logical starting point.

The first to confront these dilemmas was the CES in the middle 1930s. In its early deliberations, the CES concluded optimistically that health insurance could be established "without regard to cost" because "the insured population would include people who on average already spend from their private purses as much money as the program would require." At the same time, the CES stressed the fiscal and medical importance of casting the coverage net as widely as possible: "If a program is to be effective; if it is to reach those for whom it is designed and who need its benefits; if it is to protect the community and its citizens from the improvidence of those who are unfortunate or irresponsible, if it is to rest on a sound financial basis, it must be *required* and *compulsory*." This optimism was quickly dashed. Even as it argued for the advantages of the broadest possible coverage, the CES was forced to admit that general revenues were "not practical as a means of financing medical service benefits" and that noncontributory benefits "for everyone without regard to his ability to provide for himself, would not be practically considered in a capitalistic state." Following the logic of the unemployment and pension programs, the tentative health insurance title retreated to a contrib-

[33] "The AALL and the First Health Insurance Movement," handwritten notes; New York State League of Women Voters, "Report and Protest . . . New York League for Americanism," both in Box 209, Witte Papers; "Standards of Sickness Insurance" (1914), reel 62, American Association for Labor Legislation Papers [AALL] (microfilm); E. M. Stanton, "Some Fundamental Defects Inherent in Compulsory Health Insurance," *JAMA* (24 Jan. 1920), 272.

utory basis (although it rejected the use of copayments or deductibles on the grounds that they "would require the creation of unnecessarily complicated and expensive administrative machinery").[34]

On these terms, the proposal began to unravel. At the best of times (let alone in the midst of the Depression) many could not make the requisite contributions without some assistance from employers or the state. It would be "administratively feasible to devise a general system of health insurance for the self-sustaining group and to tie the relief cases and the medically 'dependent' group into this system, with tax payments taking the place of individual contributions," observed the CES's Michael Davis. "It would seem politically impossible, however, to legislate health insurance for self-sustaining people and to omit similar provision for some 30,000,000 persons who are below this level." The unhappy alternatives, as Davis and others saw them, were either to muddy the line between contributory and charitable care by asking the state to make some of the contributions or to narrow coverage to those who were self-sustaining anyway. This echoed the larger logic of Social Security, which pursued security for industrial workers rather than economic justice for those who remained on the margins of the labor market. Although the health insurance title did not survive in Social Security's final draft, those who hoped to reintroduce it at some later date remained convinced that "a direct earmarked contribution and the extension of the system to all who need it are likely to be mutually exclusive" and that only the former was likely to attract serious attention.[35]

For the next five years, the question of financing health was bound up in the more sweeping question of Social Security finance. Critics feared that the initial accumulation of Social Security's reserve account would have a deflationary impact in a struggling economy and, as long as receipts ran ahead of expenditures, tempt congressional extravagance. At

[34] Report of the Technical Committee on Medical Care (1938) in *President's Annual Message on Health Security*, H. Doc. 120 (76/1: Jan. 1939), p. 66; CES (Medical Advisory Board), Interim Report (Jan. 1935), Box 67, Witte Papers; CES, Preliminary Report (Sept. 1934), Box 70, Witte Papers; "Draft Abstract of a Program for Social Insurance against Illness" (1934), Box 2, CES Records; Kellogg to Witte (29 Mar. 1935), Box 12, CES Records; Barbara Armstrong memo (Sept. 1934), Box 17, CES Records; Bureau of Research and Statistics, "Memorandum on Health Insurance" (1937), pp. 55–56, Box 34, Decimal 056, Chairman's File, Commissioners' Records, SSA Records; CES, "Final Report on the Risks of Economic Insecurity Arising out of Illness" (1934), p. 39, Box 3, CES Working Papers, SSA Records.

[35] Michael Davis, "Some Relations between Health and Economic Security" (9 Oct. 1934), Box 18, CES Records; CES (Medical Advisory Board), Interim Report (Jan. 1935), Box 67, Witte Papers; Bureau of Research and Statistics, "Memorandum on Health Insurance" (1937), 58–59, Box 34, Decimal 056, Chairman's File, Commissioners' Records, SSA Records.

the same time, many Social Security advocates wanted to liberalize benefits and bump up the start date in order to solidify public support.
"Whether or not all the cost is from an 'earmarked' tax is of secondary
importance to the fact that the potential beneficiary must feel that he
has 'earned' his benefits or Insurance by paying with *his* money," argued
one Social Security staffer, "and the direct results are [that] the American
public ties together *the tax* and *the benefits*—so those who advocate more
benefits must advocate a higher tax." In turn, the 1938 Advisory Council
struggled over the question of including domestics, farmworkers, and
the self-employed, and affirmed the "family concept" of social insurance
by establishing new benefits for widows and survivors of those who died
before retirement and differential benefits for married and single workers. But with the family-wage exception, the contributory principle
clearly confined coverage. "If everybody is in from the standpoint of benefits, then everybody is in from the standpoint of contributions," argued
Advisory Council member Paul Douglas in 1939, "it is going to be difficult to have the entire population pay taxes for benefits designed for
only half the population."[36]

Reformers regrouped in the late 1940s with renewed programmatic
and fiscal optimism. "The contribution for medical care insurance will
not mean an added burden," they argued. "The American people are
now spending for physicians services and hospitalization enough to provide for all with only minor supplementation, if these payments are regu-
larized instead of falling with disastrous uncertainty." Federal Security
Agency (FSA) staff estimated that national health insurance could provide universal coverage at a cost only marginally larger than projected
private health spending, and argued that this was not a "cost" at all but
a reorganization of existing expenditures.[37] Architects of the WMD bills
toyed with various combinations of employment-based contributions,

[36] "Social Security" (1939), Box 34, Decimal 056, GCF (1939–1944), HEW Records; "Tentative summation of the present thinking of the members of the Social Security Advisory
Council" (Nov. 1938), Box 199, Witte Papers; Statement of Benjamin Anderson (10 Dec.
1937), Box 199, Witte Papers: Minutes of the Meeting of the Advisory Council, Afternoon
Session, 19 February 1938, pp. 22–27, Box 12, Decimal 025, SSB Records, Office of the
Commissioner, SSA Records; Douglas quoted in Alice Kessler-Harris, "Designing Women
and Old Fools: The Construction of the Social Security Amendments of 1939," in *U.S.
History as Women's History*, ed. Linda Kerber, Alice Kessler-Harris, and Kathryn Kish Sklar
(Chapel Hill, N.C., 1995), 102. See also Mark Leff, "Taxing the 'Forgotten Man': The Poli-
tics of Social Security Finance in the New Deal," *JAH* 70 (1983): 359–81; Robert Ball, "The
Original Understanding on Social Security: Implications for Later Developments," in *Social
Security: Beyond the Rhetoric of Crisis*, ed. Marmor and Mashaw, 25–27.

[37] "Principles of a Nation-Wide Health Program" (1945), Box 4, NAM-IRD Papers; "Estimate of Expenditures" (May 1949), Box 69:705, Series II, Falk Papers; Ewing to HST (4
Dec. 1947); "Assumptions as to Program Expansion" (1 Dec. 1947), both in POF 419F, Box
1262, Truman Papers.

earmarked income taxes, and general revenue. Some drafts included a federal contribution toward the goal of universal coverage; others, uncomfortable with muddying the logic of contributory finance, relegated noncontributory, means-tested programs to a separate title.[38] The determination of congressional sponsors and the FSA to keep the health bill out of the hands of southerners and fiscal conservatives on the House Ways and Means and Senate Finance committees further complicated the financing question. Reformers were able to avoid the finance committees (at least initially) by avoiding the tax and fiscal issues for which they were responsible, but in the long run it meant that the WMD bill, as one critic noted, "has no logical financial philosophy—[it is] a hybrid combination of free benefits and earmarked tax ... [in which] earmarking serves no purpose and has no logic."[39]

Once again, contributory finance was inextricably entangled with the question of coverage. Some pressed for universal coverage and general revenue financing but, for the most part, the debate raged around the ethical, political, and administrative relationship between contributions and benefits. The starting point, not surprisingly, was industrial coverage. "We have long recognized that when health insurance proposals approach the voting stage they may be focused on urban and industrial coverage," reasoned one reformer, "and have to be complemented for the rural areas by comprehensive measures which do not closely follow the customary insurance approach." Beyond this, reformers were torn between the administrative headache of including agricultural workers and others and the practical and political headaches of not including them. The irony, only dimly appreciated at the time, was that the "the political attractiveness and industrial area feasibility of the contributory social insurance system" directed reform away from those who needed it the most. Some clung to the hope that contributory programs might serve as a foot in the door and tried to figure out how to exact contributions from those outside industrial employment in the hope that this would leave "for reconciliation with the 'contributory principle,' only the group who (not being eligible as dependents) have incomes of less than $500 a year." Some, in an effort to buttress the bill's political chances, went so far as to twist the limited coverage of the contributory approach into a virtue:

[38] "Hearings on S. 1606," 130:16 *JAMA* (1946): 1176; "Assumptions as to Program Expansion" (1 Dec. 1947), POF 419F, Box 1262, Truman Papers; Falk, "Comments on H.R. 7534" (12 Nov. 1942), Box 60:536, Series II, Falk Papers.

[39] Willcox to Miller (13 Nov. 1945), Box 3, Altmeyer Papers; "Hearing on S. 1606," *JAMA* 130:15 (1946): 1024; Fein, *Medical Care, Medical Costs*, 46–47; *Congressional Record* 95:13 (1949): A2531–32; handwritten Gerig comments (27 Sept. 1946), Box 63:579, Series II, Falk Papers.

The belief on the part of contributors that they have earned their benefits would undoubtedly be stronger if benefits were denied to *ALL* non-contributors. Granting benefits to the dependents of contributors will doubtless do little or nothing to impair the belief in a purchased right, because support of the family by its breadwinner is so ingrained in the public thinking. But to go beyond that, and cover SOME of the poor by use of tax funds, seems almost as detrimental to the 'contributory principle' as to go the whole way and cover ALL of the poor.[40]

Reformers toyed with general revenue finance long enough to manipulate congressional committee assignments, but there was otherwise not much enthusiasm for such an approach. "A bill providing for less than universal coverage but for general revenue financing," observed Social Security's Alanson Wilcox, "would be vulnerable, if not to ridicule, at least to very severe criticism from the excluded groups." The Social Security Board saw little equity in relying on general revenues, arguing that the tax system was so rife with exemptions and loopholes that many would "escape the tax but receive the benefit." Some viewed general revenue financing as simpler and more equitable but noted glumly that "tax supported medical care . . . is associated with dependency in the minds of most people in this country. The extension of tax supported medical care would have to proceed gradually . . . from dependent to low-income groups upward, and to be held back at each stage as demands from sections of the public and of the medical profession for an income limit and a means test." The conclusion was inescapable: "Broad coverage can be more effectively maintained through the contributory principle." For these reasons, reformers saw means-tested alternatives as both a cynical legislative ploy and a serious threat to social insurance principles. Although the Taft bill focused its attention on those likely to fall between the cracks of a contributory system, it would also (to the horror of reformers) "treat as charity cases both those who are now dependent on public assistance *and* persons who are otherwise self-supporting and able to pay their medical expenses if insurance premiums are scaled to incomes."[41]

[40] Excerpt from FSA report (23 Sept. 1946), Box 63:579, Series II, Falk Papers; Willcox to Falk (18 Aug. 1949), Box 2, Decimal 11, Division of Research and Statistics, SSA Records; Harry Rosenfield, "Confidential Material on Rural Area Considerations in a National Health Bill" (Nov. 1946), Box 46, Decimal 011.4, GCF (1944–1950), HEW Records; Milton Roemer, "Universal Coverage under a National Health Insurance System" (23 Sept. 1946), Box 131, Decimal 056.1, GCF (1944–1950), HEW Records; "National Health Bill—Coverage" (6 Nov. 1946), Box 63:579, Series II, Falk Papers.

[41] Willcox to Miller (13 Nov. 1945), Box 3, Altmeyer Papers; " 'Universal' vs. 'Non-Universal' Coverage under a National Health Bill" (1947), Box 3, Decimal 011.1, Division of Research and Statistics (General Correspondence, 1946–1950), SSA Records; "Principles

As in the 1930s, there was rampant confusion as to whether contributory financing was an administrative convenience or a moral imperative. Few acknowledged, as Surgeon General Thomas Parran did in 1946, how unfair it was to "deny health services to some people merely in order that others may appreciate their entitlement more." In the shadow of the larger debate over Social Security, reformers were also uncertain whether it was the fact or the appearance of contributions that was important, offering that such contributions might be considered "legally taxes" but "morally premiums." In turn, reformers' dependence on contractual logic snapped back at them in the form of demands for exemptions. Most saw an "opting out" clause as consistent with their contractual characterization of plan and as perhaps the only way to address charges of "compulsion" or "regimentation." At the same time, most agreed that "contracting out" would invite "adverse selection, increase administrative difficulties and expense, and stimulate undesirable forms of insurance coverage which would be impossible to control." Finally, reformers were uncertain as to what should follow the passage of the WMD bill. Some hoped the social insurance system would add new benefits, new programs, and broader coverage with each passing year. Some shared this goal but feared that an undue reliance on contributory benefits would "interpose an affirmative obstacle to the attainment of the goal of universal coverage." Others shared this view, but applauded the results, arguing that any "scheme for universal coverage departs too far from the contributory principle of social insurance."[42]

Health reform languished through the 1950s as Republicans accepted the Social Security system but remained leery of its fiscal implications. The Eisenhower-era HEW dismissed earmarked taxes as "a poor idea [because] there is no necessary connection between the yield of a given earmarked tax and the need for which taxes are spent," and viewed proposals for extending medical coverage to OASI recipients as a threat to the security of both the federal budget and Social Security. Such a program would "pour more money into the attempt to purchase a relatively

of a Nation-Wide Health Program" (1945), Box 4, NAM-IRD Papers; "Comparison of Three Major Health Bills," Box 211,Witte Papers; Falk to Winslow (31 Dec. 1946), Box 3, Decimal 11.1, Division of Research and Statistics, SSA Records.

[42] "National Health Bill—Coverage" (25 Nov. 1946), Box 46, Decimal 011.4, FSA, Office of the Administrator (GCF, 1944–1950), HEW Records; "Alternatives to Comprehensive National Health Program" (Nov. 1949), Box 45, Decimal 011.4, FSA, Office of the Administrator (GCF, 1944–1950), HEW Records; Altmeyer to Ewing (31 Oct. 1947), Box 4, Altmeyer Papers; Sanders to Falk (5 June 1946), Box 3, Decimal 011.1, Division of Research and Statistics (General Correspondence, 1946–1950), SSA Records; "Population to Be Covered" (19 Jan. 1949), Box 46, Decimal 011.4, FSA, Office of the Administrator (GCF, 1944–1950), HEW Records.

inelastic set of services," argued one HEW analysis, adding that this would not only "drive prices up further and faster" but also set a danger-ous precedent by "putting the social insurance system into a service bene-fit role." Reformers and conservatives alike remained uncertain whether piggybacking health care on the back of Social Security finance was a good idea (because it disguised reform as a moderate expansion of a popular program) or a bad idea (because it might undermine the fiscal health of the pension program).[43]

The fiscal logic of contributory health programs cut two ways: on the one hand, contributory financing was politically acceptable and fiscally responsible because it kept health spending "off budget"; on the other, the contractual "right" to service benefits seemed to invite malingering, inflation, program expansion, and erosion of the larger Social Security system. For these reasons, HEW devoted much of its attention to the promise of hidden expenditures, such as federal reinsurance of private health plans or tax breaks for individuals or employers purchasing health insurance. And it set the tone for future efforts at cost-conscious reform by pointing out both the inflationary dangers of first-dollar coverage and the importance of ensuring (through copayments and deductibles) that the rights of beneficiaries were restrained by their responsibilities as con-sumers. Indeed, some began to turn the logic of social insurance inside out, arguing (as one insurer put it in 1960) that alternatives to contribu-tory finance held out the hope that "financing benefits as a matter of right could be avoided."[44]

The first stabs at a Medicare program underscored these anxieties and dilemmas. Congress, in the yawning gap between its interest in health care for the aged and its reluctance to pay for it, patched together the Kerr-Mills program. By putting the onus on the states, national legislators were able to avoid direct responsibility for determining coverage or ad-ministering means tests. And as in other instances of deference to state governments, the federal motive was programmatic and fiscal restraint rather than respect for the boundaries of American federalism. At the same time, opponents slowed the progress of Medicare by returning to the question of means testing—a point on which reformers were quite vulnerable. Means-tested alternatives such as Kerr-Mills offered better benefits to those in greater need, while contributory social insurance programs focused on the exceptional costs (usually hospitalization)

[43] Miles to Flemming (25 Apr. 1960), Box 225, Decimal 900.1, SSC (1956–1974), HEW Records; Miles to Flemming (9 Nov. 1959), Box 124, Decimal 900.1, SSF (1955–1975), HEW Records.
[44] Miles to Flemming (9 Nov. 1959), Box 124, Decimal 900.1, SSF (1955–1975), HEW Records; Minutes of the ALC-LIAA Social Security Committee (12 Apr. 1960), Box 20, Grahame Papers.

faced by those whose very ability to contribute to program costs testified to their relative security.[45]

As Medicare took shape—indeed as soon as reformers turned their attention from the Truman plan to a more modest expansion of Social Security—the solution was shaped more by administrative and fiscal concerns than by the problem it sought to address. Numerous observers pointed out that the nation's elderly were both more likely to need expensive and ongoing care and less able to meet their needs through employment-based insurance. Yet Medicare was organized not around the needs of the nation's elderly but around the ability of some of the elderly to fund postretirement care through their enrollment in Social Security. The dilemma, for reformers and opponents alike, was to reconcile the needs-based argument for Medicare with the contributions-based logic of the proposed legislation. Much of this battle was fought on the terrain of "medical indigency," the notion that many who might not otherwise qualify for means-tested assistance might nevertheless be impoverished by medical bills. More broadly, the prospect of extending benefits to all the elderly, of distinguishing between simple indigency and medical indigency, or of extending service benefits threatened both the contributory principle and its fiscal logic. "Raising social security taxes to cover the enormous and unpredictable costs of hospitalization for millions," argued the AMA's Donovan Ward, "must certainly endanger the entire system." The service-benefit departure "implies a dual obligation," the National Council on Aging warned in 1964, "to the patient and to the taxpayer or voluntary contributor."[46]

Muddier still, given the larger confusion over reserve, contributory, and "pay as you go" financing, was the logic of launching contributions and benefits simultaneously. "The idea is that health care coverage under Social Security would be a 'right' comparable to private insurance in that it would have been earned and 'paid for,' " noted a Kaiser official, "[but] this concept will become true only after the Social Security financing method has been in effect long enough that retired Social Security beneficiaries will have made substantial contributions under the new tax rate." Administration officials and congressional reformers worried that launching benefits immediately would violate the social insurance principle and endanger other Social Security programs—and for this reason insisted that Medicare be a "separate, independent, and self-sustaining

[45] "Alternatives to Comprehensive National Health Program" (Nov. 1949), Box 45, Decimal 011.4, FSA, Office of the Administrator (GCF, 1944–1950), HEW Records.

[46] Theodore Marmor, *The Politics of Medicare* (Chicago, 1970), 21; "Are 200,000 Doctors Wrong?" *JAMA* 191:8 (1965): 662; Edith Alt, "Who Is Medically Indigent?" (1964), Box 1018, Central File, 1963–1968, RG 102, Records of the Children's Bureau, National Archives.

program." The most persistent criticism on this score was that Medicare was not a contributory program at all, that current workers were shouldering the burden of providing care for current retirees, and that "if health care benefits are provided to all those *eligible* for Social Security benefits," as one critic worried, "it would appear to be inevitable that such benefits be extended to those who are *paying* for them—the workers under 65." Medicare's architects struggled to reconcile the congressional insistence that Medicare not pay benefits until it had amassed a sufficient reserve with the administration's anxiety about the "fiscal drag" caused by raising Social Security taxes without spending the money.[47]

These concerns pressed the architects of Medicare to assemble the three-layer cake of health legislation finally passed in 1965. Medicare Part A retained the features of a contributory program, although, in order to accomplish this, benefits were pared back to cover hospital charges alone. Medicare Part B embodied the growing conviction that contractual social provision was best accomplished by private and voluntary insurance. And Medicaid built on the conservative argument that public assistance be provided on the basis of present need rather than past contribution. The 1965 reforms both challenged and affirmed the principle of contributory finance. Since serious reservations remained as to whether health care could ever be accommodated as social insurance, Medicare/Medicaid was designed to ensure that health spending did not undermine the logic or finances of the broader Social Security system. The goal was to win the passage of Medicare but also to barricade it (with Part B and Medicaid) against demands for expansion. By establishing a separate trust fund, the architects of Medicare were able to ride the popularity of contributory benefits without burdening the pension program.[48] Medicare and Medicaid, in this respect, reflected broader fiscal anxieties that pressed the Great Society to rely on means-testing, off-budget contributory financing, and a patchwork of programs targeting disadvantaged urban populations. The result, as Michael Brown has argued, was a sort of truncated universalism that both perpetuated the two-track approach to social provision and invited a popular backlash against those who benefited from the new programs.[49]

[47] Fleming to Keene (24 July 1961), Box 366, Edgar Kaiser Papers; Ardell Everett, "The March to Utopia," *Weekly Underwriter* (2 Jan. 1960); "Financing Social Security and Medicare" (13 Mar. 1965), WHCF WE 15, LBJ Papers.

[48] Chamber of Commerce, "Adding Health Benefits to Social Security"; Marmor, *Politics of Medicare*, 39–40, 69; O'Brien to LBJ (27 Jan. 1964), WHCF LE/IS 75, LBJ Papers; letters in Boxes 1–33, Medicare Correspondence, Records of the House Committee on Ways and Means, 88th Congress.

[49] Michael K. Brown, *Race, Money, and the American Welfare State* (Ithaca, N.Y., 1999), 18–19.

The decade after 1965 marked a crucial turning point in the debate over health care finance. Medicare's "blank check" reimbursement policy exacerbated health care inflation at just the moment that the fiscal and political logic of postwar growth politics was beginning to unravel. Inflationary and budgetary anxieties turned political attention from coverage to costs. And competitive anxieties pressed employers to look for ways to pare back employment-based benefits. When national health insurance reemerged in the early 1970s, the task was to stem the bleeding in private plans (and perhaps mandate employment-based coverage) and subsidize coverage "for those who fall out of the competitive market for insurance" without making any new demands on the federal budget. The Nixon transition team took one look at Medicare and Medicaid in 1968 and concluded that "our position should be one of concern with an accompanying unwillingness to increase the budget." Democrats too understood that increased coverage could only come through savings in existing programs or off-budget devices like an employer mandate. After 1976 the Carter administration agreed that increased coverage was clearly secondary to "the priority that cost containment has in connection with any national health insurance proposal."[50] As important, contributory financing was seen less as a moral imperative than as a means of braking the inflationary engine of third-party finance. Into the 1960s, contributions created a "purchased right" or an entitlement to benefits. After the 1960s, contributions (in the form of copayments or deductibles) discouraged that sense of entitlement by reminding consumers that their purchased right was only partially paid for.

These dilemmas were neatly reflected in the debate of the early 1970s. Reformers fully appreciated the "inherent logical difficulty" of relying on payroll taxes but conceded that they had little choice but to make employment-based health provision the foundation of reform. The 1971 Kennedy plan tried to sever the relationship between contributions and benefits by arguing that, while payroll contributions or taxes were a lucrative and politically acceptable source of revenue, they should not also determine who received benefits. The Committee for National Health Insurance struggled to craft a formula of employer, employee, and general tax revenues, and vacillated between using payrolls or the tax system to collect the money. In the end, most reformers conceded that they could not consider using general revenues toward that end: such a "radi-

---

[50] Minutes of the Meeting of the CNHI Technical Committee (5 July 1972), Box 3, Altmeyer Papers (add.); Ehrlichman to Nixon, Box 36, File IS:1, White House Special File (Confidential Files) [WHSF], Nixon Papers; Minutes of the CNHI Technical Committee (31 Aug. 1972), Box 3, Altmeyer Papers (add.); Bernice Bernstein to Cohen (22 Feb. 1978), Box 228:2, Cohen Papers.

cal" financing mechanism was "a millstone that we should get off our neck . . . we face enough obstacles without adding this one." Political and budgetary considerations (the need to minimize "the VISIBLE price tag") recommended a reliance on employment-based social insurance, if only to "avoid tak[ing] on any avoidable battles on the financing side."[51]

Alternatives floated by the Nixon administration were less ambitious but no less confused. HEW garnered little interest with a suggestion that increased coverage might be paid for by taxing employers' contributions and the income-equivalent of benefits received, and the notion of using Medicare and a supplemental payroll tax to reach those stuck in the "medigap" between private provision and Medicaid eligibility was dismissed as "neither programmatically sound nor politically viable." HEW staffers could not decide whether to pursue the preventive benefits of first-dollar coverage or the discipline of coinsurance and deductibles and constantly fretted over the "income level [at which] we wish to make the consumer price-conscious by paying out of pocket."[52] The administration recast the financing question, focusing less on who paid the bills and more on how those bills were paid. The riddle, for midcentury reformers, had been how to provide care to those who could not contribute to program costs and could not claim benefits as a right. The riddle, for late-century health reformers, was how to restrain and regulate the demands of those who claimed those rights but who paid for them in a perversely inflationary and cost-unconscious manner. The solution was the health maintenance organization. In some respects, HMOs reaffirmed the practice of contributory finance by accepting the logic of group-based employee coverage and using coinsurance and deductibles to restore ties between contributions and rights that had been tangled by third-party

[51] Altmeyer to Falk (8 Feb.1970), Box 3, Altmeyer Papers (add.); Eveline Burnes, "A Critical Review of National Health Insurance Proposals" *HSHMA Health Reports* (Feb. 1971), 113; "Max Fine to Executive and Technical Committees" (30 Apr. 1970), Box 3 (Mss 400), Altmeyer Papers; "Minutes of the Technical Advisory Group of CNHI" (16 Dec. 1969) and (10 Mar. 1970), Box 3 (Mss 400), Altmeyer Papers; Willcox to Fine (3 Feb. 1972), Box 150:2178; Altmeyer to Falk (8 Feb. 1970) and Falk to Altmeyer (20 Feb. 1970), Box 144:2082; Joint Meeting of the Executive Committee of CNHI and HSAC (2 Aug. 1974), Box 146:2130, all in Series III, Falk Papers; Melvin Glasser to Leonard Woodcock (31 Oct. 1973); Minutes of the Joint Meeting of the Executive and Technical Committees of the CNHI (26 Feb. 1970); Joint Meeting of the CNHI and HSAC Executive Committees (10 Nov. 1972); and Joint Meeting of the Executive Committees of the CNHI and HSAC (2 Aug. 1974), all in Box 110, Part I, Series VI, Records of the United Autoworkers Social Security Department [UAW-SSD], Archives of Labor History and Urban Affairs, Wayne State University, Detroit, Mich.

[52] Weinberger to Nixon (11 Jan. 1974), Box IS:3, WHCF, Nixon Papers; "Report of the Domestic Council Health Policy Review Group" (8 Dec. 1970), Box IS:1,WHSF, Nixon Papers; "Confidential Memorandum on Paying Medical Bills" (25 Jan. 1971), Box IS:2, WHSF, Nixon Papers; Starr, *Social Transformation of American Medicine*, 393–98.

payers. In other respects, HMOs embodied long-standing doubts that health insurance could work as social insurance by arguing that service benefits could not and should not be viewed as a purchased right.

This confusion persisted in the Clinton health plan, which replayed the debate of the 1970s in a context of even more tenuous employment-based coverage and even less fiscal elbowroom. The CHP leaned heavily on the logic of contributory finance, not out of any great conviction or interest in the principles of social insurance but simply because it viewed private insurance and fiscal neutrality as the only viable starting points. The administration was careful to portray its plan as a mandate or subsidy of private insurance and to stress that its goal was not "universal coverage" but "universal *access* to coverage." The administration leaned on "premiums" because a "payroll-based contribution," as Paul Starr warned, "whatever you call it, will not be or look like a price. It will clearly be a tax" and "the Republicans will have a field day." At the same time, the Health Care Task Force confined its attention to a "budget-neutral plan" and argued that "augmenting the payroll-based system involves minimal disruption to the current system and appears to require the smallest increase in new *public* funds." Indeed, as in the Carter era, fiscal restraint and cost-consciousness overwhelmed all other aims. "I talked for a moment with the First Lady to try to underline the key importance of the purchasing co-operatives," Starr recalled, "and before I could finish a sentence she said, 'But we need cost containment.' And then she ran off."[53]

The CHP reflected the long-standing dilemmas of social insurance and health provision. Liberal reformers routinely premised their calls for national health insurance on the plight of the rural poor, the elderly, or the uninsured, but were just as routinely seduced by "contributory" or employment-based solutions that left these problems largely unaddressed. For their part, conservatives pressed means-tested alternatives but complained about the consequences, including the social implications of providing assistance to the poor and the fiscal implications of having governments assume all the bad risks. The convergence of these approaches in the 1990s left little room for meaningful reform. "Since most Americans have insurance, they think of the uninsured as 'them'— this creates an 'us versus them' mentality," reasoned the Clinton task force, "We should not even talk about '37 million uninsured' because

[53] (Quote) "Tollgate 2 Presentation" (n.d.), Box 3305; (quote) Starr to Magaziner (22 Apr. 1993), Box 3210; Starr to Magaziner (31 Mar. 1993), Box 3210; "Economic Dilemmas for Health Care Reform" (n.d.), Box 670; Starr to Magaziner (7 Feb. 1993), Box 3308, all in CHTF Records; Theda Skocpol, *Boomerang: Clinton's Health Security Effort and the Turn against Government in U.S. Politics* (New York, 1996), 39–41, 122–23.

that is not who the proposal is designed to protect."[54] The only common ground lay in relying on employment provision, but this too raised problems. Although encouraging or mandating employment-based care satisfied the fiscal motive behind contributory social policy, it also (by relying on third-party payment by employers) scrambled the political and psychological motives.

Dilemmas of the "Deserving" Citizen

The overarching consequence of both the insistence on contributory programs and the confusion over how to pay for them was reliance on employment-based, private health insurance. This was a compromise shaped by both political deference to the principle of social insurance and a practical admission that health provision was incompatible with the fiscal assumptions of social insurance and the actuarial assumptions of commercial insurance. Regardless, reformers and opponents persistently made the link between productive employment and access to health care. "Benefits based on a wage record are a reward for productive effort and are consistent with general economic incentives," concluded the 1939 Advisory Council, "under such a social insurance system, the individual earns a right to a benefit that is related to his contribution to production." Or as a Blue Cross executive saw it: "You couldn't insure the unemployed person because they had no obligations, they didn't have to go to work, they could just go to the hospital and lie down. This was uninsurable."[55] Such arguments ran parallel to the larger logic of American social provision which—in its administration, its income thresholds and benefit levels, and its often Byzantine standards for eligibility—disciplined the labor market and enforced gendered, racial, and regional norms for participation in it. Recipients of social insurance or work-based benefits, it was commonly assumed, had proved something positive: that they had worked toward the protection of themselves and their families. Recipients of means-tested assistance, by contrast, had demonstrated something negative: that they had failed the most basic expectation of a "self-sustaining" person or a "breadwinner."[56]

[54] "Talking About Health Care," (n.d.), Walter Zelman files, quoted in Skocpol, *Boomerang*, 118.

[55] "Mr. Linton's Discussion" (6 Nov. 1937), Box 9, Decimal File 025, SSB Records, Office of the Commissioner, SSA Records; Colman in Robert Cunningham III and Robert M. Cunningham, Jr., *The Blues: A History of the Blue Cross and Blue Shield System* (De Kalb, 1997), 25.

[56] Frances Fox Piven and Richard Cloward, *Regulating the Poor: The Functions of Public Welfare* (New York, 1993), 131–33; Joanne Goodwin, " 'Employable Mothers' and 'Suitable Work': A Re-Evaluation of Welfare and Wage-Earning for Women in the Twentieth Century

Work was established as the focal point of health provision by the AALL, which assumed that even nonoccupational illness was a consequence of industrial employment and that the costs of medical care for workers and their dependents could be measured in lost wages. Although the AALL reforms sputtered, their basic assumptions persisted in public and private perceptions of welfare capitalism and into the economic security debates of the early 1930s. Both CCMC and CES reformers recognized the pitfalls of attaching health provision to employment and went so far as to "condemn in no uncertain terms further consideration of insurance limited to gainfully occupied persons." But such doubts were overwhelmed by the political and administrative appeal of using payrolls to organize payment and determine eligibility. The issue was not access to care per se, but "loss of capacity to be employed," "loss of earnings," or the "costs of medical care to gainfully employed persons." The only exception to this was the family-wage extension of benefits to dependents. Although health insurance did not survive the final draft of Social Security in 1935, further consideration of the issue reflected the New Deal's larger premise that ensuring the income of "breadwinners" was "the one almost all-embracing measure of security."[57]

The dramaturgy of "work" was reinforced and reaffirmed through the late 1930s and 1940s. Indeed, social insurance logic hijacked any possibility that health care might actually be considered a right of citizenship. "The fullest measure of security rests on the assurance of opportunity to work and earn a living in an economy organized to produce abundantly," the National Resources Planning Board stressed in 1943. "To whatever extent this goal is met, social security must also include provision for continuity of income during periods of when family livelihood is threatened." The president concurred that "real social security is dependent upon providing jobs for all who are able and willing to work." For some, such sentiments pointed to the urgency of filling in gaps in employment with social insurance programs; for others, the promise of economic growth and stable employment rendered the debates of the 1930s en-

---

United States," *Journal of Social History* 29 (1995): 253–58; Ball, "The Original Understanding on Social Security," 19.

[57] CCMC, *Medical Care for the American People* (Chicago, 1932), 51; "Preliminary Draft of a Program for Social Insurance against Illness" (1934), Box 2, CES Records; CES, "Interim Report" (Feb. 1935), p. 33, Box 67, Witte Papers; CES, "Final Report on the Risks of Economic Insecurity Arising out of Illness" (1934), p. 7, Box 3 CES Working Papers, SSA Records; CES (Medical Advisory Board), Interim Report (Jan. 1935), Box 67, Witte Papers; Proceedings of the Meeting of the Medical Advisory Board, CES (29–30 Jan. 1935), pp. 150–66, Box 42:236, Series II, Falk Papers; Theodore Marmor, *America's Misunderstood Welfare State* (New York, 1990), 33–34; "An Outline of a Possible Health Insurance Approach" (1939), Box 34, Decimal 056, GCF (1939–1944), HEW Records.

tirely moot. Organized labor often saw little to choose between public programs and collectively bargained benefits: either option was "in accord with the self-respect of labor," as an AFL official argued. "The worker wants to pay his way. He will not be exposed to the stigma of charity and will get medical attention as a right and not a condescension."[58]

After 1949 private and public policies hardened the ties between productive employment and social citizenship. Indeed, the prominence of payroll-based social insurance and private insurance made it increasingly difficult to identify whether it was work-based contributions or work itself that marked employees as "deserving"—especially in the eyes of a labor movement increasingly occupied by the task of bargaining over benefits. Postwar bargaining equated benefits with wages—indeed, as the UAW toyed with a fully prepaid health plan in the mid-1950s, it rebuffed charges that "free" services might be "valued lightly" by emphasizing that "the services are earned . . . they are part of the workers' salary."[59] The distinction between Medicare and Medicaid rested on the assumption that the former was a work-based insurance program while the latter offered only means-tested "welfare medicine." And the importance of work as a source of social entitlement was reflected in the prominence of mandated work-based insurance as the starting point for reform in the 1970s and the 1990s. The goal, as the Nixon administration put it in 1971, was simply to "push private insurance into present gaps in coverage for the employed population, leaving to government the residual responsibility for the population not in the labor force."[60] Once again, an argument made on administrative or political grounds had much broader ethical and political implications, and relegated those not covered by an employer mandate to a less generous and less legitimate stream of provision.

Whether it rested on administrative convenience or moral imperative, the reliance on employment benefits had clear and debilitating consequences.[61] The piecemeal growth of employment-based care confused

[58] Alan Derickson, " 'Take Health from the List of Luxuries': Labor and the Right to Health Care, 1915–1949," *Labor History* 41:2 (2000): 181–83; I. S. Falk, "Proposed Extension of the Social Security Program," *NEJM* 230:9 (2 Mar. 1944): 243; NRPB, *Security, Work, and Relief Policies*, 1–3; "Suggested Draft of Message on Social Security Expansion (2/7/45)," Box 3, Altmeyer Papers; Fein, *Medical Care, Medical Costs*, 25–26; Henry Richardson, "Health Program for America," *American Federationist* 53:1 (1946): 19.

[59] Sheps and Drosness, "Prepayment for Medical Care," 390; (quote) "Meeting Regarding CHA" (Jan. 1957), Box 3, Community Health Association Papers, UAW-SSD Records.

[60] "Memorandum on Paying Medical Bills" (25 Jan. 1971), Box IS:2, WHSF, Nixon Papers.

[61] Katherine Swartz, "Why Requiring Employers to Provide Health Insurance Is a Bad Idea," *JHPPL* 15:4 (1990): 781; Nancy Jecker, "Can an Employer-Based Health Insurance

the mechanism for dispensing health insurance with the standard or eligibility for coverage and allowed the distribution of jobs to determine the distribution of benefits. Given both long-standing patterns of occupational segregation and discrimination (by region, skill, race, and gender) and insurers' practice of "experience rating" employee groups, job-based health insurance subverted claims based on need and widened the compensation gap between organized white male workers in the industrial North and the rest of the working class. In turn, work-based insurance privileged only some kinds of work and contributed to the invisibility of casual, agricultural, domestic, and unpaid labor.[62] As reformers conceded, accepted, and sometimes even celebrated the role of the labor market as a conduit for benefits and a determinant of eligibility, they conceded, accepted, and sometimes even celebrated the ideal of family-wage social provision as well. This was clear in the AALL's proposals and in the appeals to manly independence with which the AFL responded; in the CES's fascination with "breadwinner" social insurance; in the 1939 recasting of Social Security as a system of family protection built on differential benefits; and in the parallel trajectories of public and private provision in the postwar era, which routinely assumed that work-based coverage would (and should) reach women and children as dependents.[63]

The emergence and elaboration of work-based benefits contributed to the administrative complexity (and costs) of health provision and the dilemmas reformers faced whenever they argued for universal or categorical expansion. Through the New Deal, reformers generally agreed that it would be sufficient to encourage, subsidize, or mandate work-based social provision. While concern was increasingly raised after the 1940s about the practical and inherent limits of work-based coverage, reformers saw their job as one of supplementing private coverage rather

---

System Be Just?" *JHPPL* 18:3 (1993): 657, 662, 666–68; Peter Budetti, "Universal Health Care Coverage: Pitfalls and Promises of an Employment-Based Approach," *Journal of Medicine and Philosophy* 17 (1992): 22–23; Joni Hersch and Shelly White Means, "Employer Sponsored Health and Pension Benefits and the Gender/Race Wage Gap," *Social Science Quarterly* 74:4 (1993), 854.

[62] Report of the Technical Committee on Medical Care (1938) in *President's Annual Message on Health Security*, H. Doc. 120 (76/1: Jan. 1939), p. 66; Senate Committee on Labor and Human Resources, *Hearing: Health Insurance Portability and Accountability Act of 1996: First Year Implementation Concerns* 105:2 (Mar. 1998), 7; Kaiser memo on Wagner bill (Dec. 1944), Box 272, Henry J. Kaiser Papers, Bancroft Library; Falk to Altemeyer (16 Dec. 1947), Box 46, Decimal 011.4, FSA, Office of the Administrator (GCF, 1944–1950), HEW Records; Brown, *Race, Money, and the American Welfare State*, 16–17.

[63] Linda Gordon, *Pitied but Not Entitled: Single Mothers and the History of Welfare* (New York, 1994), 179; "Plan for the Study of Economic Security" (1934), POF 1086, Franklin D. Roosevelt Papers, FDRPL; Ball, "The Original Understanding on Social Security," 25–27; David, "Old-Age, Survivors, and Disability Insurance," 11; Robert Ball OH, p. 14, LBJPL.

than displacing it—a strategy that was routinely identified both as a practical concession to vested interests and practices and as a means of reinforcing the sanctity of the link between social provision and employment. As a NAM spokesperson suggested in the late 1980s, "we arrived at a social contract that if government would take care of the old and the poor, the private sector would take care of the working."[64]

How then could reformers argue for coverage of those whose "deservedness" did not flow from employment? The absence of universal provision invited conservatives to distinguish between deserving and undeserving and pressed reformers to identify worthy population groups that might serve as an opening for broader coverage. As a political strategy, however, this created more problems than it solved. For some, it was an exercise in juggling different kinds of claims—according to contribution, to entitlement, or to need. For others, it was a political tack dictated by the constraints imposed by race, gender, and federalism. For still others, it reflected a genuine commitment to categorical coverage, although the battle then had to be fought over who were the "worthiest" (or the better organized) of the residual population. "We have a sort of NHI [national health insurance] system, with separate programs for the aged, poor, employed middle class, veterans, military dependents, etc," as the managed competition guru Alain Enthoven observed, adding that "we are already paying for NHI but we are not getting the benefit because we have an inefficient inequitable system that results from historical accident and interest group pressure."[65] Some understood the attention to "specified populations" as an acceptable solution, especially when a compelling case for federal responsibility could be made. Others saw danger in any incremental reform. "We have gradually been made a nation of 'Gimmes,' " argued a constituent to the White House in the late 1940s, "because we see this group and that group favored, and believing as we do, that all should be treated alike, we strive for our share of the pap."

[64] AFL Social Security Dept., "Nine Good Reasons for the Forand Bill" (Mar. 1960), Box 206, Witte Papers; Memorandum: Alternative Policy Positions (20 Mar. 1961), Box 20, Grahame Papers; Altmeyer to Falk (24 Dec. 1970), Box 144:2082, Series III, Falk Papers; NAM cited in "The Battle for Health Insurance," *Fortune* 118:7 (26 Sept. 1988): 145.

[65] Schultze to Califano (27 Sept. 1965), WHCF FG 364, LBJ Papers; Falk to Altmeyer (16 Dec. 1947), Box 2, Decimal 11.1, Division of Research and Statistics, SSA Records; "Managed Competition and Its Potential for Reducing Health Expenditures" (23 Dec. 1992), Box 4001, CHTF Records; First Progress Report of the Interdepartmental Committee to Coordinate Health and Welfare Activities [ICHWA] (12 Feb. 1936), and Second Progress Report (12 Feb. 1936), Box 12; "Health and Welfare Activities of the Federal Government" (6 July 1937), Box 13; Franks Hines to Josephine Roche (11 Oct. 1937), Box 12, all in ICHWA Records, FDRPL; Franz Goldmann, "Public Policy in Organizing Medical Care," *AAAPSS* 273 (1951): 63–64; Alain Enthoven, "Notes on National Health Insurance" (16 May 1977), Box 489, Edgar Kaiser Papers.

The arguments of the AMA were peppered with warnings about entering wedges, feet in the door, camel's noses, and Trojan horses. "What one section of the population gets from the federal government, the rest are likely to want in the near future," reasoned the doctors in 1956, "so what is the next step? Government hospital and medical care for the dependents of veterans?—for industrial workers?—for white-collar workers?— for farmers?—for old people?—for everyone with an income under $5000 a year?—for the entire population?"[66]

The poor almost always emerged as the first target of assistance. But though most agreed that the poor were needy, they rarely agreed that the poor were also deserving: means-tested programs served as both a minimal concession of state responsibility and a means of marking off welfare or welfare medicine as less legitimate commitments. Health care was unique in this respect, because conservatives clung to the notion that health care was a commodity rather than a right, only belatedly conceded that there were any gaps between personal responsibility and medical charity, and objected strenuously to public coverage of those "who theoretically can pay something." Doctors and others insisted that health care was a consumer good subject to consumer preferences. And reformers and their opponents battled over the appropriate income threshold at which public assistance would become available. Reformers, who hoped that social insurance would eventually subsume social assistance, objected to means testing. But this was not simply a matter of pressing for expansive programs organized around a relatively high income threshold, because it was also important that such thresholds be low enough to avoid offending "self-sustaining" persons by including them. For its part, the CES struggled to find a level of income that was high enough to ensure sufficient income for the public plan, but low enough to exclude "the well-to-do people [who] are much more exacting and much more fussy with respect to the type of medical services which they expect, with respect to the type of hospital accommodation which will meet their needs, medical or esthetic, and so on."[67]

After 1935 this debate increasingly revolved around the uncertain measure of "medical indigency." Under Kerr-Mills, this threshold varied widely by state, often including not only both an income and tangible asset test but an estimate of "contributions which a son, daughter or estranged spouse should be making to the applicant." Indeed, fifteen

[66] NAM, "Proposed Policy Recommendation" (Dec. 1970), Box I:103, NAM Records; O'Donnell to HST (20 Nov. 1945), PPF 200, Box 257, Truman Papers; "Socialized Medicine and Socialism by Way of the Veterans Administration," *JAMA* 162:9 (1956): 865.

[67] Rashi Fein, "Health Care Cost: A Distorted Issue," *American Federationist* 82:6 (1975), 15; (quotes) Medical Advisory Board minutes (29 Jan. 1935), 110–16, 174, Box 67, Witte Papers.

states adopted Kerr-Mills means tests so rigid that most already receiving public assistance could not qualify. As Kerr-Mills was recast as Medicaid, HEW worried about both the burden and the propriety of maintaining different thresholds for conventional (Aid to Dependent Children) and medical assistance—and state standards varied widely (eligibility for a family of four ranged from $2,400 in annual income and $800 liquid assets on Oklahoma to $6,000 in income and $3,000 assets in New York). Health interests argued that, in order to protect the legitimacy of private insurance, public assistance should kick in only after medical expenses had pushed an individual or family below the poverty line. In revisiting the question in 1974, the Kennedy-Mills bill proposed an even harsher distinction between contribution and indigency that counted (among other things), income, liquid assets, life insurance proceeds, and casual employment earning more than $30.[68]

Social insurance widened the gap between need and deservedness. Time and time again, reformers used the circumstances of the indigent and underserved as an argument for reform but then drafted proposals that treated the poor as a "residual population." Through the postwar years, reformers routinely admitted that their principal concern was not the poor or the uninsured, but the anxieties of those who might become poor as a consequence of medical expenses or who might lose their insurance. Eager to avoid confrontations with organized medicine, reformers also routinely restricted their attention to the costs of hospitalization. As a result, means-tested alternatives to national health insurance put forth in the 1940s, the 1960s, and the 1970s actually offered much broader coverage for the poor—an irony that medical conservatives never tired of pointing out. Indeed, confusion over the nature of medical indigency and its place in reform efforts was largely responsible for the emergence, especially after 1965, of the "medigap" between those who claimed private coverage and those who qualified for public programs.[69]

Another tack was the attempt to extend coverage to the elderly—a group, as Theodore Marmor observes, "presumed to be both needy and deserving because, through no fault of their own, they had lower earning capacity and higher medical expenses than any other adult age group." At the same time, the post-65 population was itself an artifact of private

---

[68] "Criteria for a Good Bill," *The Nation* 194 (17 Feb. 1962), 134–35; "The Dynamite in the 1962 Elections," *American Federationist* 69:2 (1962): 6; "Medicare: The Major Defects," *The Nation* 200 (28 June 1965): 699; draft: The Problem of Extending Health Coverage to the Uninsured (22 Jan. 1966), Box 23, Grahame Papers; "National Health Insurance: Diagnosing the Alternatives," *American Federationist* 81:6 (1974): 7.

[69] Berkowitz, *Mr. Social Security,* 236–37; CCMC, *Medical Care for the American People,* 6–9; James Tallon and Rachel Block, "Changing Patterns of Health Insurance Coverage: Special Concerns for Women," *Women and Health* 12:3 (1987): 123.

employment and private coverage. The elderly needed more care be-cause they were old, but the fact that they had trouble meeting the costs of that care rested on prevailing patterns of risk rating and employment-based coverage. For reformers, this made the elderly an attractive bet. Age was an easy and universal criteria for eligibility. There was no ques-tion, among the retired population, of access to work-based programs. And at least after 1935, Social Security had already established the na-tion's elderly as deserving of state attention. It was for these reasons that, after the late 1940s, reformers focused on the modest goal of providing hospitalization insurance to OASI recipients. "It will benefit and attract a most deserving group in the population," as FSA administrator Oscar Ewing argued in 1952, "which other groups will be loath to attack."[70]

Opponents, by contrast, collapsed the issues of elderly and indigent care. In this view (captured by the AMA's 1964 Eldercare proposal) the nonindigent elderly were no more deserving of care than the rest of the self-sustaining population. The AMA warned of "an enormous perma-nent mechanism, imposing heavy additional taxes on all working people for all the years of their working lives, so that everybody—the well-off as well as the poor, the proud as well as the humble, the cheaters as well as the deserving—would be taken into a compulsory government system." The AMA resented the inclusion of anyone willing or able to pay his or her doctor's bills, argued that conventional income thresholds over-stated the poverty of the elderly by ignoring savings or assets, and hoped that private group coverage would eventually offer more systematic re-tiree benefits. Even erstwhile allies in the labor movement were leery of seniors' demands, at least insofar as they threatened competing claims. Nelson Cruikshank, the AFL-CIO's social insurance expert, saw in Medi-care an "irresponsible" echo of the Depression-era Townsend movement (a campaign for generous old-age pensions)—"a sort of gerontocracy that would plague the government for one handout after another."[71] As fiscally-anxious stabs at reforming Medicare in the 1980s and 1990s would make clear, the deservedness of the elderly was always compro-mised by the reach of indigent programs on the one hand and the exten-sion of employment-based programs on the other.

At times, reformers (and opponents) adopted a "lifeboat strategy" of concern for mothers and children. The target of such efforts was really just children: women were considered only as mothers and then only as

---

[70] Marmor, *Politics of Medicare*, 15; " 'Medicare,' the Cure That Could Cause a Setback," *Fortune* 67:5 (May 1963): 133; Fein, *Medical Care, Medical Costs*, 54; statement by Oscar Ewing (25 June 1951), Box 211, Witte Papers; "Draft Memorandum for the President" (11 Feb. 1952); and "Conway Memo" (30 July 1951), POF 286A, 931, Truman Papers.

[71] "Are 200,000 Doctors Wrong?" 663; Marmor, *Politics of Medicare*, 61–62; "Some Obser-vations on Financial Assets of the Aged," *JAMA* 171:9 (1959): 1228–31; "Health Insurance

a necessary vehicle for delivering care or financial assistance to the child. The CES, for example, left little doubt that benefits under Social Security's Aid to Dependent Children title

> are not primarily aids to mothers but defense measures for children. They are designed to release from the wage earning role the person whose natural function is to give her children the physical and affectionate guardianship necessary not alone to keep them from falling into social misfortune, but more affirmatively to rear them into citizens capable of contributing to society.

"The public would condemn benefit payment on behalf of working wives," as a 1942 survey of social insurance argued typically. "In the case of wives with children in their care, however, it was felt that the situation was somewhat different," and the survey even suggested that "only a wife with a child in her care be regarded as dependent." The deservedness of children was largely unquestioned; they could neither be expected to participate in contributory programs nor be held at fault for the failure of their parents to do so.[72] Liberals routinely defended the principle of "starting gate equality," and pointed out the perverse inequities of lavishing care on the well-insured elderly while (even at the peak of private coverage) as many as a quarter of all children went without stable access to care.[73] For their part, conservatives elevated children by dismissing or demonizing virtually all other claimants, although they were often leery of state encroachment on familial responsibility: one opponent viewed the national health insurance proposals of the late 1940s as a precursor to "the radical reorganizing of family life in America," in which politicians would use reproductive services "to establish 'quotas' for the baby crop in the same way that the Agricultural Department theorists set 'quotas' for farm production."[74]

For these reasons, maternalist efforts to expand coverage often fragmented it instead.[75] Elite women reformers in and around the Children's

---

for the Aged," *JAMA* 170:6 (1959): 689–92; Cruikshank quoted in Richard Harris, "Annals of Legislation: Medicare," *New Yorker* (16 July 1966): 51.

[72] ICHWA, "Draft Report and Recommendations" (Jan. 1939), Box 5, Oscar Chapman Papers, HSTPL; CES quoted in Gwendolyn Mink, *The Wages of Motherhood: Inequality in the Welfare State, 1917–1942* (Ithaca, N.Y., 1995), 132; Report of the Interbureau Technical Committee, "Dependents' Benefits in Social Insurance" (Nov. 1942), Box 68:699, Series II, Falk Papers.

[73] Ronald Dworkin, "Will Clinton's Plan Be Fair?" *New York Review of Books* 41 (13 Jan. 1994): 20–25; Douglas Diekma, "Children First: The Need to Reform Financing Health Care Services for Children," *Journal of Health Care for the Poor and Underserved* 7:1 (1996): 4–8.

[74] "Dan Gilbert's Washington Letter" (Dec. 1948), reel 7, Michael Davis Papers (microfilm), HSTPL.

[75] Linda Gordon, "Putting Children First: Women, Maternalism, and Welfare in the Early Twentieth Century," in *U.S. History as Women's History*, ed. Kerber, Kessler-Harris, and Sklar, 65, 72–73.

Bureau, for example, often found themselves defending discrete maternal programs (such as the Sheppard-Towner Act in the 1920s, or the Emergency Maternity and Infant Care program of the 1940s) against retrenchment or expansion.[76] The architects of Social Security ducked universal coverage in favor of (Title V) provision for maternal and child health. Some at the FSA were quite taken with the idea of a "Children's Health Act" as an alternative to the more expansive reforms pressed in 1948 and 1949, but also worried that such a strategy (alongside employment benefits and veterans' programs) might splinter the constituency for universal programs. After 1965 reformers repeatedly floated the option of "kiddycare," and the Nixon administration's "Family Health Insurance Plan" went so far as to peel off poor families with children for special attention while leaving the rest under Medicaid. In recent years, concern for children's health has often come at the expense of other health programs or as a means of bypassing "undeserving" adults altogether (the 1997 State Children's Health Insurance Program or SCHIP, offers federal grants for the coverage of children in working families with incomes too high to qualify for Medicaid but too low to afford private coverage).[77]

In such efforts, as Linda Gordon suggests, maternalism was both a tangle of assumptions about women's appropriate private and public roles and a strategy by which reformers "held up children in front of them, plump little legs and adorable wide eyes inducing a suspicious gatekeeper to open a door to the public treasury." The strategy often backfired: celebration of children as especially deserving always suggested that their parents were less so, making it difficult to deliver assistance to children at all. However compelling the arguments for meeting the health needs of young children, reformers and opponents alike have always assumed that provision via parental (usually paternal) breadwinners was a natural and laudable feature of social insurance—while provision via parental (usually maternal) recipients of social assistance was an unfortunate necessity. As a result, children have always fared badly in the United States on virtually every measure of social or health policy.[78]

As categorical targets of political attention or sympathy, children, the elderly, and the poor were all defined primarily by their relationship to

[76] Gordon, *Pitied but Not Entitled*, 254–62; "Principles to Be Considered . . . for an Emergency Maternity and Infant Care Program" (May 1951), Box 3, SSB Records, Office of the Commissioner, SSA Records.

[77] Pace Memorandum (4 Apr. 1949), POF 7N, Box 82, Truman Papers; "The Children Are Still Waiting," *The Nation* 219 (28 Sept. 1974): 275–76; Berkowitz, *Mr. Social Security*, 265; "National Health Insurance Act of 1971," Box 198:1, Cohen Papers; "Retreat from National Health," *The Nation* 226 (11 Feb. 1978): 144–45; Report of the 1964 Task Force on Health (Nov. 1964), Box 1, Task Force Reports, LBJPL; Nancy McKenzie and Ellen Bilofsky, "Shredding the Safety Net," *Health/PAC Bulletin* 21:2 (Summer 1991): 9.

[78] Gordon, "Putting Children First," 65–66, 71, 76 (quote), 85.

the labor market and work-based health benefits. Different arguments surrounded one other target of federal health policy: the nation's veterans. Veterans' care reflected an entitlement or "deservedness" that flowed from the fulfillment of an exceptional civic obligation. "Military service," as the NRPB concluded in 1942, "has long been recognized as establishing a claim against the government, and pensions and special insurance rights have been a part of our system for years." This was especially true of health benefits that (unlike employment, housing, or education programs) were often a direct compensation for service-related injuries or disabilities. Yet veterans' programs in the United States were largely confined, before 1945, to the provision of pensions and a scattering of veterans' homes and hospitals. Arguments for special attention to veterans' needs did not fly very far in the 1930s when both Hoover and Roosevelt put off the payment of a bonus to World War I veterans— Roosevelt telling the American Legion bluntly that "the fact of wearing a uniform" was not enough to place veterans in "a special class of beneficiaries over and above other citizens."[79]

This reticence collapsed during World War II. The sheer scale of mobilization created immense demands for health services. The Children's Bureau lobbied for an expansive program of maternity care in overcrowded military and industrial centers and ultimately settled for coverage of military families under the Emergency Maternity and Infant Care (EMIC) program. "Congress takes the view," the Social Security Board concluded, "that maternity and infant care is a right attached to service in the armed forces"—an argument that even the AMA found difficult to challenge. In turn, the anticipated prosperity of the postwar era easily accommodated both expansion of the Veterans' Administration (VA) hospital system and the broader GI Bill.[80] For reformers, veterans' care was a puzzle. Some sought to ride the popularity of veterans' benefits and wondered if "any useful argument could be made in behalf of the health insurance program out of this situation?" Others saw universal coverage as a pipedream and proved willing to hear any arguments for special consideration. For its part, the VA played both sides, suggesting to reformers that the VA was "a ready made, long established and well recognized test area for . . . a complete national health program," while assuring opponents that veterans' coverage would deflect more expansive reform. By 1944–45, the administration had largely accepted the

---

[79] NRPB, *Security, Work, and Relief Policies*, 3; Roosevelt quoted in Theda Skocpol, "The G.I. Bill and U.S. Social Policy," *Social Philosophy and Policy* 14:2 (1997): 103–4.

[80] "Federal Aid for Maternity Care," *JAMA* 120:1 (1942): 47–58; "Memorandum on Consultations Re: EMIC" (4 Apr. 1951), Box 3, Records of the SSA, Office of the Commissioner, SSA Records; Daily to Lenroot (12 Mar. 1951), Box 3, SSB Records, Office of the Commissioner, SSA Records.

view that veterans were "entitled to special consideration" and cobbled together a discrete welfare state for them.[81]

Opponents appreciated the political status of the VA and applauded the fact that it eroded the urgency for reform and demobilized an important reform constituency. But they also questioned the assumption that military service conferred expansive entitlements. As early as 1933, *Fortune* assailed VA spending as "the sacred white elephant of the U.S. Budget . . . hallowed, untouchable, taboo to unfriendly hands" and argued for distinguishing "deserving sheep" from the "undeserving goats" demanding a steady diet of pensions, bonuses, and health benefits. Others, reflecting the views of reformers, worried that the VA could just as easily invite expansion as contain it. "We had so many enthusiasts for our brand of government medicine," recalled VA medical director Paul Magnuson, "that I was scared for a while that we had . . . given aid and comfort to those who wanted to bring all medicine under government control." Opponents proved quite willing to play on VA successes as well, arguing (for example) that national health insurance "would be grossly unfair to millions of veterans already entitled to free care." This argument echoed labor's anxieties about "double taxation." "Compulsory health insurance would impose an unjust tax on the veteran's paycheck," agreed the American Legion, "*for medical care to which he is now entitled free of charge as a reward for service to his country.*"[82]

Such ambivalence persisted through the postwar era. In 1950 congressional conservatives added dependent care to basic VA coverage, reasoning that a more expansive veterans' welfare state would erode or fragment support for universal programs. In a 1953 survey of veterans' care, however, the AMA called for restraint on the grounds that "a consideration of this problem must of course be predicated upon a concern for the health of the entire population and not just a particular segment" and that "lifelong care should not evolve alone from the very normal

[81] Springarn Memo for Elsey (24 Aug. 1950), OF 286A, Truman Papers; Ida Merriam to Harry Rosnfield (9 Dec. 1946), Box 3, Decimal 11, Division of Research and Statistics, SSA Records; (quote) Memorandum on Interview with General Bradley (Jan.? 1946), PSF, Box 140, Truman Papers; Draft of Statement by the President (4 Sept. 1943), POF 1710:2, FDR Papers; Edwin Amenta and Theda Skocpol, "Redefining the New Deal: World War II and the Development of Social Provision in the United States," in *The Politics of Social Policy in the United States*, ed. Margaret Weir, Ann Orloff, and Theda Skocpol (Princeton, N.J., 1988), 81–94, 107–8.

[82] "P-E-N-S-I-O-N," *Fortune* 7:1 (Jan. 1933): 34, 41; Magnuson in "The Health 'Bible' Still Gathers Dust," *American Federationist* 67:8 (1960): 24; NPC, "Compulsion: The Key to Collectivism" (1949), p. 37, SHSW Pamphlets; American Legion Resolution (11 Feb. 1950), File 81A-H7.2, Box 183, Records of the House Committee on Foreign and Interstate Commerce, Records of the House of Representatives; Summary of Hearings (3 May 1946), Box 3, Decimal 11.1, Division of Research and Statistics, SSA Records.

incident of fulfilling the duties required of every citizen." For the AMA and others, the VA remained a "Trojan horse of ominous dimensions" due largely to its gradual acceptance of non-service-related coverage and the accompanying expansion of facilities. When the Johnson administration tried to close or reorganize nineteen VA hospitals in early 1965, it faced a bitter backlash from both veterans' groups and Congress. Without fail, opponents of the reorganization plan cited the sanctity of military entitlement and blasted the administration for cutting veterans' benefits at a time when benefits were being made available to millions of "less-deserving" citizens. Similar confrontations, cutting across party lines, arose periodically in the post-Vietnam era; legislators blasted any effort to restrain VA spending as the violation of a sacred trust. "Recently there has been a lot of discussion about the health care delivery system in our country—about pending legislation that is being called the 'patients' bill of rights,' " as presidential hopeful John McCain reminded an American Legion audience in 1999, "but what about a 'veterans' bill of rights'?"[83] At the same time, however, medical conservatives led a push to privatize the VA and displace service benefits at VA facilities with vouchers for conventional private insurance. In all, arguments for the exceptional "deservedness" of veterans were not easy to sustain before or beyond the exceptional circumstances of the late 1940s.

The debate over health insurance was never (save in the rosiest musings of reformers) a debate about universal coverage. Instead, it was a more complex attempt to identify deserving or convenient population groups and to sell the limited notion of contributory, contractual "insurance" for wage earners. This debate exposed both the general limits of the American system of social insurance and the particular dilemmas of including the provision of health benefits in that system. Arguments for health coverage were based on a tangle of competing and often contradictory claims, including the rights of citizenship, the needs of patients, the return on contributions, the responsibilities of breadwinners, and the compensation of "deserving" citizens. At various junctures, reformers and their opponents offered versions of all of these arguments. Reformers sought to expand coverage on categorical grounds, some because they believed that less-than-universal coverage was just and proper, some

[83] Brown, *Race, Money, and the American Welfare State*, 129; "To Socialized Medicine and Socialism by Way of the VA," *JAMA* 162:9 (1956): 860 (1953 AMA report cited at 860); "The Medicare Program," *JAMA* 171:11 (1959), 1485–87; "Memorandum of the Events Relating to Proposed VA Hospital Closings" (January 1965), WHCF VA 11; letters and telegrams in WHCF VA12–15s, LBJPL; "Veterans—Hospital Closings" clippings, Box 72, Democratic National Committee Records, LBJPL "Battle for Veterans' Vote Heats Up," *Washington Post* (9 Sept. 1999); #A8.

because they viewed piecemeal coverage as the only practical solution, and some because they hoped to use unarguably deserving populations as an entering wedge for universal coverage. Over time, fragmented coverage—as a policy goal or a strategic gambit—remained fragmented and undermined arguments for universality. As firms and industries erected discrete private welfare systems, they created a further tangle of private claims and expectations and responsibilities. More broadly, every argument for a particular or categorical claim to health coverage carried with it, at least implicitly, arguments against a host of other claims. And every effort to identify those left behind stigmatized their failure even as it sought to meet their needs.

4

Socialized Medicine and Other Afflictions: The Political Culture of the Health Debate

Over the course of the twentieth century, the language and culture of American politics shaped the aspirations of reformers, animated the arguments of their opponents, and set the terms and the boundaries of public discourse. This is not to say, as is often casually concluded, that a popular aversion to statist solutions doomed the prospects for national health insurance. Periodic measures of public support suggest quite the opposite: most Americans did not view a system of national health insurance as at all incompatible with their beliefs about the responsibilities of individuals or the role of government. In any case, it is a mistake to attribute such generic beliefs to "Americans" without regard to either disagreements among them or changing historical circumstances. The keywords of American political culture—republicanism, liberalism, individualism—have proved quite plastic, animating in equal measure, for example, Andrew Carnegie's Gospel of Wealth and the struggles of Carnegie's workers, Hoover's "American Individualism" and Roosevelt's New Deal, the civil rights protests of the 1960s and the recalcitrance of southern segregationists.[1]

What was important was not the generic language of American politics but the ability of health interests to give this language a particular meaning and urgency. Sometimes, these interests sincerely believed their apocalyptic fears of state medicine; at other times, they manufactured and manipulated such fears. "The Americanism part of it is a joke," a member of the New York League for Americanism conceded during the AALL debate. "The League for Americanism was organized primarily to kill off health insurance and other such fool legislation. . . . You can go ahead and stir up sentiment on Americanism and other men will follow

[1] Gary Gerstle, "The Protean Character of American Liberalism," *American Historical Review* 99:4 (1994): 1045–47; Louis Hartz, *The Liberal Tradition in America* (New York, 1955); Dorothy Ross, *The Origins of American Social Science* (New York, 1990), 29–34, 140; John Laslett, "Sombart and After: American Social Scientists Address the Question of Socialism in the United States," in *Why Is There No Socialism in the United States?* ed. Jean Heffer and Jeanine Rovet (Paris, 1988), 45–46; Aaron Wildavsky, "Resolved, That Individualism and Egalitarianism Be Made Compatible in America: Political-Cultural Roots of Exceptionalism," in *Is America Different? A New Look at American Exceptionalism,* ed. Byron Shafer (New York, 1991), 120–22; Michael Rogin, *The Radical Specter: The Intellectuals and McCarthy* (Cambridge, Mass., 1967), 9–31, 261–82.

along after you."[2] Reformers, in 1915 and beyond, spent as much time and effort responding to or defusing such charges as they did crafting legislative solutions. In doing so, they often reinforced such sentiments and narrowed future alternatives. Arguments that national health insurance was "contrary to the spirit of our institutions and the deep-rooted instincts of our people" or that it threatened the "inherent rights and sanctity of the individual" were routinely echoed by reformers anxious to assure the public of their own commitment to "maintaining a uniquely American system."[3] The language of politics did not determine or confine policy, but it did nurture an atmosphere in which state intervention and public social provision were easily dismissed or demonized.[4]

Some of these elements of the health debate are touched upon in other chapters. We have seen how American liberalism nurtured a weak sense of social citizenship and how an antistatist culture persisted despite the remarkable growth of state institutions; and we will see how racial assumptions and racial interests discouraged the pursuit of universal provision and how, over time, only certain kinds of state intervention (those that disguised their real costs by subsidizing "private" provision) were seen as legitimate. In this chapter we turn to other cultural and ideological premises of the health debate. Why did mobilization for war, a catalyst for national social policies in other capitalist democracies, not have the same effect in the United States? How did various interests assess, and employ in American health politics, the health systems of other countries? In what ways did gender politics reify and reinforce the politics of voluntarism and individualism? Why was the health debate increasingly marked by the conviction that health care was a commodity rather than a right and how did this conviction shape the politics of the medical profession?

Fighting for Security: War and the Politics of Health

Both world wars followed flurries of reform in which public health programs were considered but ultimately put off. For reformers, mobilization offered an important opportunity, in part because concerns about

---

[2] New York State League of Women Voters, "Report and Protest . . . New York League for Americanism," in Box 209, Edwin Witte Papers, State Historical Society of Wisconsin [SHSW], Madison, Wis.

[3] Quotes, in order, from P. Tecumseh Sherman in Roundtable on Social Insurance, Chamber Proceedings (Apr. 1931), p. 479, Box I:7, Chamber of Commerce Papers, Hagley Museum and Library, Wilmington, Del.; NPC, "Compulsion: The Key to Collectivism" (1949), p. 7, SHSW Pamphlets; "Talking Points" (n.d.), Box 1172, Records of the Clinton Health Care Task Force [CHTF], National Archives, College Park, Md.

[4] Alice Kessler-Harris, "In the Nation's Image: The Gendered Limits of Social Citizenship in the Depression Era," *JAH* 86:3 (Dec. 1999): 1256–60.

growth of the federal state were muted and in part because military drafts served as a damning index of public health. And international involvement set American social policies against the example and experience of other nations. All of this raised the stakes for reformers and opponents alike, and caricatured the ways in which both could champion liberal values toward quite opposite ends.[5]

Health examinations for military service, especially in 1917–18, were one of the most expansive public health initiatives to date, and reformers seized on the results as further argument for compulsory health insurance. A deferral rate approaching one-third of enlistees was, as George Creel of the administration's Committee on Public Information argued, "at once a warning and a national disgrace." The New Jersey Health Commission agreed that "health protection . . . has been raised by the war from a position deserving of humanitarian consideration to one demanding action if we are to survive as a nation," adding that "our *laissez faire* industrial policy has been at least partly responsible for the fact that half of our young men cannot qualify physically when the army calls." While medical conservatives disputed the figures or ascribed them to racial or personal failings, reformers blamed uneven or inadequate access to basic medical services.[6] This debate replayed itself in the 1940s, by which time conservatives could also float discretionary solutions, including postwar hospital construction or improvements in veterans' care.

More broadly, the politics and political culture of mobilization offered reformers a real opening, both because public health could be linked to national security and because federal management of the war effort often trumped philosophical or constitutional concerns about new national programs. The Children's Bureau, for example, forged an alliance with the AALL and the Milbank Fund in 1915 and used "preparedness" as grounds to argue for more expansive health programs. The bureau and others reprised this strategy in the 1940s, using the popular portrayal of workers as "production soldiers" to argue for civilian medical services commensurate with those enjoyed by the military. "We have come to

[5] Robert Westbrook, "Fighting for the American Family: Private Interests and Political Obligation in World War II," in *Power as Culture,* ed. T. J. Jackson Lears and Richard Wightman Fox (New York, 1993), 135–60; Nancy Fraser and Linda Gordon, "Contract vs. Charity: Why Is There No Social Citizenship in the United States? *Socialist Review* (1992): 45–67; Paul Starr, *The Transformation of American Medicine* (New York, 1982), 253–57, 286–89; James Morone, *The Democratic Wish: Popular Participation and the Limits of American Government* (New York, 1990), 257–65; Elizabeth Fones-Wolf, *Selling Free Enterprise: The Business Assault on Labor and Liberalism* (Urbana, Ill., 1994).

[6] Creel quoted in Gwendolyn Mink, *The Wages of Motherhood: Inequality in the Welfare State, 1917–1942* (Ithaca, N.Y., 1995), 15; N.J. Health Commission quoted in "The Draft and Health Insurance," *The Survey* 39 (2 Mar. 1918): 608.

recognize that any person who makes his contribution to our national [economic] life," as the National Resources Planning Board reasoned hopefully, "is entitled to protection against the necessary interruptions in income." Indeed, reformers hoped that various aspects of wartime health care, including the Emergency Maternity and Infant Care program and the military experience of medical professionals, might serve as springboards for reform.[7]

Such hopes were dashed. Opponents were keenly aware of the threat of state expansion posed by the war, and they too stepped up their efforts and their rhetoric. The AMA urged its members to use "politicized medicine" and "state-managed medicine" alongside its conventional specter of "socialized medicine" and gravely noted the retreat of Canadian and British doctors under the pressures of the war. Most starkly, medical conservatives promoted a ruggedly individualist version of American war goals and identified social policy with totalitarian enemies. In 1917 health insurance was a product of both "German conceptions of state policy" and "the plans and purposes of the International Socialist Movement"; a quarter century later, opponents claimed that health reform was "born in Germany—and is part and parcel of what our boys are fighting overseas." A Kentucky medical society warned that national health insurance would "make the Surgeon General of the United States a medical dictator . . . as much so as a Nazi dictator . . . conditions proposed in the measure are comparable to National Socialism, a condition against which seven million Americans are fighting." And Oklahoma doctors went so far as to resolve that the Holocaust "could never have happened if Bismarck had not clandestinely murdered the free spirit of medicine [with] . . . compulsory health insurance."[8]

Such sentiments swamped efforts to employ democratic internationalism and domestic mobilization toward more progressive ends. This pat-

---

[7] Linda Gordon, *Pitied but Not Entitled: Single Mothers and the History of Welfare* (New York, 1994), 104–5; "Workers' Health in War," *American Federationist* 49:7 (1942): 12–14; NRPB, *Security, Work, and Relief Policies* (Washington, D.C., 1942), 3.

[8] "The National Emergency as a Pretext for Compulsory Health Insurance," *JAMA* 116:4 (1941): 310–11; "Socialized Medicine as a Slogan," *JAMA* 114:14 (1940): 1364; "The Movement Toward Compulsory Health Insurance in Canada," *JAMA* 121:11 (1943): 880; quotes (in order) from Frederick Hoffman, *Facts and Fallacies of Compulsory Health Insurance* (Newark, N.J., 1917), 7, 12; "Check and Double Check on Compulsory Sickness Insurance" (1946) in AMA Kit on Health Insurance, Box 43, Decimal 011.4, General Classified Files [GCF] (1944–1950), RG 235, Department of Health, Education, and Welfare [HEW], National Archives; Geraldine Sartain, "California's Health Insurance Drama," *Survey Graphic* 34:11 (Nov. 1945): 45; Memo: "Doctors Threaten to Quit" (Oct. 1943), Box 50:368, Series II, Isidore Falk Papers, Sterling Library, Yale University; Oklahoma State Medical Assoc. to HST (7 July 1947), President's Official File [POF] 286A, Box 930, Harry S Truman Papers, Harry S. Truman Presidential Library [HSTPL], Independence, Mo.

tern was neatly captured by the contest over the meaning of the Four
Freedoms floated by President Roosevelt in 1943. Reformers pointed to
the British Beveridge Plan and argued that expansion of Social Security
constituted "a political litmus test for all who seek or hold public office
to determine whether they are sincere when the pay homage to the four
freedoms and promise to help build a better world." The National Lawyers Guild agreed, and cited "the deep yearning of men and women
everywhere to achieve that freedom from want which is one of the Four
Freedoms at stake in the global conflict in which we are engaged."[9] Opponents countered that "it would be the supreme tragedy of the nation's
history if these young men were spoiled by a system of cradle-to-the-grave
benefits. All their fine courage and high ideals would be smothered by
entering into a Lazy Man's Paradise." Indeed while some invoked the
four freedoms as a postwar prescription for social and economic security,
they were more commonly and insistently interpreted as a proscription
of the state. Returning soldiers "will want security," argued the Ohio
Chamber of Commerce, "but the good old-fashioned kind of American
security—the security of opportunity. They certainly will not want the
paternalistic type of security found in Europe, based upon a despotic
system against which they are fighting on the far-flung battlefields of the
world." The AMA was particularly fond of this argument and, as late as
1949, AMA president Donovan Ward used it in private appeals to legislators: "I am calling on you as a believer in the principles of democracy
and free enterprise and the much publicized 'Four Freedoms' to stand
firmly against any legislation which has a tendency to subjugate American medicine."[10]

Reformers abandoned such rhetorical flourishes with the war's end,
but opponents stuck with them. The National Physicians Committee
(NPC) clung to the example of the German health system, arguing in
1948 that "the bureaucracy that was built to service the system became
the single greatest source of strength for Adolph Hitler in his ruthless
rise to power." A year later, the NPC intoned that "the decisions of the

---

[9] (Quote) George Addes, secretary-treasurer UAW, "The Plot against the W-M-D Bill"
(17 Feb. 1944), Box 60:519, Series II, Falk Papers; *Labor's Monthly Survey* (Dec. 1942) in
POF 142:1, Franklin D. Roosevelt Papers, Franklin D. Roosevelt Presidential Library
[FDRPL], Hyde Park, N.Y.; (quote) National Lawyers Guild, "The New Wagner-Murray-
Dingell Social Security Bill" (1944), Box 60:520, Series II, Falk Papers.

[10] (Quotes) Ohio Chamber of Commerce, "A Death Thrust . . . " (1943), POF 4351:2,
FDR Papers; memo: "Doctors Threaten to Quit" (Oct. 1943), Box 50:368, Series II, Falk
Papers; Elizabeth Wilson, *Compulsory Health Insurance* (NICB: Studies in Individual and Col-
lective Security, 1947), 93; Oklahoma State Medical Assoc. to HST (7 July 1947), POF 286A,
Box 930, Truman Papers; "Wagner-Murray-Dingell Bill," *JAMA* 123:1 (1943): 36; "Does
American Medicine Need a Dictator?" *JAMA* 123:9 (1943): 564; (quote) Ward to Guy Gil-
lette (17 Mar. 1949), Box 1, Donovan Ward Papers, University of Iowa Special Collections,
Iowa City, Iowa.

United Nations and the signing of treaties of peace are of passing consequence" alongside the health question, adding that the "splitting of the
atom and the development and control of atomic energy are of lesser
importance. In this matter we are dealing with the essence which is the
Soul of Man." In the 1948–49 debate, the AMA infused its advertising
with references to the Korean War, arguing that "the sacrifices of our
fighting men will be futile if, here at home, we lose permanently the
basic freedoms which have made this nation great." By contrast, efforts
by the Federal Security Agency to use Korea-era draft deferrals in arguing
for the "the complementary relationship between progress toward basic
social objectives and the demands of military security" fell on deaf ears.[11]

Although popular support for national health insurance persisted,
conservative appeals to the goals and sacrifices of the war contributed
to labor's willingness to accept employment benefits as a surrogate for
national policy and narrowed political attention to provision for veterans. And ordinary Americans routinely echoed the conservative equation
of national health insurance with German experience or Soviet design.
The Wagner-Murray-Dingell bill, as one constituent warned President
Harry Truman, would be "a direct infringement against our liberties—
which we have recently fought a bloody and cruel war to preserve." Such
allusions also peppered reactions to private coverage. When the Pennsylvania Railroad adopted a commercial health insurance plan for nonop-
erating employees in the early 1950s, for example, workers (many of
whom already had Blue Cross coverage) responded with a barrage of
letters complaining of the company's high-handedness. "My husband
fought in World War II and also in the Korean conflict so that the United
States would be free of such tyranny," argued one worker. "It is not the
American way to have to take something that the individual does not
need or want."[12]

"Keystone in the Arch of the Socialist State": Medicine's Cold War

While medical conservatives were able to hijack the liberal and democratic rhetoric of the war efforts, allusions to the German origins or
threat of national health insurance were relatively short-lived. Between

[11] NPC, "Wake Up America" (1948), Box 33, Oscar Ewing Papers, HSTPL; (quote) NPC,
"Compulsion: The Key to Collectivism" (1949), p. 8, SHSW Pamphlets; (quote) AMA ad in
Editor and Publisher (Sept. 1950), in Box 209, Witte Papers; FSA Fact Sheet (1 June 1946),
Box 60, Caroline Ware Papers, FDRPL; (quote) FSA memo (3 Dec. 1951), Official File
419F, Box 1267, Truman Papers.

[12] Florence Nelson to HST (20 Nov. 1945), President's Personal File [PPF] 200, Box 257,
Truman Papers; (quote) Martha Deutsch to Travelers (26 Feb. 1955), Chas. Campbell to
Travelers (n.d.), Box 849:9, Pennsylvania Railroad Papers, Hagley Museum.

the wars, and especially after 1945, the AMA and others preferred the broader specter of "socialized medicine." Medical conservatives never missed a chance to refer to the National Socialism of Hitler's Germany, but they more often attributed the idea of "cradle-to-grave" benefits to a generic "red fascist" menace—the "German-Japanese-Russian philosophy."[13] Opponents focused popular and political attention on the threat of compulsion or centralized political control over the professions. And reformers often found themselves either occupied with defusing such charges, or searching vainly for euphemisms ("Health Security" was a favorite) in order to avoid loaded words like "compulsory" or "national" or "medical."

Anxieties about socialized medicine, and the willingness to exaggerate and traffic in them, ran parallel to the broader history of American anti-communism and peaked first in the World War I era. "The propaganda for compulsory health insurance through the American Association for Labor Legislation," a pamphlet printed and distributed by Prudential Insurance warned, "represents rather the plans and purposes of the International Socialist Movement than the aims and ideals of the overwhelming majority of American wage earners."[14] Business interests echoed this reasoning and its implication that state control over other professions and industries was sure to follow. Such arguments were both unapologetically apocalyptic and internally inconsistent; like so much of the era's red scare, they simultaneously warned of impending class conflict and denied that the United States was a class society. And such arguments relied heavily on their endorsement by the leadership of the AFL, whose stance in the AALL health debate reflected both voluntarist opposition to political solutions and a bid for political credibility.

Through the 1920s, health care remained at the forefront of antiradical politics. The Sheppard-Towner Act, which slipped by the AMA's attention in 1921, became a lightning rod for New Era red-baiting. This campaign was animated not only by antiradicalism but by gender politics as well. Organized medicine turned the future of Sheppard-Towner into a confrontation between male professional control and a "radical federal bureaucracy of social workers." In the postsuffrage decade, conservatives (including patriotic women's organizations) routinely portrayed politically active women as bolshevist dupes. Social reformers and public health advocates in and around the Children's Bureau figured prominently in the infamous Spider Web charts that tied domestic reformers into a sprawling socialist network. This was the "worst form of commu-

---

[13] "Check and Double Check on Compulsory Sickness Insurance" (1946) in AMA Kit on Health Insurance, Box 43, Decimal 011.4, GCF (1944–50), HEW Records.
[14] Hoffman, *Facts and Fallacies*, 12.

nism . . . the feminist phase," one conservative women's group declared in petitioning Congress, charging that Sheppard-Towner was aimed at "arousing women against men, wives against husbands [by] providing community care for children, legitimate and illegitimate."[15]

The red scare surrounding Sheppard-Towner had scarcely abated when it was rekindled by the Committee on the Costs of Medical Care. "The alignment is clear," editorialized *JAMA* in response to the CCMC's final report. "On one side [are] the forces representing the great foundations, public health officialdom, social theory—even socialism and communism—inciting to revolution; on the other side, the organized medical profession of this country urging an orderly evolution guided by controlled experimentation." Medical conservatives responded in much the same way to the Inter-departmental Committee on Health and Welfare Activities' 1938 Washington Health Conference and, two years later, Republican candidate Wendell Wilkie solicited doctors' support by promising to stand firm against "Senator Wagner, Miss Roche, and the horde of reds, pinks, and yellows assembled in the so-called Washington Health Conference." By the late 1930s the easy equation of any public health initiative with socialized medicine suffocated even the most modest proposals. "Any plan can be damned by the label that is given to it," lamented a public health official. "I have had the employment of two school nurses in the City of Quincy, Illinois labeled bolshevism."[16]

During the war, opponents substituted the "coercion and regimentation of a national socialistic fist" for the socialist threat—but the arguments were essentially the same and were animated by both the postwar culture of anticommunism and the persistent threat posed by the WMD bill. In 1943 the NPC answered reformers with pamphlets like "Abolishing Private Medical Practice or Prelude to Centralized Control of the Professions and of Industry." In 1945 the editors of *Medical Economics* dubbed WMD a "milestone on the road to medical serfdom." But medical McCarthyism really picked up steam after 1948 as WMD wound its way through Congress and anticommunist posturing increasingly dominated partisan politics. The AMA's infamous Public Education Campaign put

[15] Robyn Muncy, *Creating a Female Dominion in American Reform, 1890–1935* (New York, 1991), 124–57 (quote at 128); Kim Neilsen, "UnAmerican Women: Anti-Radicalism, Gender, and the First Red Scare" (unpublished ms., 1999), 185–98 (Woman Patriots quoted at 187).

[16] Odin Anderson, "Compulsory Medical Insurance, 1910–1950," *AAAPSS* 273 (1951): 109; (quote) "The Committee on the Costs of Medical Care," *JAMA* 99:23 (1932): 1950, 1952; Wilkie quoted in W. B. Russ, "Medical Practice and the New Deal" (1940) in POF 511a, FDR Papers; (quote) Medical Advisory Board, Minutes of Meetings (29 Jan. 1935), p. 112, Box 67, Witte Papers; Forrest Walker, "Americanism versus Sovietism: A Study of the Reaction to the Committee on the Costs of Medical Care," *BHM* 53 (1979): 489–504.

the socialist threat front and center. "First you have to give the program a bad name," as Clem Whitaker recalled, "and we're going to call it 'socialized medicine' because the idea of socialism is very unpopular in the United States." AMA publicists even manufactured a quote from Lenin—"Socialized Medicine is the keystone to the arch of the Socialist State"—and used it as a punchline in a slough of pamphlets and advertisements. In turn, the AMA sponsored the distribution of a wide range of anticommunist literature, including a million and a half copies of John Flynn's 1949 tract *The Road Ahead*. Republicans echoed the AMA line, accusing the Truman administration of "hatching sly schemes that are propelling us faster and faster down the Russian road."[17]

The core argument of medical McCarthyism was that national health insurance rested (in the words of the NPC) on the "strange and untried system of *compulsion*." In part this argument built upon the war-era battle over the meaning of the four freedoms. "I think WE in America have had quite enough Regimentation," one constituent wrote Edwin Witte in 1943, "and should I need medical aid I certainly don't propose to have the Surgeon-General of the United States, the President of the Untied States, Mr. Wagner, Mr. Murray, nor Mr. Dingell tell me what doctor I can call in . . . nor any Professor of Economics down in Washington to handle my case for me." And in part it reinforced postwar perceptions of health care as either a consumer good or a private benefit. "We vigorously oppose legislation designed to create State Medical care with its vast extension of a parasitic bureaucracy," one conservative group petitioned Congress in 1949 "which could result in a Socialistic State in violation of the principles set forth in the constitution of the United States."[18]

As in postwar labor and foreign policy, conservatives used anticommunism not only to dismiss the prospect of reform but to impugn the motives and loyalties of reformers. In 1949, the NPC derisively listed those who had testified on behalf of the WMD bill as "16 federal payrollers, 11 party-line fronts, 12 left-wing politicos, 15 social workers, 6 labor

[17] (Quote) S. Heubner in Roundtable on the Future of Insurance, Chamber Proceedings, 30th Annual Meeting (Apr. 1942), p. 281, Box I:9, Chamber of Commerce Papers; (quote) Plumley Memorandum Re: NPC (23 Sept. 1943), Box 60:524, Series II, Falk Papers; (quote) "The New Wagner-Murray-Dingell Bill," *Medical Economics* (July 1945), preprint in Hagley Museum Imprints; Whitaker quoted in Oscar Ewing OH, p. 181, HSTPL; Harry Becker Address (25 June 1950), Box 212, Witte Papers; (quote) Republican National Committee, "The Truth about Socialized Medicine" (1949), SHSW Pamphlets.

[18] Quotes (in order) from Statement of Senator Hill before Senate Committee on Labor and Public Welfare (24 May 1949), Box B:11, William Davis Papers, SHSW; Ethel ? to Edwin Witte (1 Dec. 1943), Box 210, Witte Papers; General Society of Sons of the Revolution to Sam Rayburn (15 Aug. 1949), File 81A-H7.2, Box 183, Records of the House Committee on Foreign and Interstate Commerce, RG 233, Records of the House of Representatives, National Archives.

groups, 2 chiropractors and osteopaths or the bureaucrats, the politicians seeking to extend power, the professional 'do-gooders', Communist Front organization representatives attempting to fundamentally alter the American conception of our institutions." The AMA tallied WMD supporters as "The Federal Security Agency, All who seriously believe in a Socialistic State, Every Left wing organization in America . . . especially organized propaganda groups . . . , some AFL and CIO leaders . . . The Communist Party [and] some well-intentioned but misinformed people." Congressional Republicans parroted these charges and launched loyalty investigations of key Social Security staffers. "American communism holds this program as a cardinal point in its objectives," Representative Forest Harness (R-Ind.) argued, "[and] in some instances, known Communists and fellow-travelers within federal agencies are at work diligently with Federal funds in furtherance of the Moscow party line in this regard." As in the larger pattern of McCarthyism, suspicion was often tantamount to guilt. In the early 1950s the AMA's Elmer Henderson criticized the "pinkish pigmentation" of the Committee for the Nation's Health simply because "many of [its] officers, directors, and most vocal members have been listed in the files of the House Unamerican Activities Committee for subversive connections or activities."[19]

Such charges not only chilled debate but raised the personal and political stakes for reformers. After 1946 congressional Republicans pressed the FBI to investigate a "conspiracy" of health insurance advocacy in the Federal Security Agency and the Social Security Administration. And a Senate subcommittee launched its own investigation of I. S. Falk and others at Social Security, charging them with (among other things) "subversive" contact with the International Labor Organization and the export of socialized medicine to occupied Japan. Although the officials involved successfully fought the charges, reformers became increasingly sensitive to any appearance of radicalism. The Social Security Administration quietly established a Business Advisory Group to balance its labor contacts. By its own estimate, the FSA exhausted much of its energy in 1948–49 deflating charges of socialized medicine and viewed the 1952 President's Commission on the Health Needs of the Nation as "a project which *really* was set up to get the President off the hook of being in favor of 'socialized medicine,' with which he was being tarred and feathered."[20]

[19] (Quote) NPC, "Compulsion: The Key to Collectivism" (1949), pp. 27, 49, SHSW Pamphlets; (quote) AMA, "The Voluntary Way Is the American Way" (1948), Box 206, Witte Papers; (quote) Forest Harness, "Forcing Socialized Medicine on America by Use of Federal Employees and Government Money" (Sept. 1947), reel 6, Michael Davis Papers, HSTPL; Henderson quoted in CNH Release (27 Feb. 1951), Box 142, Ware Papers.

[20] See responses in National Health Program, 1948 and 1949 folders, Boxes 43 and 44, Decimal 011.4; and "Notes on Preparing Health Insurance Correspondence" (1949), Box

In the early years of the Medicare debate, medical conservatives back-pedaled from the apocalyptic anticommunism of the 1940s and stressed instead the threat of state compulsion. The AMA's public relations consultants advised that the public had tired of "socialized medicine" but promised that "compulsion" still resonated. "It is well understood by students that the apogee of welfare statism is reached when government assumes the responsibility for the health care of the individual," agreed the HIAA. "When the mind of man has been so conditioned by socialist propaganda that he will surrender to government the right to make decisions concerning his health care, he has been readied for the yoke of totalitarianism." Clearly such sentiments still resonated. "Perhaps I cannot understand such thought processes because I do not understand socialism," one doctor wrote the White House in 1960. "I do not understand it, but I can surely recognize it, even in creeping form." At least in part to assuage such anxieties, arguments for Medicare were extraordinarily careful to underscore the plan's private roots and extraordinarily deferential to private interests on key points of program design and implementation."[21]

For a variety of reasons, anticommunist arguments and imagery were less prominent through the 1970s and after. The Vietnam War undermined the efficacy and the wisdom of leaning too heavily on such heavy-handed abstractions. Conservatives were increasingly able to employ budgetary and inflationary anxieties to the same effect. And as many business interests now clamored for state intervention in health care, they found such sweeping arguments less helpful. This is not to say, however, that such arguments were not trotted out when they were useful. Much of the attraction of insurance reform, employer mandates, HMO

44, Decimal 011.4, GCF (1944–1950), HEW Records; Monte Poen, *Harry Truman versus the Medical Lobby* (Columbia, Mo., 1979), 105; Misc. documents re FBI investigation, Box 49:331–43, Series II, Falk Papers; CNH Legislative Memorandum (17 Feb. 1948), Box 142, Ware Papers; (quote) Ewing to Truman (8 Nov. 1951), Box 5, Decimal 011, GCF (1951–1955), HEW Records; (quote) Milton Kayle OH, p. 97, HSTPL; David Stowe OH, p. 94, HSTPL; see also Healing Arts Committee Spot Announcements (1950), OF 103, Box 575, Truman Papers; Alan Derickson, "The House of Falk: The Paranoid Style in American Health Politics," *AJPH* 87 (1997): 1836–43; Jan Pacht Brickman, " 'Medical McCarthyism': The Physicians Forum and the Cold War," *Journal of the History of Medicine* 49 (1994): 398–99.

[21] Richard Harris, "Annals of Legislation: Medicare," *New Yorker* (16 July 1966), 40; (quote) Report of the Special Committee on Continuation of Coverage (16 May 1960), Box 18, Orville Grahame Papers, University of Iowa Special Collections; (quote) Vincent to Eisenhower (29 Aug. 1960), Box 225, Decimal 900.1, Secretary's Subject Correspondence (1956–1974), HEW Records; Task Force on Health and Social Security, Report to President-Elect Kennedy (January 1961), Box 4, Arthur J. Altmeyer Papers (1970 supplement), SHSW; Perkins to Pond (19 Feb. 1961), Box 225, Decimal 900.1, Secretary's Subject Files (1955–1975), HEW Records.

development, and the like continued to rest on fears of direct state inter-vention—accompanied by an unabashed clamor for indirect interven-tion (subsidies, tax breaks, "mop-up" programs). When health reform reared its head again in the early 1990s, opponents drew on a deep his-tory of anticommunist health politics—pointing out the irony of per-sisting with statist solutions after the collapse of the Soviet model, warn-ing of the dangers of "eternal police surveillance" represented by Clinton's short-lived promise of a "health security card," and raising once again the specter of state medicine encroaching on the rights of patients and providers. Although the hyperbole of the cold war had faded, such sentiments persisted in public debate and public policy—particularly sur-rounding the championship of market solutions such as managed com-petition or Medical Savings Accounts. "We need a new 'Health Care Dec-laration of Independence,' " Presidential hopeful Steve Forbes argued in 1999: "No American should be forced into government-run-health care programs or forced into managed care and HMO programs against their will."[22]

Un-American Activities: Britain and Canada in American Health Politics

The specter of socialism was as predictable as it was effective and drew on powerful assumptions about the material and ideological roots of American exceptionalism. The challenge for medical conservatives, how-ever, was more complex. Proposals for universal health coverage, after all, owed much more to the example of democratic capitalist peers—especially Great Britain and Canada—than to that of Germany or the Soviet Union. Alongside the routine aspersions of "Prussian" or "social-ized" medicine, accordingly, the AMA and others sustained an ongoing campaign against a pantheon of national health insurance systems which, by the 1960s, were in place in virtually every first- and second-world country except South Africa.

During the Progressive Era, the AALL leaned heavily on foreign expe-rience in drafting its plan, which John Commons trumpeted as an amal-gam of "the best possible points of the British and German systems." Such arguments were almost immediately undermined by the outbreak of war, which made appeals to European leadership increasingly suspect. Opponents lashed out at both the German example and the American reformers inspired by it. "At last," one observer noted in 1920, "the ger-manophilic glasses were struck from our eyes." Opponents of the AALL

---

[22] Steve Forbes, *A New Birth of Freedom* (Chicago, 1999), 86–90.

plan were quick to equate German policy with a generic threat of "foreign bureaucracy" and to suggest that "the ultra paternalistic governments of Europe and the pauperized conditions of the laboring and lower classes there have necessitated a resort to this heroic treatment of uplift by force." What the AALL was "proposing for democratic America," one doctor argued, was "a system as truly paternalistic as any now in effect in king-ridden Europe."[23]

Attention also turned to the British health system. In much the same way that the AALL had tried to import British reform ideas and practices after 1911, the AALL's opponents, led by the National Civic Federation and the New York League for Americanism, moved to import British opposition. In a practice that would last for decades, medical conservatives employed foreign correspondents to feed the medical and mainstream press a steady diet of horror stories about the fate of patients and practitioners under British (and later Canadian) health insurance. The ideological assumptions and tactics of American conservatives were not far removed from those of British conservatives but, for a variety of reasons, were far more influential. The relative success of American opponents reflected profound racial anxieties (and their reflection in partisan politics) about the prospect of any universal social programs: social insurance, as one doctor argued, was peculiarly suited for those nations "consisting of a homogenous race of people." And the ambivalence of the American labor movement on the question painted reformers into a lonely corner by making it possible for opponents to gleefully argue that the working people the AALL sought to protect were—at least as represented by the AFL—not interested. For these reasons, as Daniel Rodgers suggests, "ideological materials common throughout the North Atlantic economy were given a distinctive spin in the United States."[24]

After World War I, foreign experience was clearly to be avoided rather than emulated. The AMA trafficked heavily in dismal accounts of the

[23] Daniel Rodgers, *Atlantic Crossings: Social Politics in a Progressive Age* (Cambridge, Mass.: 1998), 251–53 (Commons quoted at 252); (quote) M. L. Harris, "Effects of Compulsory Health Insurance," *JAMA* (10 Apr. 1920): 1042; Hoffman, *Facts and Fallacies,* 7; Ronald Numbers, "The Specter of Socialized Medicine," in *Compulsory Health Insurance: The Continuing American Debate,* ed. Ronald Numbers (Westport, Conn., 1982), 6–7; NCF, *Compulsory Health Insurance: Annual Meeting Addresses, 1917* (New York, 1917), 22; (quote) Executive Committee of the New York Board of Trade, "Shall Health Insurance Be Made Compulsory by Law?" (1916), reel 62, American Association for Labor Legislation [AALL] Papers (microfilm); (quote) C. W. Garrett memo (1916), reel 62, AALL Papers.

[24] New York State League of Women Voters, "Report and Protest . . . New York League for Americanism," in Box 209, Witte Papers; "The A,B,C of British Health Insurance," *The Survey* 40 (1 June 1918): 263–64; (quote) "Abstract of Remarks by Dr. C. E. Mongan," *BMSJ* (4 Jan. 1917): 38; Rodgers, *Atlantic Crossings,* 255–59 (quote at 259).

British health system and ran a regular "letter from London" in *JAMA* under the banner "the evils of medical socialism." Though not necessarily enamored with their National Health System, many British doctors were sharply critical of the AMA's foreign correspondence. In 1935 the chair of British Medical Association charged that the AMA's reports from London were ridiculous caricatures and that his own comments had been interpolated in an "unfair and misleading way" or italicized as "an unworthy trick." The AMA jealously guarded its role as the American doctors' source of information on other health systems, routinely quashing efforts by state medical societies to launch their own foreign studies.[25] Not surprisingly, by the time the CCMC reported its findings in 1932 and the New Deal considered health insurance in 1934–35, popular knowledge found little to admire north of the border or across the Atlantic. Reformers, reluctant to borrow from or point to foreign experience, carefully avoided any such references. "Would it be possible to leave out that awful word 'Saskatchewan' plan?" asked one CES member in early 1935. "Couldn't it be given an American name? That nearly kills it to start with." "We can call it the American plan," suggested another, "versus what many people have gradually come to believe is a very undesirable foreign plan." Some thought medical opinion on the issue so poisoned that "in spite of the theoretical advantages of an inclusive plan for health insurance, the attention of a great proportion of practicing physicians in this country has been repeatedly called to the faults and defects of health insurance as utilized in other countries. They have slight knowledge of its merits or advantages. In consequence, health insurance in many parts of the country would not have the guidance and cooperation necessary to insure its success." For those who insisted that reformers look first to the successes and failures of foreign systems, such blinders proved immensely frustrating. "I cannot see to save myself any particular province in discussing the general philosophical basis and value of health insurance," conceded Edgar Sydenstriker of the Public Health Service, "when apparently the people who discuss it don't know a damn thing about it."[26]

World War II set the arguments of reformers and opponents in stark contrast. Just as each laid claim to the true meaning of war-era tropes like the four freedoms, each also laid claim to the meaning and import

---

[25] *JAMA* 97:19 (1933): 1396; "The American Medical Association," *Fortune* 18:5 (Nov. 1938), 166; "Doctors and Dollars," *Today* (16 Feb. 1935), Box 209, Witte Papers; "Medical Groups Drive for Health Insurance," *Social Security* (June–July 1934): 3.

[26] (Quotes) Medical Advisory Board [CES], Minutes of Meetings (29 Jan. 1935), pp. 40, 116, Box 67, Witte Papers; (quote) Dr. Farran, "A Coordinated Plan to Achieve Health Security" in Medical Advisory Board, Minutes of Meetings (29 Jan. 1935), p. 82, Box 67,

of war-era developments in Allied social policy—especially the British Beveridge Plan. Initially, reformers lauded the British initiative and drew liberally from it. But this was a risky tack. Opponents quickly and easily lumped the Beveridge Plan in with Soviet and Nazi health policies, all of which shared "certain social philosophies which look to central government for the organization and administration of most phases of communal and individual existence." When the press dubbed the war-era drafts of the WMD bill the American Beveridge Plan, reformers found the reference "unfortunate" and "too foreign." Accordingly, the closest thing to an American Beveridge Plan—the 1942 National Resources Planning Board report, *Work, Security, and Relief Policies*—tied the future of American social policy not to a more expansive definition of social citizenship but to the deus ex machina of full employment.[27]

After 1945 opponents cast their nets more widely, dismissing Soviet and Canadian and Western European social policies as generic examples of "statism and other un-American trends." Opponents further muddied such distinctions by linking British and Canadian health policies to leftist subversion in those countries—as when they portrayed health care reform (in the United States and beyond) as a pet project of the International Labor Organization and "other international agencies with interlocking directorates" (ironically, American reformers were instrumental in the early years of the "Saskatchewan" plan that launched the Canadian health system). And opponents often drew upon conservative anxieties about postwar internationalism and foreign aid. The AMA's Elmer Henderson, for example, scored the WMD bill in 1949 for parroting the "discredited system of decadent nations which are now living off the bounty of the American people."[28]

Stung by charges of socialized medicine and outflanked by the AMA's portrayal of Canadian and British policy, reformers regrouped in the 1950s around the lesser goal of hospitalization coverage for the elderly and the conviction that future efforts be promoted as resolutely Ameri-

---

Witte Papers; Sydenstriker quoted in Proceedings of the Meeting of the Medical Advisory Board, CES (29–30 Jan. 1935), p. 238, Box 42:236, Series II, Falk Papers.

[27] (Quote) New York Academy of Medicine, *Medicine and the Changing Order* (New York, 1947), 208; (quote) Woofter to McNutt (19 Feb. 1943), Box 10, Decimal 011.4, General Reclassified Files (1939–1944), HEW Records; Rodgers, *Atlantic Crossings*, 494–500.

[28] (Quote) State Medical Society of Wisconsin to American Legion (18 Nov. 1949), printed in *Capital Times* [Madison, Wis.], clipping in Box 211, Witte Papers; (quote) NPC, "Compulsion: The Key to Collectivism" (1949), SHSW Pamphlets; "Labor's Program to Socialize Medicine Internationally," *Medical Economics* (1945); Michael Grey, *New Deal Medicine: The Rural Health Programs of the Farm Security Administration* (Baltimore, 1999), 176–77; "What Are We Arguing About?" ADA Pamphlet, in Box 211, Witte Papers; "Statement on the Truman Health Plan," *JAMA* 140:1 (1949): 114.

can solutions. "We are not a people to be bought off by Bismarck seeking to perpetuate an empire," J. Douglas Brown of the Advisory Council on Social Security argued in 1956. "Nor were we a class-divided society that sought a leveling kind of wholesale relief. Rather we wanted our government to provide a mechanism whereby the individual could prevent dependency through his own efforts. . . . To us social security was a social mechanism for the preservation of individual dignity, not for the insurance of the political status quo." Much of the championship of private insurance was animated by the notion that it was a private and contributory—and hence American—form of provision. "It would be national folly," the AMA's Edward Annis argued in 1963, "to abandon New World progress and embrace the regressive methods of the Old World."[29]

At the same time, medical conservatives were increasingly cautious in invoking the British example. "I wonder if it has ever occurred to the members of this audience that the United States is the only major nation in the world that does *not* have a national compulsory system of state payment for medical care," a public relations consultant asked the AMA in 1961. "If the system is really as bad as it is usually pictured here, would fifty-nine nations have adopted it? Wouldn't the conservative party in some nation rally all those discontented people to its cause by proposing to abolish the low-quality, high-cost system?"— adding bluntly that he would not advise raising the specter of state compulsion and runaway costs "if you have an audience, or an opponent, who knows how foreign systems are run." Not surprisingly, such arguments were a source of some bewilderment to foreign observers. In 1958, when Ontario followed Saskatchewan's lead in establish a provincial hospitalization plan, the HIAA wrote Canadian bankers to solicit condemnations. The response was tepid. "I'm not sure what the word 'socialization' means," replied one. "It seems to me that hospital insurance is being regarded by a growing number of Canadians in the same category as unemployment insurance benefits, old age pensions, and other social security measures."[30]

After the passage of the Canada Health Act in 1968, Canada crowded out Britain in both the aspirations of reformers and the sights of opponents. For reformers, the Canadian example was a more relevant and appealing one. The Canadian system, which combined single-payer (government) funding with locally elected hospital boards and freedom of

[29] Brown quoted in Theda Skocpol and John Ikenberry, "The Political Formation of the American Welfare State in Historical and Comparative Perspective," *Comparative Social Research* 6 (1983): 88; (quote) Edward Annis, "Government Health Care: First the Aged, Then Everyone," *Current History* (Aug. 1963): 106.

[30] Harris, "Annals of Legislation: Medicare," 43; J. Wadsworth [Canadian Bank of Commerce] to Grahame (2 Oct. 1958), Box 29, Grahame Papers.

choice for providers and patients, was less of a political or cultural threat than the British "panel" system (which controlled provision through local committees). And perhaps most important, the Canadian system demonstrated—at a time when American health costs were beginning to spiral out of control—that universal coverage dampened health costs. At the same time, reformers remained leery of leaning on foreign examples. "We do not propose a system of nationalized or socialized medicine, nor a system borrowed from other nations," stressed the AFL-CIO's Walter Reuther in 1969. "We propose to create a system uniquely American which will harmonize the best of American health care while insuring meaningful freedom of choice."[31]

Opponents began to invoke the Canadian system (or a crude carica-ture of it) in much the same way they had invoked the British system since 1911. In the early 1970s the Nixon White House went out of its way to solicit both British and Canadian conservatives "to point out the difficulties of a Kennedy-type health bill." In the 1990s the AMA and the business press recycled often dubious anecdotal evidence of waiting lines and cross-border surgery—much of which was eagerly exported by the Ontario Libertarian Party or Vancouver's far-right Fraser Institute. *The Economist* (after trotting out all the usual stories) conceded, "There is little hard evidence to support them." Much of the Canadian criticism of Canada's system was routinely and cynically taken out of context. "The rhetoric of underfunding, shortages, excessive waiting lists, and so on," Canadian health economist Robert Evans reminded Congress, is simply "an important part of the process by which providers negotiate their share of public resources—including their own incomes." Although the AMA and insurers kept up a steady campaign against the "Canadian op-tion," business interests proved more ambivalent. *Business Week*, for ex-ample, maintained the fiction that a single-payer system would cost too much money as "governments get intimately involved, politicizing the process and adding bureaucracy" while also acknowledging that a single-payer system might "serve some profoundly conservative principles," adding that "no other plan would do more to preserve the two traditional bedrocks of American medicine: the freedom to choose your own doctor and the autonomy of physicians to care as they see fit."[32]

[31] Ruether quoted in Hickman to Fine (17 Mar. 1969), Box 144:2091, Series III, Falk Papers; Christopher Potter and Janet Porter, "American Perceptions of the British National Health Service: Five Myths," *JHPPL* 14 (1989): 341–65.

[32] Morgan to Cavanaugh (16 Mar. 1971), Box HE:1, White House Central File [WHCF], Richard M. Nixon Papers, National Archives; *Economist* (15 June 1991), 27; *BW* (9 Mar. 1992), 52; *BW* (21 Mar. 1994), 82. See also *NYT* (29 June 1989); *Fortune* (1 July 1991); Enthoven in *JAMA* (15 May 1991), 2535; Sammons letter to *NYT* (28 May 1989); *Vancouver Sun* (13 Mar. 1992), B7; "Debating Canadian Health Model," *NYT* (29 June 1989); "Health

The ability of medical conservatives to shape popular understanding of the British and Canadian health systems reinforced the basic message of medical McCarthyism and confined political attention to those solutions that could be presented as acceptably "American." Reformers looked to lessons from abroad only to have those lessons thrown back at them. Although popular support for a single-payer system remained steady, so did the conviction that foreign transplants would not do well in American soil. This not only made substantive reform more difficult, but pressed incremental reform in often surprising directions, as the larger goals of increased coverage or cost control were distorted by the political necessity of accommodating private coverage, nurturing competition among providers or insurers, or maintaining the peculiarly American distinction between contributory social insurance and charitable state assistance.

"A Thrust at American Manhood": Gender and the Health Debate

Behind both attacks on other national health systems and the exhortations to self-reliance and individualism that accompanied them lay the persistent assumption of the "family wage." Although the wider welfare debate remained torn between deeply gendered notions of contractual social insurance and charitable state assistance, the provision of health care fit comfortably in neither category. Opponents of health reform equated state assistance with the inability of male breadwinners to provide for their families. And reformers often reinforced such sentiments by championing solutions that organized health care provision around male employment. This meant not only that women enjoyed uneven access to health care but that notions of feminine dependence and masculine independence were woven into the rhetorical fabric of health politics as well.

During the AALL debate of 1914–20, health reformers understood the efficiency and health of male breadwinners to be the first concern of private employment and public assistance. As I. M. Rubinow argued in 1915, compulsory health insurance could "prevent the destruction of wage-working families as consuming units." In turn, reformers' emphasis on securing male incomes opened the door for opponents to argue that

Care in Canada," *Washington Post* (18 Dec. 1989); Ronald S. Bronow et al., "The Physicians Who Care Plan," *JAMA* (15 May 1991): pp. 2511–15; Evans in *NEJM* 320:9 (1989): 571–77; Colin Gordon, "The American Politics of Canadian Health Care," *Canadian Dimension* (Dec. 1992): 17–20.

such security questioned the independence and masculinity of male workers. This was the core of the AFL's voluntarism. "There must necessarily be a weakening of independence of spirit and virility," as the federation's Grant Hamilton argued in 1917, "when compulsory insurance is provided." And it was the clarion call of medical conservatives in 1915–19, who argued that the AALL would "substitute for American thrift and the American spirit of manhood independence, a pauperizing, bolstering, paternal system which would not in the least encourage virility of character but foster and perpetuate the habit of weakness and dependence."[33]

Such sentiments sharpened after 1921 when, for a brief time, Sheppard-Towner shunted health care to the "maternal" track of social policy. Reformers and opponents alike understood maternalism as an entering wedge for broader social programs. "Maternity Legislation leads to Socialism," one critic charged, continuing, "Socialism leads to Bolshevism; Bolshevism leads to Anarchy." For some, even the noble task of "saving the children" inspired fears that the state would displace fathers and husbands. Opponents worried that the even the act's narrow educational mission might include "birth control, use of contraceptives, sex-hygiene, endowment of motherhood, wages for mothers, State support of children, economic independence of women from husbands, free love, etc." And professional anxieties prompted organized medicine to dig in against the intrusion of the "old maids" or "office-holding spinsters" who, in its view, populated the Children's Bureau. Indeed the gendered claims that made Sheppard-Towner possible in 1920 doomed its chances for renewal by the decade's end. The strategy of pressing maternal interests narrowed rather than expanded the ambit of social policy. Officials at the Children's Bureau even objected to the use of the word "welfare" in proposals to extend Sheppard-Towner because they thought the term "undefined and its meaning altogether uncertain" and because they recognized the stigma it had acquired in debates animated by the promise of social insurance.[34]

[33] (Quote) I. M. Rubinow, "Social Insurance and the Medical Profession," *JAMA* (30 Jan. 1915), 381; Grant Hamilton [AFL], "Proposed Legislation for Health Insurance," in U.S. Department of Labor, *Proceedings of the Conference on Social Insurance*, Bureau of Labor Statistics Bulletin 212 (Washington, D.C., 1917), 568; Gwendolyn Mink, "The Lady and the Tramp: Gender, Race, and the Origins of the American Welfare State," in *Women, the State, and Welfare*, ed. Linda Gordon (Madison, Wis., 1990), 92–122; Executive Committee of the New York Board of Trade, "Shall Health Insurance Be Made Compulsory by Law?" (1916), reel 62, AALL Papers.

[34] (Quote) Senate Brief in *BMSJ* (2 June 1921), 575; Massachusetts Civic Alliance to James Davis (18 Feb. 1921), Box 233, Central File, 1921–1924, RG 102, Records of the

As the Depression recast Progressive ideas, reformers refocused their attention on the security of male breadwinners. Maternalism survived in Social Security's social assistance titles but only as a last resort for those not accommodated by family-wage male employment and the act's social insurance titles. As early as the CCMC report of 1932, reformers viewed male employment and the benefits that flowed from it as the best form of health provision. The CCMC devoted much of its attention to industrial medical plans on the understanding that "care may often be extended to dependents and that the aim in each case should be to consider the entire family as the unit for which medical services is provided." This reasoning echoed through the CES's health studies and its broader approach to social security. As Grace Abbot of the Children's Bureau argued, "the security most men seek is for their families, for their children, rather than for themselves." Early drafts of a health insurance title specified that "selection of the population eligible to insurance should be based on family, as distinguished from individual, units though the funds may be raised in terms of gainfully employed persons." Through the CES deliberations, staff routinely crossed out terms like "insured population" or "individual" and penciled in "family."[35]

Through the late New Deal and the 1940s, reformers and opponents voiced maternalist or family-wage assumptions in different ways and for different reasons. Some argued for social insurance–based health provision as a logical extension of the family-wage premises of the Social Security system. A draft of Roosevelt's 1939 health message began: "Like every other husband or father, I've known what sickness and the costs of medical care could do to the family budget." In 1943 the AFL lobbied for WMD on the grounds that "every free man has the right to a chance to build up a good home, to give his children education, to get ahead himself and equip his family for a good life." And, while FSA reformers worried constantly about the inefficiency and fragmentation of wage-based programs, they nevertheless routinely confined their attention to "a worker and his family."[36]

Children's Bureau, National Archives; Nielsen, "UnAmerican Women," 185–95; Muncy, *Female Dominion*, 132–43; (quote) Grace Abbott, "Memorandum for the President" (5 Feb. 1930), Box 422, Central File, 1929–1932, Records of the Children's Bureau.

[35] (Quote) CCMC, *Medical Care for the American People* (Chicago, 1932), 110; (quote) Abbott to Altmeyer (18 July 1934), Box 47, Records of the Committee on Economic Security [CES], RG 47, Records of the Social Security Administration [SSA], National Archives; (quote) "Preliminary Draft Abstract of a Program for Social Insurance against Illness" (1934), Box 2, CES Records; (quote) CES, "Risks to Economic Security Arising out of Ill Health," Box 2, CES Records.

[36] Draft of President's Message (May 1939), Box 45:281, Series II, Falk Papers; *Labor's Monthly Survey* (Oct. 1943) in POF 142:1, FDR Papers; FSA recommendations for 1950

In the end, such assumptions proved much more appealing and effective for opponents. The AMA lumped postwar proposals in with the war-era EMIC program and concluded starkly that federal health initiatives amounted to little more than "a proposal that the family be destroyed and that the state take care of the children and of the mothers in childbirth." The Ohio Chamber of Commerce blasted WMD as "a death thrust at state sovereignty, at national solvency, at American manhood, [and] at postwar recovery." "It is high time for Americans to get some of the brawn of their pioneer forebears," argued one benefits consultant, "and quit being dainty, steam-heated, rubber-tired, beauty-rested, effeminized, pampered sissies." Or, as a guide for health insurance sales agents put it: "It is easy to see why the need for accident and health insurance is so widespread. . . . Money builds a home for a man; it helps to raise his family and to make him somebody in the eyes of his wife, his family, and his community. . . . You want to be able to convince your prospect that his ability to earn money should be insured."[37]

After 1949, reformers narrowed their attention to two issues irretrievably confined by the logic of the family wage: the prospect of expanding Social Security to include health coverage for the elderly, and the politics of subsidizing or sustaining the growth of private job-based health insurance. In this public-private welfare state, only men could consistently make claims as citizens; women's claims, by contrast, reflected the failure of men to fulfill their private obligations. Opponents argued that health care was a matter of private provision and private consumption, and that coverage of any but the truly destitute posed a threat to gender and familial relations. The inclusion of health coverage under Social Security, as one insurer argued in 1954, would be above all a blow to "the responsible American citizen, the family man."[38]

The trajectory of private employment and private benefits upended many of these assumptions. As postwar growth slowed, American employ-

---

State of the Union Address (2 Nov. 1949), POF 419F, Box 1264, Truman Papers; Miles to Staats (26 Nov. 1947), POF 419F, Box 1262, Truman Papers.

[37] (Quote) Morris Fishbein, "Medicine in the Postwar World," *NEJM* 235:21 (21 Nov. 1946), 742; (quote) Ohio Chamber of Commerce, "A Death Thrust . . . " (1943), President's Official File 4351:2, FDRPL; (quote) Mahoning Valley Industrial Council, "Clinic on Health in Industry" (1940), Box 21, National Association of Manufacturers [NAM] Industrial Relations Department [IRD] Papers, Hagley Museum; NPC Pamphlet, reel 11, Davis Papers; (quote) Jerome Miller, *Selling Accident and Health Insurance* (New York, 1940), 4–5.

[38] Carole Pateman, "The Patriarchal Welfare State," in *Democracy and the Welfare State*, ed. Amy Guttmann (Princeton, N.J., 1988), 240–41; Nancy Fraser, "Struggle over Needs: Outline of a Socialist-Feminist Critical Theory of Late-Capitalist Political Culture," in *Women, the State, and Welfare*, ed. Gordon, 211–14; (quote) Statement of Rulon Williamson (15 Apr. 1954), Box 28, Grahame Papers.

ers increasingly questioned the logic and resented the costs of job-based health insurance. At the same time, women (by choice and necessity) flooded into the jobs created and re-created by a deindustrializing economy. In turn, discrimination by insurers, persistent patterns of job segregation, and employer anxieties combined to undermine benefit provision in the new economy. Not surprisingly, employers, insurers, and reformers—at least in part because women claimed a higher percentage of the labor market and a much higher percentage of new hires—made less and less of the sacred connection between private employment and familial provision. Instead, as we have seen, employers, insurers, and reformers shifted their attention from the point of provision to the point of consumption; from the rights of workers to the responsibilities of consumers.

Women's increased participation in the labor force encouraged a variant of maternalism that, alongside the backlash against the welfare state, often bypassed women altogether. As women moved into low-wage, no-benefit service employment, attention turned to public provision for children. At their best, such programs represented a commitment to the principle of starting-gate equality in the absence of truly universal programs. But in practice such programs reflected a haphazard set of assumptions and realities: since many women were working (or, in the wake of welfare reform, *should* be working), they were no longer an appropriate target of public assistance or conduit for public assistance flowing to their children; but since women's jobs were unlikely to include health coverage, their children remained uncovered. In a sense, working women ceased to be treated as dependents of male breadwinners, yet never enjoyed the independence that rested on decent wages and employment-based benefits.

From the Country Doctor to the HMO: The Market in Health Politics

Another reflection of the health care debate's preoccupation with private, masculine, and "American" solutions was the prevailing assumption that providers and patients could and should be considered producers and consumers in a medical marketplace. Such terms meant different things to different interests and were employed, in different contexts, by both conservatives and reformers. Above all, the marketplace analogy was an argument against reform. As embattled entrepreneurs, doctors could appeal to public sympathy and forge alliances with other economic interests in efforts to stave off regulation or intervention. By portraying patients as consumers, medical conservatives could portray health care provision not as a right but as a choice akin to buying clothes or cigarettes. And by extending the market metaphor, they could confine political attention to the rights and responsibilities of producers and consumers and avoid the question of who had the opportunity or resources to participate in the market in the first place. For their part, reformers parroted such language when it proved useful, even if doing so made universal programs more elusive. Arguments for social insurance borrowed heavily on notions of individual responsibility and consumption. Reform efforts, especially after 1949, often focused on artificial barriers (such as a dearth of providers or restrictive underwriting) to the production and consumption of health care. And especially after the mid-1970s, many viewed a combination of market discipline and consumer protection as the only solution to the twin crises of collapsing coverage and spiraling costs.

Over time, such assumptions proved complex and often quite contradictory. Organized medicine was never entirely comfortable portraying doctors as producers, especially when it came at the expense of professional status or prestige. Professionalization through the late nineteenth and early twentieth century was, in many ways, a strategy for protecting doctors from the implications of crass self-interest or ambition. The AMA's position, in effect, was that doctors were independent entrepreneurs vis-à-vis the state, entitled to autonomy from state regulation; but that they were selfless professionals vis-à-vis their patients, willing to provide care without regard to their compensation. This tension shaped medical politics throughout the twentieth century and proved especially troubling at a number of key junctures—including the AMA's antitrust battle in the late 1930s, its efforts to come to terms with private insurance in the 1940s and 1950s, and its confrontation with HMOs in recent years.[39] For reformers, this was also dangerous rhetorical territory. The language of the marketplace facilitated conventional appeals for state intervention (in efforts to break medical society prohibitions on group practice in the 1930s and in the drive for "consumer rights" in recent years, for example) but also conceded considerable political ground. Increasingly, reformers lowered their sights from citizens' rights to consumers' rights, from access to basic care to access to private insurance, from the ideal of health care as a public good to the availability of health care as a private commodity.

Such arguments were complicated by the peculiar character of the modern health care market in which classical expectations of supply and demand invariably faltered. Supply is controlled largely by professional

---

[39] Deborah Stone, "The Doctor as a Businessman: The Changing Politics of a Cultural Icon," *JHPPL* 22:2 (1997): 535; John McArthur and Francis Moore, "The Two Cultures and the Health Care Revolution," *JAMA* 277:12 (1997): 985–89.

monopolies and a mix of public and private hospitals. Demand is shaped by the fact that consumers (patients) do not usually *want* to purchase health care and often rely on sellers (doctors and hospitals) to gauge their needs. Over the course of the twentieth century, new technologies and methods of production made most goods cheaper but made health care more expensive; as consumption of most goods was democratized, health care became an expensive luxury. With the emergence of employment-based private insurance, conventional assumptions about economic behavior were further scrambled by the presence of large institutional consumers and third-party payers. Some argued that insured individuals, having established coverage, lost any incentive to control their consumption; others argued that employers, who were paying for care but not receiving it, had every incentive to minimize their purchases and shuffle the burden to employees. Since the 1970s, confusion has reigned over the question of whether a "health care market"—in the classical sense of a self-regulating mechanism for allocating resources—can or should exist. "Fundamental economic principles," *Scientific American* editorialized in 1993, ". . . put efficient, competitive health care markets in the same class as powdered unicorn horn." Yet at the same time, public policy has been increasingly swept up by market solutions that promise to emancipate consumers and providers by introducing competition and to protect consumers and providers by managing that competition.[40]

As modern medical practice emerged in the early twentieth century, organized medicine clung to a nineteenth-century entrepreneurial ideal. "Physicians expected to compete with each other for patients just as small-town merchants competed for customers," Donald Madison has suggested. "For both, competition was the natural expression of individual initiative in a liberal society." Doctors embraced some forms of cooperation (such as medical societies) but shunned others (group or contract practice). In confronting the AALL, not surprisingly, doctors reacted like any economic interest facing state intervention: they were instinctively leery of political encroachment, while at the same time drawn to the prospect that reform might broaden coverage and stabilize incomes. "People want security, so do physicians," reasoned one doctor. "Physicians want to be paid for what they do."[41] But doctors did not em-

[40] Nancy Tomes, "Merchants of Health: Medicine and Consumer Culture in the United States, 1900–1940," *JAH* 88:2 (2001): 526–27; *Scientific American* cited in Robert Evans, "Going for the Gold: The Redistributive Agenda behind Market-Based Health Care Reform," *JHPPL* 22:2 (1997): 428; Uwe Reinhardt, "Economists in Health Care: Saviors, or Elephants in a Porcelain Shop?" *AER* 79:2 (1989): 337–39; Thomas Rice, "Can Markets Give Us the Health Care System We Want?" *JHPPL* 22:2 (1997): 383–426.

[41] Donald Madison, "Preserving Individualism in the Organizational Society: 'Cooperation' and American Medical Practice, 1900–1920," *BHM* 70:3 (1996): 442–45 (quote at

brace the political, economic, or managerial character of the emerging corporate order. The result, persisting well beyond the Progressive Era, was a profound tension between professional status and property rights. On the one hand, doctors routinely defended their professional responsibility to provide a certain level of charity care and avoid crass material competition. During World War I, medical conservatives invoked the Prussian menace of "efficiency, applied science, and Compulsory Insurance proudly exhibiting the crude art of their Krupp masterpiece of materialistic individualism." On the other hand, organized medicine routinely insisted on the right of doctors and patients to sell and buy health care free from political interference. "The State or Nation has as much right to pay my grocery bill as to pay that under discussion," sniffed one medical journal. The AMA, employing a consumer analogy that would become one of its stock arguments, agreed that "more is paid for 'movies' and 'rum' than is paid for medical attendance and treatment."[42]

Such sentiments, and their contradictions, animated the debates of the 1930s and 1940s. The AMA and others continued to equate the purchase of medical care with a host of other choices made by consumers: "The very people who accumulate vast amounts for Christmas savings which are dispensed for trifles during a holiday week, who pay regular installments for pianos, automobiles, radios, electric refrigerators, jewelry, and fur coats because of appeals made to them through advertising, find themselves unprepared when the illnesses which they should know are inevitable come on them." Conservatives objected to the implication of any relationship between income and access to care on the grounds that "the same could be said of spendable incomes and the costs of travel, shelter, clothing and everything else." By this reasoning, reform was little more than an attempt by "sociologists and politicians [who] feel that if these people will not spend their incomes 'properly' of their own accord, we should compel them to." In the medical marketplace, as one doctor argued in 1943, people went without care "not because they can't afford it but because they don't want it."[43]

---

445); Ronald Numbers, "The Third Party: Health Insurance in America," in *The Therapeutic Revolution: Essays in the Social History of American Medicine,* ed. Charles Rosenberg and Morris Vogel (Philadelphia, 1979), 177–81; "Memorandum re Doctors" (1918), reel 63, AALL Papers; (quote) Charles Mayo [AMA] address (1917), reel 62, AALL Papers.

[42] Madison, "Preserving Individualism," 480–81; (quote) Andrew Downing, "Lest We Forget," *BMSJ* (17 Apr. 1919): 440–41; (quote) A. H. Quessy Senate Brief in *BMSJ* (2 June 1921): 576; AMA official quoted in James G. Burrow, *AMA: Voice of American Medicine* (Baltimore, 1963), 147; "Malingering" (1914?), reel 62, AALL Papers; "Report of the Committee on Social Insurance," *JAMA* (17 June 1916): 1974.

[43] JAMA quoted in Douglas Parks, "Expert Inquiry and Health Care Reform in New Era America: Herbert Hoover, Ray Lyman Wilbur, and the Travails of the Disinterested Experts" (Ph.D. diss., University of Iowa, 1994), 277; (quote) Harold Maslow, "Brief Sketch

The insistence that health care was simply a consumer good was especially prevalent in the immediate aftermath of the war. Again opponents threw health care in with a long list of spending choices. "If we are going to give free medical care to all people," Senator Taft asked, "why not provide them with free transportation, free food, free housing, and free clothing—all at the expense of the taxpayer?" AMA officials claimed to see no distinction between compulsory medical care and the compulsory financing of "food, clothing, recreation, and haircuts." Such arguments typically employed the most frivolous of purchases as a means of both satirizing reformers' aims and underscoring consumers' often dubious choices. "When do we get free ice cream and marbles?" asked one character in "The Sad Case of Waiting Room Willie," a comic book sponsored by the AMA. "I wanna free doll carriage and roller skates!" demanded another. In 1949 the Republican National Committee charged that the Democrats would soon be "promising free toupees and beauty treatments to everyone in America, at the taxpayer's expense." Or as the *Cincinnati Enquirer* editorialized: "If it is the Government's business to finance medical care, it is likewise the government's business to impose a toothbrush tax on everyone and have toothbrushes issued from government warehouses; to impose umbrella and overshoe taxes, and require that everyone wear GI umbrellas and overshoes on rainy days; to impose a religious tax and build Government churches which everyone would be required to attend, and so on, ad infinitum." In addition to lampooning the idea of public provision, this argument also reinforced the notion of individual responsibility for one's health by invoking consumers' apparent preference for "a daily pack of cigarettes" or their freedom to "choose their own liquor stores."[44]

While contemptuous of efforts to distinguish health care from other consumer purchases, such arguments did have to confront the rising costs of medical services. "For persons who are not indigent or medically indigent," argued a Brookings Institution report in 1948, "the question

---

of the AMA Position on the Medical Problem," Box 208, Witte Papers; (quote) J. Weston Walch, "On the Witness Stand: The Facts about Health Insurance" (1939), 15, Hagley Imprints; Dr. Follansbee in Roundtable Conference on Medical Care (Afternoon Session, 14 Nov. 1943), Box 65, Witte Papers.

[44] Taft quoted in *Medical Economics* (1946) clipping, Box 210, Witte Papers; other quotes (in order) from; Frank Dickinson, "An Analysis of the Ewing Report" AMA Bulletin no. 69 (1949): 11; "The Sad Case of Waiting Room Willie" (1949), POF 286A, Box 931, Truman Papers; RNC, "The Truth about Socialized Medicine" (1949), SHSW Pamphlets; *Congressional Record* 95:13 (1949): A2533 (reprint of *Cincinnati Enquirer*); AMA, "Compulsory Health Insurance: A Message from your Doctor" (1950), Box 212, Witte Papers; Marie Seale to HST (19 Nov. 1945), POF 286A, Box 930, Truman Papers. See also "Roundtable Session on National Health Insurance," p. 176 (Madison, Wis., Nov. 1949), Box 206, Witte Papers.

is not whether they can afford adequate medical care if they want to give it the necessary priority but how they wish to finance it." The answer, which acknowledged cost barriers without conceding on the issue of private consumption, was credit financing. "If these families had to pay cash for their automobiles, for their electric refrigerators, or for their television or radio sets, many would not be in a position to buy them," one doctor reasoned. "Is it fair to say because they cannot pay cash for these items they cannot afford them? Because this same group cannot pay for a major illness at the time it occurs, is it just to assume that they cannot afford to pay for it?" For others, credit financing—at least for items other than medical care—was also the culprit. "After indulging in all sorts of luxuries to the limit of our income, after indulging in all the credit plans for this or that," a Blue Cross official complained in 1949, "a certain element of our population excuses their improvidence by blaming the cost of medical care."[45]

Reformers were torn between the ethical pitfalls and the strategic advantages of treating health care as just another item in the family budget. Many were involved in health politics precisely because they viewed health care as nothing less than a fundamental right of citizenship. "It is no answer to say that we are getting the kind of medical care we pay for," Grace Abbott argued in 1934. "Health is not in the same category as rugs or automobiles." Yet many also conceded ground on this point, either because they feared the moral hazard of free and universal provision or because they thought it necessary to meet opponents halfway. Arguments for social insurance simultaneously challenged and accepted the assumption that health care was a consumer good. In arguing that health reform would merely rearrange private expenditures, the CES and others eased budgetary concerns at the expense of a broader commitment to public provision. And in arguing that social insurance could replicate the discipline of private purchases—"the psychological element in the patient paying a little something if he can because he really thinks it is there and he respects it"—the CES and others eased fears of malingering but underscored the opponents' assumption that patients could and should behave like cost-conscious consumers.[46]

[45] (Quote) George Bachman and Lewis Merriam, *The Issue of Compulsory Health Insurance* (Washington, D.C., 1948), 38; (quote) Leland McKitrick, "Medical Care for the American People: Is Compulsory Health Insurance the Solution?" *NEJM* 240:25 (23 June 1949): 998–99; (quote) Paul Hawley [Blue Cross] in "Roundtable Session on National Health Insurance," p. 177.

[46] Abbott memo for Altmeyer (18 July 1934), Box 47, CES Records; "Abstract of a Program for Social Insurance against Illness: Preliminary Draft" (1935), p. 46, Box 67, Witte Papers; Medical Advisory Board, Minutes of Meetings (30 Jan. 1935), p. 454, Box 67, Witte Papers.

The reformer's confusion on this point, however, paled beside organized medicine's efforts to juggle competing self-images and their political implications. The doctors' instinct, evident in their response to Sheppard-Towner and the CCMC, was to portray themselves as independent and competitive producers. "You must credit [us] with having some knowledge of what medicine is," argued one medical advisor to the CES, " . . . and what it is that makes men ambitious, and what the competitive scheme is as compared with this scheme." Another doctor dubbed any effort to displace private practice as "a disavowal of the basic principles of life," arguing that "this would seem to be the aspiration of those who would by some weird alchemy of so-called social reform remove forever from life the necessity for struggle and combat." For many, both private and public health insurance threatened to "destroy the competition there is now between doctors . . . if any such leveling program as an insurance scheme comes into effect you will have taken away from the doctor that incentive to rise." In making such arguments, doctors and others invoked the social benefits of free enterprise in both relations between providers and patients and competition among providers. "The doctors fight the Federal Compulsory Socialized System of health insurance because they wish to preserve their freedom," one AMA official argued in 1948, ". . . after all, what is the objection of union labor to the Taft-Hartley Act but a fight to retain what they feel is their freedom?"[47]

But organized medicine could not simply champion free enterprise and challenge public solutions. Because doctors, especially after the mid-1940s, also faced the encroachment of other private interests, they had to champion a particular view of free enterprise. The doctors' stance was "comparable with the competition between the independent storekeeper and the chain store," Social Security officials noted in 1937. "In both cases those whose interests are hurt find that what is against their interests is also against the interests of the public, and in one case as in the other, opposition parades in fine phrases—the interloper is unethical and his competition unfair." The result, through the 1930s and 1940s,

---

[47] (Quote) Medical Advisory Board, Minutes of Meetings (30 Jan. 1935), p. 241, Box 67, Witte Papers; David Rothman, "A Century of Failure: Health Care Reform in America," *JHPPL* 18:2 (1993): 278–80; (quote) Nathan Van Etten, "An Economic Problem for 1935," clipping from Philadelphia County Medical Society in Box 207, Witte Papers; "What Is Socialized Medicine?" (1938?), Box 8, President's Interdepartmental Committee to Coordinate Health and Welfare Activities, FDRPL; (quote) Dr. Follansbee in Roundtable Conference on Medical Care (Afternoon Session, 14 Nov. 1943), Box 65, Witte Papers; (quote) Rember [AMA] to Schoonard (22 Dec. 1948), Box 43, Decimal 011.4, GCF (1944–1950), HEW Records; Stafford County Medical Society to Rep. Marrow (15 Mar. 1949), File 81A-H7.2, Box 182, Records of the House Committee on Foreign and Interstate Commerce, RG 233, Records of the House of Representatives.

was an almost Jeffersonian defense of the nobility of the small proprietor. The CCMC minority report dismissed group practice as "suggestive of the great mergers in industry" and a retreat to the drudgery of "mass production methods." Critics accused the New Deal of plotting to "establish a bureaucratic, organized wholesale business in human misery with central control and many branch establishments," or of treating medical practice like "a sort of glorified factory." And the Republican National Committee dismissed the Truman-era plan as an "assembly line medical program."[48]

Such sentiments persisted through the 1940s and beyond, but they were less and less grounded in reality, especially as doctors retreated on group practice and prepayment. For organized medicine, private insurance remained a riddle. Although the AMA condemned any form of group practice as the leading edge of socialism through the 1920s, support of voluntary insurance and group plans under medical control emerged as necessary defenses against "socialized" medicine. Private insurance also fortified the carefully constructed cultural wall between professional status and self-interest: doctors could now operate in a setting in which money rarely changed hands between provider and patient. At the same time, however, doctors remained leery of the interposition of a third party between themselves and their patients. Doctors now claimed less control over billing—especially with the increased use of fee schedules and capitation (per patient rather than per service) payments. And doctors now faced another decision maker whose interests were distinct from either the personal choices of the patient-consumer or the professional judgments of providers.[49]

[48] (Quote) Bureau of Research and Statistics, "Memorandum on Health Insurance" (1937), p. 15, Box 34, Decimal 056, Chairman's File, Commissioners' Records, SSA Records; (quote) CCMC, *Medical Care for the American People*, 154; (quote) F. F. Borzell, "Organized Medicine and Social Insurance," clipping from Philadelphia County Medical Society in Box 207, Witte Papers; (quote) "A Critical Analysis of Sickness Insurance," *JAMA* 29:4 (1934): 58–59; (quote) RNC, "The Truth about Socialized Medicine" (1949), SHSW Pamphlets; Harold Maslow, "Brief Sketch of the AMA Position on the Medical Problem," in Box 208, Witte Papers.

[49] Dr. Van Etten in Roundtable Conference on Medical Care (Afternoon Session, 14 Nov. 1943), Box 65, Witte Papers; Minority Report in CCMC, *Medical Care for the American People*, 167; Memoranda on Attitudes of the AMA (10 Feb. 1944), Box 45:284, Series II, Falk Papers; Alan Siegel, *Caring for New Jersey: A History of Blue Shield of New Jersey, 1942–1986* (Montclair, N.J., 1986), 10–12; Paul Starr, "Transformation in Defeat: The Changing Objectives of National Health Insurance," in *Compulsory Health Insurance: The Continuing American Debate*, ed. Ronald Numbers (Westport, Conn., 1982), 115–43; Frank Dickinson, "A Brief History of the Attitude of the American Medical Association toward Voluntary Health Insurance," AMA Bureau of Medical Economics, Research Bulletin 70 (1949); Numbers, "The Third Party," 181–83; "A Critical Analysis of Sickness Insurance," *AMA Bulletin* 29:4 (Apr. 1934): 67–68; Stone, "The Doctor as a Businessman," 539–41.

The ideal of entrepreneurial medicine also posed real political risks. The problem, at least in part, was that the AMA insisted on having it both ways. When the state threatened to displace private medicine, doctors were quick to portray themselves as small producers subject to onerous regulation. But when private third parties such as insurers reared their heads, doctors eschewed the "competitive commercialism" of contract practice and claimed professional status. Doctors objected to the "commercialization" and "competition" and crass "solicitation of patients" encouraged by group practice. "Medical service is not a commodity," the AMA argued in 1935. "It is primarily a relation between physician and patient." The AMA and local medical societies retreated frantically from free enterprise arguments when, in the late 1930s, their efforts to quash lay-controlled group health plans drew the attention of federal antitrust prosecutors. Suddenly, the District of Columbia Medical Society (the target of the suit) and the AMA were forced to take the position that medical care was *not* a commodity in order to argue that prohibitions on group practice did not constitute a "restraint of trade." In the wake of the antitrust case (which the AMA lost), organized medicine defined private practice less as an entrepreneurial ideal than as a simple alternative to socialized care.[50]

In the 1940s and beyond, doctors' collective self-perception was important to the ways in which they framed and pursued political demands—even if this fierce individualism bore little resemblance to the actual practice or organization of medical care. While the producer-consumer ideology of fee-for-service care persisted into the 1950s and 1960s, doctors increasingly ceded control over the provision, or at least the organization, of care to commercial insurers. And individual consumers were displaced by institutional consumers: organized labor and employers. Despite all of this, the AMA and others continued to employ the arguments forged in the 1920s and 1930s—at times in response to threats of state intervention, and at times in defense of a system of private insurance that posed a parallel, or even graver, threat to professional autonomy.

The simple consumerist equation remained a favorite political tack. "If a family can afford a daily pack of cigarettes or a weekly movie," the AMA reasoned in 1951, "that family can buy the finest health insurance in the world." The AMA spent a great deal of time in the 1950s tracking medical spending alongside spending on alcohol, tobacco, recreation,

[50] (Quote) AMA Bureau of Medical Economics, "Some Phases of Contract Practice" (1934), pp. 18–19 and (quote) Bureau of Medical Economics, Statement on Sickness Insurance (1935?), Box 67, Witte Papers; Magee Address, Box 53, Frank Kuehl Papers, SHSW; J. Weston Walch, "On the Witness Stand: The Facts about Health Insurance," 13; Memoranda on Attitudes of the AMA (10 Feb. 1944), Box 45:284, Series II, Falk Papers; Siegel, *Caring for New Jersey,* 10–12.

and jewelry in order to point out both relative inflation and consumer "choices." The Chamber of Commerce argued that "apparently, many people want other things far more than they want medical care. For example, we spend in total more for TV sets, cosmetics, recreation, [and] tobacco." Faced with the persistence of this argument and the political failure of the late 1940s, the 1952 presidential commission called for some experiments in group payment but concluded that "for those able to work and earn enough to pay for their own care, opportunity to do so is, in the American scene, the most desirable plan." And not surprisingly, such arguments permeated both the meager political initiatives of the Eisenhower administration and the early Medicare debate. HEW's Marion Folsom objected to offering tax credits for health insurance on the grounds that this would amount to "federal subsidy" of "an item of personal consumption." And critics of social insurance–based coverage for the elderly were quick to spin out a now familiar scenario: "What is the biggest financial burden of old folks? Simple: Food. Why not free food for all over 65? Lodging can become a problem. Why not a nationwide program of federal housing, free to all over 65? Deaths, wills, estates, and inheritances are inevitable and very close to the aged, no less a problem than medical care. Why not free legal service to all over 65? (Or does that touch a nerve? Imagine any member of a law-making body sponsoring a bill for free *legal* care for the aged!)"[51]

Such arguments also reflected and reinforced doubts about the propriety of funding health care through social insurance. "In this bill we are establishing a precedent wherein the social security program will be used to provide the payment of specific personal needs," Senator John Williams (R-Del.) lamented in 1965, " . . . having established that precedent, it would be but a short step to a program next year, say, for a program earmarked specifically for the payment of rent, and perhaps the next year other payments earmarked specifically for the payment of clothing purchases, and then one for food only, or transportation, or even entertainment."[52] The Chamber of Commerce agreed that

[51] AMA quoted in New York State Bar Association, Report of Committee on Federal Legislation (26 Jan. 1951), Box 33, Ewing Papers; Statement of Charles Scott, Box 57, Records of the President's Commission on the Health Needs of the Nation [PCHNN], HSTPL; (quote) "The Economic Position of Medical Care, 1929–1953," *JAMA* 159:1 (1955), 41–46; (quote) Chamber of Commerce, "Free Health Care for Everyone?" (1955), Box 206, Witte Papers; (quote) "First Draft: Health of the Aging" (26 June 1952), pp. 21, 27, PCHNN, Box 74, Witte Papers; Folsom to Perkins (21 Oct. 1954), Box 235, Decimal 901, Federal Security Agency, Office of the Administrator (GCF, 1951–1955), HEW Records; (quote) Vincent to Eisenhower (29 Aug. 1960), Box 225, Decimal 900.1, SSC (1956–1974), HEW Records.

[52] *Congressional Record* 111:12 (1965): 16147.

the initiation of Social Security Benefits in the form of services rather than in the form of cash would be a fundamental departure from accepted American principles. It would, in effect, deny to every beneficiary the right to make decisions for himself. . . . This complex of conflicts is rooted in the initiation of a Social Security benefit in the form of *services* rather than in the form of cash. These fundamental conflicts are inevitable in any proposal to graft a benefit in the form of federally-dictated consumer *expenditures* onto a system of benefits in the form of consumer cash income.[53]

Although contributory social insurance was, in many respects, a concession to notions of individual consumption and responsibility, many also saw it as an escape from the "natural discipline" of the market. "Patients who need close attention," the AMA's Edward Annis warned, "have to compete for the doctor's time with the whole gamut of people who have only minor complaints, imaginary ailments, trivial requests, or just a desire to 'cash in' on whatever benefits are available."[54] Such arguments shaped not only national health politics but also the day-to-day attitudes and assumptions of working Americans. As early as the 1950s, covered workers both celebrated the virtues of private coverage and chafed at its restrictions. When the Pennsylvania Railroad changed insurance carriers, for example, the response was swift and strident: "As a citizen of the United States I do not believe that any one person or group of persons can tell me what kind of insurance gives my family and myself the best coverage. . . . Further, [I am also] proceeding on the theory that a purchaser has a right to know the price he is expected to pay on an article before accepting it." Or, as another argued, the switch was in "direct disregard of the constitution of the United States . . . MAKING me take a Health and Welfare Insurance plan I am not interested in. After all, you or anyone working with your company wouldn't buy a pair of shoes without seeing them or trying them on to see if you like them or if they fit."[55]

The prominence of collectively bargained private health insurance plans after the late 1940s recast the consumption of care. Third-party employers and insurers not only realized the long-standing fears of organized medicine but also scrambled the incentives and logic of the medical marketplace. But the basic cultural assumptions—including the sanctity of contractual social provision and the producer-consumer relationship—held fast. As private health insurance drifted into a state of crisis, business argued that copayments and deductibles were needed to dampen costs and utilization, that "the regular hospital plan should

---

[53] Chamber of Commerce, "Adding Health Benefits to Social Security: Are There Basic Conflicts? (June 1963), Hagley Imprints.

[54] Annis, "Government Health Care: First the Aged, Then Everyone," 107.

[55] Raymond Cannon to Travelers Insurance (25 Feb. 1955), Box 849:9, PRR Papers.

not endeavor to do any more than simply help take the sting out of the employee's medical expenses." As the principal consumer of health care (and yet not the recipient of services), business argued that health care was mismanaged, inefficient, and overutilized.[56] This lament, originally a reaction to the precedent of private provision in the 1940s, was increasingly animated by the inflation of health care costs.

Through the 1970s and beyond, the old consumerist arguments were turned inside out. More and more, it was employers—and not the AMA—who played the consumer card, especially as a way of arguing for more influence over coverage or utilization or reimbursement. As employers and insurance companies began questioning patterns of provision, organized medicine retreated from its long-standing argument that private purchasers would or should contribute to any natural equilibrium in health care markets—arguing, for example, that patients and third-party payers should defer to doctors as "the only ones with the capacity to pass judgement" on the quality or propriety of medical care.[57] On the sidelines of this tug-of-war between providers and payers, reformers also began to use the language of "consumer control" or "consumer choice." Although many were leery about such a rhetorical turn, it drew on the new interests in consumer rights integral to the social movements (including the women's health movement) of the 1970s. And it was often the only way to confront the institutional actors (hospitals, insurers, employers, and the state) who dominated health markets.[58]

Such confusion persisted into the 1980s and 1990s as market solutions increasingly dominated health care debates. The logic of such solutions has always been in doubt because health care has always lacked the basic characteristics of a conventional "free" market. The historical conceit of the market reformers, in this sense, was that there was a golden age of competition to which everyone could return.[59] The rhetoric of free or managed competition ran far ahead of its actual accomplishments, and

[56] Sears and GE Executives in NICB Proceedings, "Getting the Most for Your Insurance Dollar" (Jan. 1953), p. 164, Box I:43, NICB Papers, Hagley Museum; Minutes of the NAM Employee Health and Benefits Committee (30 Nov. 1962), Box IV:109, NAM Papers, Hagley Museum.

[57] AMA official quoted in Eveline Burns, "A Critical Review of National Health Insurance Proposals," *HSHMA Health Reports* (Feb. 1971): 119.

[58] David Vogel, "The 'New' Social Regulation in Historical and Comparative Perspective," in *Regulation in Perspective*, ed. Thomas McGraw (Cambridge, Mass., 1981), 155–86; Garrick Cole to Dorothy Garrison (9 July 1971), NWRO Statement (July 1971), both in Box 23, George Wiley Papers, SHSW; Stone, "Doctor as a Businessman," 543–44.

[59] Eli Ginzberg, "The Grand Illusion of Competition in Health Care," *JAMA* 249:14 (1983): 1857–59; David Wilsford, *Doctors and the State* (Durham, N.C., 1991), 19–20; William Glaser, "The Competition Vogue and Its Outcomes," *The Lancet* 341 (27 Mar. 1993): 805–12; Evans, "Going for the Gold," 428–65.

most interested parties embraced the marketplace only insofar as it served to camouflage more prosaic battles over costs or resources. Business interests applauded "competitive" reforms as consistent with the wider deregulatory logic of Reaganomics and because they promised to dampen health inflation by introducing providers and patients to the discipline of the market. By the same token, however, business was afraid that extending such reforms to public programs might throw more of the health care burden onto private shoulders.[60] Doctors were drawn to such solutions as a logical extension of their defense of free enterprise medicine. Yet while continuing to view patients as price-conscious consumers, the AMA was wary of granting the same status to employers or insurers.[61] Not surprisingly, most viewed their own position as natural or virtuous and argued that the health care crisis could and should be solved by imposing the rigors of the market on someone else.

The HMO revolution magnified and distorted the imagery of the marketplace. Though often presented as a neoclassical deference to (or unleashing of) the consumer, "managed competition" was aimed more at changing the behavior of providers, at "stimulat[ing] a course of change in the health industry that would have some of the classical aspects of the industrial revolution," HMO guru Paul Ellwood put it, "conversion to larger units of production, technological innovation, division of labor, substitution of capital for labor, vigorous competition, and profitability as the mandatory condition of survival." What this meant, in practice, was that doctors were expected to consider not only the health of the patient but the efficiency or solvency of the actuarial pool to which the patient belonged. The consumers disciplining the market, in this respect, were not the patients receiving care but the insurers paying the bills. Market enthusiasts used abstractions like "consumer choice" to promise more control over medical decisions to patients, and HMOs used titles like "gatekeeper" or "financial manager" to promise that control to doctors—while both tried to distract attention from the tangle of constraints and incentives imposed on both. The HMO, as Deborah Stone has suggested, did not so much resolve the persistent tension between professional stature and economic self-interest as it tilted the cultural balance between the two. The genius of the HMO was not that it imposed new market incentives but that it celebrated them, and encouraged patients and providers to do the same.[62]

---

[60] Cathie Jo Martin, "Markets, Medicare, and Making Do: Business Strategies after National Health Care Reform," *JHPPL* 22:2 (1997): 558–59.

[61] "Effects of Competition in Medicine," *JAMA* 249:14 (1983): 1864–68.

[62] Ellwood quoted in David Himmelstein and Steffie Woolhander, "The Corporate Compromise: A Marxist View of Health Policy," *Monthly Review* (May 1990): 26; Stone, "The Doctor as a Businessman," 533–34, 541–45, 551–53.

Perhaps the most telling marker of late twentieth-century health politics, in this respect, was the willingness of organized medicine to contemplate unionization. On its surface, this was hardly surprising. As providers increasingly worked as salaried employees in large institutional settings, they acquired both the incentive and the legal standing to enter into collective bargaining. At the same time, efforts to win rights as workers put an unusual spin on the tension between doctors' professional and commercial status. In the 1940s and 1950s, doctors routinely embraced the equation of medical practice with other commercial enterprise; now doctors resented the HMOs' assumption, as one noted bitterly, that providers should follow their rules "just like a car dealer has to agree to sell and service all of a manufacturer's models." The AMA, for its part, took great pains to emphasize that this was simply an assertion of professional autonomy: "This is not for all physicians. This will not be a traditional labor union. Your doctors will not strike or endanger patient care. We will follow the principles of medical ethics every step of the way." What was remarkable in all of this was not that organized medicine was condoning or pursuing collective bargaining for its members but that—given the long-standing equation of private medicine and private enterprise— doing so made them so uncomfortable. "We need another tool, and a collective bargaining unit, formed under the auspices of our professional association, our AMA, is one of them," one AMA delegate argued:

> It will not be the right tool for every situation and for every physician, but it will help for some to level the roles of physicians and employers on the new playing field. It will shrink the beam, as an enduring local presence of private sector advocacy, grounded in our profession. Who better to do this than our AMA, for the essence of organized medicine is the care of our patients, first and foremost. Our loyalty is to our patients, and we work for their well being, not our own. If other entities outside of medicine create the physician CBU [collective-bargaining unit], we run the risk of alien values displacing those of our profession. And isn't collective negotiation a subset of collective action, a concept that underpins our advocacy activities at all levels?[63]

The anxieties of doctors and patients generated a backlash against managed care but did little to stem its progress. By the 1990s competition—despite its dubious logic and motives and record—was the central

---

[63] Steven Greenhouse, "Angered by HMO's Treatment, More Doctors Are Joining Unions," *NYT* (4 Feb. 1999); M. Serafini, "Physicians, Unite!" *National Journal* 1999, 31 (23):1524—35. Quotes from John Armstrong, "Professionalism on a New Playing Field," (June 1999), archived at http://www.ama-assn.org/meetings/public/annual99/ profess.htm, accessed May 2000; and Statement of Randolph D. Smoak, Jr. (June 1999), archived at http://www.ama-assn.org/advocacy/statemnt/990623s.htm, accessed May 2000.

organizing premise for reformers and their opponents alike. For opponents, championing competition was a way of both jockeying for position with other health interests and keeping the state at bay. For reformers, the politics of competition was more complex. Certainly many recognized, as one member of the Clinton task force put it, that "health care ranks among the necessities of life . . . it is not an optional commodity, like a Walkman, a tie, or a scarf." Yet the Clinton administration persistently understood health reform, before and after 1994, as a problem of patient or consumer rights.[64] This understanding reflected both the administration's strategic and budgetary retreat from the goal of expanding coverage to that of simply stabilizing coverage, and its acceptance of deeply seeded (if also deeply flawed) cultural assumptions about the private consumption of health care. And this understanding was especially apparent in the late 1990s, as Democrats confined their attention to the issue of patient or consumer rights within HMOs. While appropriately outraged at certain HMO practices, the political and legal flurry surrounding the "Patient's Bill of Rights" offered nothing to the growing percentage of Americans with no coverage whatsoever.[65]

[64] (Quote) Group no. 17 Draft, "A New Health Care System," Box 1183, CHTF Records; "Talking about Health Care" (n.d.), Walter Zelman files, quoted in Theda Skocpol, *Boomerang: Clinton's Health Security Effort and the Turn against Government in U.S. Politics* (New York, 1996), 118; "Ethical Guidelines for a New Health Care System" (Mar. 1993), Box 1183, CHTF Records.

[65] Democratic Policy Committee, "Patients before Profits," archived at http://dpc. senate.gov/patients_rights/, accessed May 2000.

5

Health Care in Black and White: Race, Region, and Health Politics

T HE American welfare state has always been, at root, a Jim Crow welfare state—disdainful of the citizenship claims of racial minorities, deferential to a southern-controlled Congress, and leery of the racial implications of universal social programs. At the same time, racial distinctions have rarely been explicit, masquerading as anxieties about "Americanization" in the Progressive Era, as administrative distinctions between agricultural and domestic and industrial workers in the New Deal, as deference to private labor markets and employment-based benefits in the 1950s, as concessions to federated governance through the Great Society and beyond, and as a backlash against dependency and the pathology of the inner city in more recent years. Public debate has rarely acknowledged such racial assumptions directly but has nevertheless been shaped by them. In health care, these patterns of discrimination and segregation have been both more complex and more pervasive—in large part because health (unlike other arenas of social provision) has been governed less by public policy than by private providers, employers, and insurers.

Race has shaped health provision in a number of important ways. Most starkly, private and public health care institutions until the 1960s echoed the segregation found in other public and private services. Hospitals in the South either maintained "colored" wards (often an attic, a basement, or a separate building) or supported the establishment of a "black hospital" that would tap off black patients and black health professionals. Scarcely 5 percent of southern hospitals, surveyed in the wake of the *Brown v. Board of Education* decision in 1954, were integrated. Such segregation was common in the North as well, often closely resembling patterns of residential segregation. And it was largely condoned by state and federal policy: the VA hospital system remained segregated into the 1950s; the Hill-Burton Act of 1946 maintained a separate but equal clause that was not seriously challenged until the 1960s; and the federal government proved reluctant to use the combination of Medicare and the Civil Rights Act to desegregate southern hospitals after 1965.[1]

---

[1] Vanessa Gamble, *Making a Place for Ourselves: The Black Hospital Movement, 1920–1945* (New York, 1995), 152–53, 186; David McBride, *Integrating the City of Medicine: Blacks in*

Institutional segregation was reinforced (and sometimes accomplished) by professional segregation, as patient access to hospitals often hinged on the professional affiliation or admitting privileges of attending physicians. African-American health professionals suffered first, in this respect, in access to medical education. Before the late 1960s only two medical schools (Meharray Medical College and Howard University) and meager quotas at some northern universities offered medical education to African Americans. Internships or residencies were few and far between, crowding black professionals into often-stigmatized public care settings: freedmen clinics, charity hospitals, health departments, and (later) Medicaid practice. Indeed, as hospitals increasingly became the focal point for health provision, black physicians lost ground as professional status depended more and more on clinical training, accreditation, standardization, and hospital privileges. Medical societies remained formally segregated into the early 1950s, effectively barring black professionals from local hospital privileges, contact with public health agencies, and continuing education. By the middle 1950s, all but one (Louisiana) of the state societies had desegregated, but county societies were slow to follow suit. Well into the 1960s, only a slim percentage of black professionals had applied for membership.[2]

By and large, public policy replicated (or refused to challenge) these background inequities. Since the 1870s, the South has proved both disproportionately powerful in federal politics and disproportionately anxious about the implications of federal power. National social policies threatened the South's low-wage advantage. And southern interests were loath to socialize private patterns of assistance whose benefits (depen-

---

Philadelphia Health Care, 1910–1965 (Philadelphia, 1989), 147–59; P. Preston Reynolds, "Hospitals and Civil Rights: The Case of Simkins v. Moses H. Cone Memorial Hospital," *Annals of Internal Medicine* 126:11 (1997): 898; Paul Cornerly, "Segregation and Discrimination in Medical Care in the United States," *AJPH* 46 (Sept. 1956): 1075; "Discrimination: Hospitals, 1942–1946," Part 15A, reel 5:0766–0886, NAACP Papers (microfilm).

[2] Edward Beardsley, *A History of Neglect: Health Care for Blacks and Mill Workers in the Twentieth-Century South* (Knoxville, Tenn., 1987), 77–80; Eric Bailey, "Health Care Use Patterns among Detroit African Americans: 1910–1939," *JNMA* 82:10 (1990): 722; Michael Byrd and Linda Clayton, "The 'Slave Health Deficit': Racism and Health Outcomes," *Health/PAC Bulletin* 21:2 (Summer 1991): 25–26; Gamble, *Making a Place for Ourselves*, 30, 36–37; United States Commission on Civil Rights [USCCR], *Health Facilities and Services* (Washington, D.C., 1963), 136–40; W. Montague Cobb, "The National Health Program of the NAACP," *JNMA* 45:5 (1953): 333–34; Cornerly, "Segregation and Discrimination in Medical Care," 1077–1079; McBride, *Integrating the City of Medicine*, 85–117; Robert Cunningham, "Jim Crow, M.D.," *The Nation* 174 (7 June 1952): 548–49; Algernon Jackson, "Public Health and the Negro," *JNMA* 15:4 (1923): 256–59; Frank Kennedy, "The American Medical Association: Power, Purpose, and Politics in Organized Medicine," *Yale Law Journal* 63 (1954): 938–41; "Report on Civil Rights Compliance, Atlanta Hospitals" (1966), Box 53, Office Files of Douglas Cater, Lyndon Baines Johnson Presidential Library [LBJPL], Austin, Tex.

dence in the agricultural economy) were more tangible and important than those of northern welfare capitalism. Southerners, in turn, were able to weave these parochial interests into the very fabric of federal politics. For much of the twentieth century, the southern congressional delegation (strengthened by institutional seniority, control over the committee system, and other perks of one-party rule) enjoyed an effective veto over federal reform, and routinely won concessions in the design and administration of social policy. Although the political and economic logic of the "solid South" eventually collapsed, the consequences of its confrontation with federal power in the New Deal era remain with us. This combination of racial anxiety and political advantage proved particularly sensitive to the universalist implications of national health programs. Southerners persistently worked to exclude African Americans from coverage, tap into federal funds without sacrificing local practices, and ensure that charity programs remained under the local control.[3]

Patterns of economic discrimination and disadvantage also shaped health provision. Medical and hospital services remained essentially private commodities whose quality and availability depended on one's ability to pay. Services available to the poor were stigmatized both by their very nature (as charitable rather than contributory programs) and by the fact that their clientele reflected the racial skew of poverty in the United States. The emergence of employment-based benefits as a surrogate for national policy left most African Americans and Latinos behind—in part because they were underrepresented in the unionized industrial economy, in part because employment-based benefits (like Social Security) did not reach casual or domestic or agricultural workers, and in part because the family-wage logic of public and private social insurance evaporated under circumstances in which nonwhite women often had better employment prospects than nonwhite men. Employment benefits not only attenuated racial inequality but also undermined the legitimacy of the welfare medicine for which blacks and Latinos were

[3] Gavin Wright, *Old South, New South: Revolutions in the Southern Economy since the Civil War* (New York, 1986), passim; Landon Storrs, "Gender and the Development of the Regulatory State: The Controversy over Restricting Women's Night Work in the Depression-Era South," *Journal of Policy History* 10:2 (1998): 179–94; Lee Alston and Joseph Ferrie, "Labor Costs, Paternalism, and Loyalty in Southern Agriculture: A Constraint on the Growth of the Welfare State," *Journal of Economic History* 45 (1985): 99–102; Alston and Ferrie, "Resisting the Welfare State: Southern Opposition to the Farm Security Administration," in *The Emergence of the Modern Political Economy*, ed. Robert Higgs (Greenwich, Conn., 1985); Ira Katznelson, Kim Geiger, and Daniel Kryder, "Limiting Liberalism: The Southern Veto in Congress, 1933–1950," *Political Science Quarterly* 108 (1993): 284–97. On the southern political advantage, see V. O. Key, *Southern Politics in State and Nation* (New York, 1949); David Potter, *The South and the Concurrent Majority* (Baton Rouge, La., 1972); Kevin Cox, "The Social Security Act of 1935 and the Geography of the American Welfare State" (paper presented at a meeting of the Association of American Geographers, Atlanta, 1993), 13–19.

disproportionately eligible. Finally, the poverty of public goods and services throughout much of the rural South and Southwest and the nation's inner cities often meant that the issue of formal segregation paled in settings where basic services—a hospital, a public health clinic, a doctor accepting Medicaid patients—did not even exist. In Mississippi in 1948, to offer one example, there were only five general hospital beds for every 100,000 blacks in the state—at a time when four beds for every 1,000 citizens was considered adequate.[4]

All of this became part of the very language of social provision, which was always marked, as Frances Fox Piven and Richard Cloward stress, by the "deep imprint of racism, and the complex political distortions it nourished." In health care, as in other facets of social policy, a parade of distinctions—some direct, some oblique but clearly racialized—marginalized or stigmatized black and Latino Americans. Progressive reformers routinely portrayed African Americans more as a risk to public health than as a target of public health programs. Amid more recent anxieties about welfare reform and health costs, reformers and opponents commonly cite the pathology of the inner city—handgun violence, drug abuse, family dysfunction—as both a partial explanation for the American health crisis and an argument against adopting "European" solutions. In turn, all of these assumptions are exaggerated by the peculiar anxieties that accompany health and public health policy. Especially in the early years of the twentieth century, opponents of health reform (in much the same way that some conservatives would respond to the AIDS crisis) argued that disproportionate rates of disease and infant mortality in the African-American community reflected little more than evolutionary design. "The ultimate extinction of the colored race was just a matter of time," argued one southern health official in 1917. "Why seek to check the effect of the forces of nature?" This posed a stark challenge to reformers (black and white), whose plea that "germs know no color line" confirmed segregationist fears even as it challenged them. "Vital statistics are interpreted in terms of ethnography, and mortality returns are taken as a measure of racial fitness," lamented one reformer in 1916; "pathology has become the handmaid of prejudice and the laboratory of civic oppression."[5]

<hr/>

[4] USCCR, *Health Insurance: Coverage and Employment Opportunities for Minorities and Women* (Sept. 1982), 15–38; Linda Gordon, *Pitied but Not Entitled: Single Mothers and the History of Welfare* (New York, 1994), 111–14; Beardsley, *History of Neglect*, 36–37; Cornerly, "Segregation and Discrimination in Medical Care," 1074–75; George Cannon, "Adequate Medical Care of the Individual and Family," *JNMA* 41:1 (1949): 18.

[5] Frances Fox Piven and Richard Cloward, *Regulating the Poor: The Functions of Public Welfare*, rev. ed. (New York, 1993), 423; Margaret Stecker, "A Critical Analysis of the Standard Bill for Compulsory Health Insurance" (1920?), Box V:9, National Industrial Conference Board [NICB] Papers, Hagley Museum and Library, Wilmington, Del.; Beardsley, *History*

These racial underpinnings set the American welfare state apart. Western European welfare states were forged in a context of racialized nationalism, in which racial categorization ran parallel to colonialism and citizenship. The question of incorporating racial minorities arose only with post-1945 patterns of emigration and decolonization—well after the establishment of national welfare states. In the United States, by contrast, deeply racialized contests over citizenship predated the welfare state and were reflected in it. Once established, western European welfare states shared a commitment to centralized administration (leaving little room for local variation or discrimination) while relying in varying degrees on labor market participation or citizenship to organize claims. The U.S. welfare state, by contrast, combined deference to labor markets with decentralized administration in such a way as to exaggerate and perpetuate the racial distinctions inherent in each.[6] All of this meant not only that African Americans and Latinos would remain second-class citizens of the American welfare state, but that many white Americans came to count health care (and especially private health benefits) as a "wage of whiteness" to be defended against erosion by universal programs.

This tangle of assumptions and practices and institutions vastly complicated the cause of health reform. In one respect, racial inequality contributed compellingly to arguments for universal provision, and African-American health reformers stressed connections between civil rights and universal social programs. At the same time, most white reformers avoided the issue and accepted incremental strategies that privileged family-wage coverage for white male industrial workers. Black professionals often supported segregated facilities as an immediate solution to the paucity of basic services and professional opportunities. Over time, the efforts of black professionals and public health advocates to build and sustain their own institutions and opportunities made integration a riskier venture.[7] More broadly, progress toward universal coverage was frustrated by the logic by which reformers herded all those left behind by employment- and Social Security–based programs into means-tested public alternatives, and then stigmatized or punished beneficiaries for the mere fact of their eligibility. This persistent racial divide guaranteed that a less-than-universal welfare state, under any budgetary or fiscal stress, was more likely to shrink than to expand.

---

of Neglect, 25, 130–32; Gamble, *Making a Place for Ourselves*, 136–37; Susan Smith, " 'Sick and Tired of Being Sick and Tired': Black Women and the National Negro Health Movement" (Ph.D. diss., University of Wisconsin, 1991), 119–21; C. V. Roman, "The Medical Phase of the South's Ethnic Problem," *JNMA* 8:3 (1916): 151.

[6] Robert Lieberman, "Race, State, and Inequality in the United States, Great Britain, and France" (unpublished ms., 1999), 10–11, 26–27, 45.

[7] McBride, *Integrating the City of Medicine*, 17–21, 84.

The consequences for health have been tangible and tragic. On the most common measures of public health—infant mortality and life expectancy at birth—black and Latino Americans have lagged significantly and persistently behind white Americans. Although overall infant mortality rates dropped dramatically over the course of the twentieth century, black rates (44 per 1,000 in 1950, 21 in 1980) remained consistently double the rates for whites (27 in 1950, 11 in 1980). The race gap in life expectancy at birth narrowed from fourteen years (47 white, 33 black) in 1900 to eight (69 white, 61 black) in 1950 but closed no further in the next forty years. Although access to basic health services improved in the twenty years after World War II, the slow collapse of public social programs and private health insurance in more recent years has contributed to both a deterioration of public health and a widening of the racial gap. Even when the effects of differential resources and insurance coverage are accounted for, persistent racial differentials in access, rates of use, and outcomes remain.[8]

Race and Health Provision before the New Deal

Through the early years of the twentieth century, the single most important cause and consequence of health segregation was dismal access to basic care. For this reason, black health activists and professionals, as well as some liberal foundations, devoted considerable time and effort to public health education and services.[9] In northern settings, these public health campaigns were animated by fears that migrants from the South posed a community health risk: "Jim Crow laws," an official of the Rosenwald Fund intoned in 1928, "have never successfully been set up for the germs of tuberculosis, pneumonia, typhoid, or malaria."[10] In most respects, such efforts had no practical or political connection to the debate over health insurance, which focused almost exclusively on the means of paying for care. At the same time, the health insurance debate did reflect, by explicit reference or implicit indifference, racial expectations and assumptions.

---

[8] Mitchell Rice, "On Assessing Black Health Status: A Historical Overview," *Urban League Review* 9:2 (1985–86): 9–10; Beardsley, *History of Neglect*, 11–41; "The Emerging Health Apartheid in the United States," *Health/PAC Bulletin* (Summer 1991): 3–5; David Barton Smith, "Addressing Racial Inequalities in Health Care: Civil Rights Monitoring and Report Cards," *JHPPL* 23:1 (1998): 75–76.

[9] See Susan Smith, *Sick and Tired of Being Sick and Tired: Black Women's Health Activism in America, 1910–1950* (Philadelphia, 1995).

[10] McBride, *Integrating the City of Medicine*, 33–40, 56–66 (Rosenwald official quoted at 75).

Consider the American Association for Labor Legislation campaign. The AALL focused its efforts on state-level legislative campaigns in a few northern states, confirming the southern low-wage competitive strategy and conceding to southern anxieties about federal intrusion. The AALL approached the problem as one of overcoming the financial barriers to care in industrial settings and ignored the paucity of basic health resources outside the urban North. And the AALL echoed the Progressive assumption that the targets of social assistance were lesser citizens and that those targets could be ranked—in racial, cultural, and religious terms—by biological standards of potential and productive citizenship. "All honest labor is honorable in the United States, and our most preferred class embraces the decent and thrifty, whether rich or poor," argued the New York Board of Trade in 1915. "Our lower class consists of those, rich or poor, whose voluntary habits of life have developed in them the baser elements of character." The National Civic Federation wondered how any insurance program would work as long as "there are three distinct levels of poverty—the level of the white native born, that of the immigrants, and that of the colored race—each with its own level of wages, opportunity and industrial education." African Americans and Latinos (the latter subject to both nativist anxieties and Jim Crow segregation in the South and Southwest) occupied the lowest tier. More bluntly, some opponents argued—on social Darwinist grounds—the folly of even the AALL's narrow definition of universal provision.[11]

Such assumptions were underscored by the parallel debate over maternal health. As an alternative to the AALL bill, many opponents supported a limited program of infant and child care (as the National Industrial Conference Board put it) "for the future of the race." At the same time, many reformers worried about the race and gender implications of expanding (or narrowing) coverage to include maternity benefits for wives or working women. Florence Kelley of the National Consumers' League, for one, objected strenuously to maternal coverage and categorized the "men whose wives notoriously work for wages" as "alcoholics, the mentally defective, men suffering from hookworm, tuberculosis, cancer, recognized insanity, epilepsy, and the disabling forms of venereal disease," "Negroes," and "the unskilled unorganized aliens, particularly the non-English speaking ones"—adding that maternity benefits would only encourage the procreation and immigration of "the kind of men who make

---

[11] Executive Committee of the New York Board of Trade, "Shall Health Insurance Be Made Compulsory By Law?" (1916), reel 62, American Association for Labor Association [AALL] Papers (microfilm); Frederick Hoffman, "Race Traits and Tendencies of the American Negro" (1916?) as cited in Smith, *Sick and Tired*, 8; NCF quoted in Daniel Rodgers, *Atlantic Crossings: Social Politics in a Progressive Age* (Cambridge, Mass., 1998), 258.

their wives and children work." To the degree that Kelley and other Progressives recognized and sympathized with the plight of those left behind by industry-based family-wage benefits, they still concluded that racial assumptions made organizing or funding universal health programs nearly impossible. Whether one attributed the circumstances of blacks and immigrants to their uneven education and assimilation or to systematic discrimination, noted Kelley, it remained "doubtful whether the great mass of white tax-payers will care to subsidize [them]."[12]

Consider the racial implications of World War I–era military service. While some reformers tried to make use of the dismal index of health provided by the draft, others used stark racial differences to reinforce the argument that blacks and immigrants were less intelligent, less healthy, and less deserving. Accordingly, social provision for World War I veterans was meager by both international standards and in comparison to the relative largesse of Civil War pensions. This restraint was, in part, a reaction to the corruption of the Civil War system and the institutional inability of the federal government to make the transition from patronage-based benefits to a conventional welfare state. But more important, it suggested how the idea of martial entitlement evaporated in a racially and ethnically heterogeneous military. The war reinforced opposition to provision for "unfit" men, deepened the maternalist conflation of social assistance and Americanization, and hardened the conviction that public welfare demeaned the manly and racial independence of its recipients— making "the white man the equal of the Indian," one doctor argued, "a ward of the State or nation." Some dragged in the racial logic of the red scare in reasoning that "social insurance, the child of Russia, [had been] . . . adopted by the German Empire, an empire consisting of a homogenous race of people." And some countered the reformers' claim that health insurance was no more pernicious than public education by insisting that compulsory education applied only to children; "it does not apply to unlettered immigrants who come here in late childhood and who often continue to live on in their dark world of spiritual and material ignorance."[13]

The tension between race- and service-based arguments for social provision spilled into the post–World War I era, especially in debates about

---

[12] "A Substitute for Compulsory Health Insurance" (1920), Box V:9, NICB Papers; Kelly, "Memorandum on the Maternity Features of the Proposed Act" (1915), reel 62, AALL Papers.

[13] Gwendolyn Mink, *The Wages of Motherhood: Inequality in the Welfare State, 1917–1942* (Ithaca, N.Y., 1995), 21–23, 56–58; quotes (in order) from "A. H. Quessy Senate Brief," *BMSJ* (2 June 1921): 576; "Abstract of Remarks by Dr. C. E. Mongan," *BMSJ* (4 Jan. 1917): 38; Andrew Downing, "Lest We Forget," *BMSJ* (17 Apr. 1919): 437–38. On the Civil War

the care of veterans. The congressional committee charged with sketching out a hospital system for World War I veterans concluded almost immediately that, at each turn, "one of the great American problems—that of race—obtruded itself more and more." Nowhere was this more evident than in the battle over the establishment of a national black veterans' hospital at Tuskegee. Vanessa Gamble has shown that the Tuskegee hospital was, most directly, a concession to white southern demands that veterans' care respect the racial boundaries of Jim Crow. Black veterans keenly resented the segregation of their care, which they viewed as one of many potent contradictions between the democratic rhetoric of wartime service and the racial realities of the South. While insisting on strict segregation of patients, white southerners also objected to the hiring of black health professionals—a position that, in order to protect the white medical profession, forced segregationists to favor a "mixed" system of white providers and black patients. In turn, black professionals broke ranks with the National Association for the Advancement of Colored People (NAACP) over the same issue, the former arguing that the professional gains offered by fully segregated institutions had "more to recommend it than loud mouthed preachment against segregation in the abstract," and the latter insisting that "segregation is a great enough evil when it exists over the protests of those jim-crowed, it is both an actual and a moral disaster when Negroes for the sake of jobs themselves ask for it." Although war contributed to the growth of social programs in other national settings, it tended—in the context of American race relations—to fragment social policy, divide Progressives, and mock any suggestion of equality or equal sacrifice.[14]

Consider the racial assumptions and practices woven through the Sheppard-Towner Act. The controversy surrounding Sheppard-Towner reflected the fundamental ambivalence of pro-natalist policies in the racialized American setting. Sheppard-Towner was concerned less with the provision of benefits than it was with the behavior of mothers; it was "an entering wedge for Americanization" (as Frances Perkins, then of the New York Consumers' League, put it) aimed at the "prejudices and superstitions of primitive peoples." And (like the welfare programs to follow) Sheppard-Towner conceded administration to the states in a way

---

system, see Theda Skocpol, *Protecting Soldiers and Mothers: The Political Origins of Social Policy in the United States* (Cambridge, Mass., 1992), passim.

[14] Gamble, *Making a Place for Ourselves*, 70–104 (White Committee quoted at 73), (NMA and NAACP quoted at 102–3); Steven Reich, "Soldiers of Democracy: Black Texans and the Fight for Citizenship, 1917–1921," *JAH* 82:4 (1996): 1478–1504; Ann Orloff and Theda Skocpol, "Why Not Equal Protection? Explaining the Politics of Public Social Spending in Britain, 1900–1911, and the United States, 1880s–1920s," *American Sociological Review* 49 (1984): 728–29; Mink, *Wages of Motherhood*, 13–24.

that virtually guaranteed it would do little to address the rural (and especially African-American) crisis of infant and maternal mortality. Some southern states ignored the act, because they were hard pressed to put up state funds for federal matching or because they feared that any concerted effort to make maternity safe was tantamount to "race suicide." In southern states where maternal programs flourished between the wars, their motives were deeply compromised by class and race. In North Carolina, for example, local officials promoted contraception on crassly eugenic grounds (although, at the same time, local public health activists and clients often welcomed and shaped such programs). Similar sentiments were reflected in parallel and successor programs of mother's aid or mother's pensions: annual per capita spending on mother's aid (1931 figures) ranged from $0.82 in New York to $0.03 in Louisiana. Indeed, 96 percent of the recipients of mother's pensions in the late 1920s and early 1930s were white, and some black belt states counted no black recipients at all.[15]

Health insurance proposals, such as that of the AALL, reflected the racial boundaries of a social insurance system whose first concern was the stability of white, male, and northern industrial wages. And scattered public health programs, such as Sheppard-Towner, reflected the racial underpinnings of a federal system that invited southern interests to shape national law to local customs. Although Progressive social policy initiatives were blunted before the advent of the New Deal, the fact that basic principles of coverage, financing, and administration were hammered out during the heyday of Jim Crow had enormous implications. Although the nation's public health crisis remained rooted in the rural South and Southwest, assessments of health care needs (outside public health circles) and prospective solutions focused on barriers to financial access in northern industrial settings. The Committee on the Costs of Medical Care, for its part, based the bulk of its conclusions on its 1928–31 survey of 38,000 "white persons" in 8,600 families.[16] This reflected the Progressive assumption that industrialization and urbanization were primarily responsible for the inability of individuals or families to provide

---

[15] "A Substitute for Compulsory Health Insurance" (1920), Box V:9, NICB Papers; Mink, *Wages of Motherhood*, 70–73 (Perkins quoted at 54); Miriam Cohen and Michael Hanagan, "The Politics of Gender and the Making of the Welfare State, 1900–1940: A Comparative Perspective," *Journal of Social History* 24 (1991): 473–74; Beardsley, *History of Neglect*, 137; Johanna Schoen, "Fighting for Child Health: Race, Birth Control, and the State in the Jim Crow South," *Social Politics* (Spring 1997): 90–113; Children's Bureau, *Mothers' Aid, 1931* (Washington, D.C., 1931), 13–14, 15, 17, 26; Grace Abbott to Elmer Batt (4 Sept. 1929), Box 422, Central File, 1929–1932, RG 102, Records of the Children's Bureau, National Archives.

[16] CCMC, *Medical Care for the American People* (Chicago, 1932), 6.

for themselves, the practical concession that agricultural workers and southern citizens were beyond the reach of federal programs, and the pernicious tendency to view the state of black public health as behavioral rather than economic.

The Racial Limits of the New Deal, 1933–1950

The New Deal underscored not only the racial boundaries of public policy but also the ways in which those boundaries were reinforced by the peculiar influence of southerners in national politics and policed by federalist deference to local administrative control. The Democratic South did not oppose either the New Deal or the precedent set by new federal programs as a matter of principle. As a desperately poor outpost of the party in power, the South welcomed the flow of federal funds under conditions in which racial order and state autonomy were protected. In the creation of Social Security, this meant ensuring that national programs were either less inclusive (excluding the bulk of the black southern labor force) or less national (allowing local authorities to control the terms of public assistance). By the middle 1930s, the terms of southern cooperation were beginning to unravel. The New Deal's drift to labor and social policy after 1935 posed a more direct and tangible threat to southern race relations and the region's low-wage competitive strategy. Southerners needed the New Deal less and feared its implications more—especially as the federal war effort was less able or willing to put off civil rights issues for the duration. In all, as Robert Lieberman has concluded, southerners "saw and understood the racial implications of creating a national welfare state that assigned the industrial working class to national policies and those at the margins of the industrial economy to parochial ones."[17]

By the time the New Deal gave serious attention to health reform in the late 1930s, southerners were digging in their heels against the conditions that were increasingly attached to federal funds. "Under no circumstances would I vote [for the bill]," one southern senator argued in 1939

[17] J. N. Baker [Alabama state health officer], "The Wagner Health Bill," *JAMA* 112:16 (1939): 1596–99; Alston and Ferrie, "Labor Costs, Paternalism, and Loyalty," 96–97; Robert Lieberman, *Shifting the Color Line: Race and the American Welfare State* (Cambridge, Mass., 1998), 23–66, 36–38, 48–56 (quote at 53); Jill Quadagno, "From Old Age Assistance to Supplemental Security Income: The Political Economy of Relief in the South, 1935–1972," in *The Politics of Social Policy in the United States*, ed. Margaret Weir, Ann Orloff, and Theda Skocpol (Princeton, N.J., 1988), 238–39; Katznelson et al., "Limiting Liberalism," 284–86, 289–97.

hearings on hospital funding, "if I thought the federal government could go down into Louisiana, Mississippi . . . and take charge of the hospitals of that state because forsooth they gave few dollars toward their upkeep." Similar sentiments shaped the southern response to the Truman health plan ten years later. The question of expanding Social Security to include health insurance came at a time when southern legislators were increasingly leery of federal intrusions and increasingly free of the fiscal bind that had underwritten their cooperation in the 1930s. Southern Democrats refused to endorse the postwar health bills, broke ranks with northern Democrats in sinking efforts to elevate the Federal Security Agency to cabinet status, and ultimately turned their backs on the national party altogether in 1948. "I realize that [FSA administrator] Jack Ewing is no communist . . . I also understand the political wisdom of his fight for Negro rights," conceded one southern senator. "But I'll be darned if I'm going back home and explain all of that. I'll just vote to kill the plan." The consequences of southern resistance, and federal deference, were clear. There was "no need trying to save Negroes from being lynched or to educate them for sound citizenship," the NAACP's Louis Wright observed in 1939, "if the country is going to let them rot and die as a result of the murderous neglect of health on the part of agencies solely because of race or color."[18]

At the root of the southern response was the intersection of race and class that confined the majority of southern blacks to low-wage agricultural labor. The circumstances of southern labor and the anxieties of southern landowners and employers reflected not simply the fact of low wages but also a tangle of legal controls over the rights and mobility of agricultural workers. Agricultural labor was organized largely around the paternalism of landowners who, under variations on the sharecropping system, induced loyalty by contracting for workers' food and housing as well. Federal policy posed a multifaceted threat: higher wages, as one southern executive put it, clearly favored "northern industrialists backed by labor and the President against the South and its industrial develop-

[18] Senator quoted in "Abstract of Hearings," *JAMA* 112:23 (1939): 2439; Warren Whatley, "Labor for the Picking: The New Deal in the South," *Journal of Economic History* 63:4 (1983): 905–8; Katznelson, Geiger, and Kryder, "Limiting Liberalism," 284–86; Edwin Amenta and Theda Skocpol, "Redefining the New Deal: World War II and the Development of Social Provision in the United States," in *The Politics of Social Policy in the United States* ed., in Weir, Orloff, and Skocpol, 102–3; Falk to Davis (27 Jan. 1949), reel 8, Michael Davis Papers (microfilm), Harry S. Truman Presidential Library [HSTPL], Independence, Mo.; Monte Poen, *Harry Truman versus the Medical Lobby* (Columbia, Mo., 1979), 122, 164–66, 176–77; Mink, *Wages of Motherhood*, 140–44; senator quoted in William Pemberton, *Bureaucratic Politics: Executive Reorganization during the Truman Administration* (Columbia, Mo., 1979), 118; Address of Louis Wright (1939), Part 1, reel 10:0512, NAACP Papers.

ment." Although Southerners won agricultural exemptions to most wage and social insurance programs, this also meant (as southerners argued in hearings on the National Recovery, Social Security, and the Fair Labor Standards acts) that such laws would entice black Americans away from the agricultural economy or the region. And the availability of public assistance, including both Social Security's Title IV and a raft of Depression-era relief programs, loosened the hold of southern paternalism.[19] Over time, southern resistance to federal social policy softened as many of the fears expressed in the 1930s and 1940s (migration north, agricultural mechanization spurred by the collapse of the agricultural labor market, the aging of the southern population, civil rights activism spurred by federal programs) were realized. Importantly, the template cut during the New Deal continued to shape agricultural labor markets as the locus of low-wage agriculture shifted to the Southwest and its largely Latino workforce.[20]

The South had not only compelling reasons to dig in against federal policy, but also the political tools to do so. Southern Democrats represented both a critical component of the New Deal and a ruling minority in a region marked by the systematic disenfranchisement of blacks—a combination that made the era's Democratic Party, as Ira Katznelson has observed, "a marriage of Sweden and South Africa."[21] In the South, one-party rule meant essentially private control over political representation and routine deference to local elites in the administration of the law. In Washington, the fruits of one-party rule included all the advantages of incumbency, an effective regional veto in the Senate (whose state-based representation and tradition of unlimited debate worked to the advantage of filibustering southerners) and disproportionate seniority in Congress (especially on the Ways and Means and the Finance committees). Even at the height of the New Deal, southern Democrats were able to control the flow of legislation through the committee system, kill offending legislation on the Senate floor, or secure regional concessions.

[19] Alston and Ferrie, "Labor Costs, Paternalism, and Loyalty," 95–117; Alston and Ferrie, "Resisting the Welfare State"; Whatley, "Labor for the Picking," 905–8; Marc Linder, *Migrant Workers and Minimum Wages* (Boulder, Colo., 1992), 156–59; (quote) Rogers to Graham (18 June 1935), file II:404:4, Westmoreland Coal Papers, Hagley Museum; Jill Quadagno, "Welfare Capitalism and the Social Security Act of 1935," *American Sociological Review* 49 (1984): 643–44; Lucy Mason, "Objections to Minimum Wage Discrimination against Negro Workers (29 Aug. 1933), reel 101, National Consumer League Papers (my thanks to Landon Storrs for bringing this to my attention).

[20] Richard Young and Jerome Burstein, "Federalism and the Decline of Prescriptive Racism in the United States," *Studies in American Political Development* 9 (Spring 1995): 13–32; Quadagno, "From Old Age Assistance to Supplemental Security Income," 237–63.

[21] Katznelson quoted in Lieberman, *Shifting the Color Line*, 24.

The South's principal victory in the formative years of the New Deal was the exclusion of agricultural and domestic labor from coverage under the National Recovery, Agricultural Adjustment, Social Security, National Labor Relations, and Fair Labor Standards acts—leaving fully 90 percent of the southern black workforce untouched by the new federal programs. Although some New Dealers hoped to gradually include farmworkers, southerners in Congress used the 1939 Social Security reforms to broaden the exemption to nearly half a million additional workers in farm-based agricultural processing in an effort, as one Social Security official saw it, "to relieve the entire agricultural industry of any legislative restrictions." Many argued that the motives for exclusion were administrative rather than racial, but the administrative argument (stressing the low ratio of employers to employees and the absence of conventional payrolls in agricultural settings) was made most forcefully and consistently by southerners, and the Committee on Economic Security made little effort to overcome it. The implications of the agricultural exclusion were also quite clearly specific to the South and Southwest— regions whose economies were dominated by agriculture, whose agriculture systems were peculiarly labor intensive, and whose agricultural labor markets were organized around low wages, tenancy, harsh legal controls, and violence. The practice of agricultural exclusion was firmly in place once the New Deal turned its attention to health care. In the debate over the Truman plan, labor interests made it quite evident that they "would probably go along with a modified measure if the compromises meant united Democratic backing of the bill"—that is, if southern Democrats were granted the agricultural exclusion. For their part, many reformers saw the agricultural extension as uniquely debilitating to their cause, because though the burden of unemployment and the retirement were arguably consequences of industrialization, barriers to adequate health care remained largely a rural problem.[22]

[22] Young and Burstein, "Federalism and the Decline of Prescriptive Racism," 24–25; Alston and Ferrie, "Labor Costs, Paternalism, and Loyalty," 107–13; Quadagno, "From Old Age Assistance to Supplemental Security Income," 238–39; Katznelson, Geiger, and Kryder, "Limiting Liberalism," 284–86, 289–97; Gareth Davies and Martha Derthick, "Race and Social Welfare Policy: The Social Security Act of 1935," *Political Science Quarterly* 112:2 (1997); Lieberman, *Shifting the Color Line*, 41–44; Linder, *Migrant Workers and Minimum Wages*, 130–31, 134–35, 159–65; Medical Advisory Board, Minutes of Meetings (29 Jan. 1935), pp. 140–52, Box 67, Edwin Witte Papers, State Historical Society of Wisconsin [SHSW], Madison, Wis.; (quote) Eleanor Dulles, "Conference with Mr. Fowler on Agricultural Workers" (23 Apr. 1940), Box 32, Decimal 054.11, Records of the Social Security Board [SSB], Office of the Commissioner, RG 47, Social Security Administration [SSA], National Archives; Kenneth Finegold, "Agriculture and the Politics of U.S. Social Provision: Social Insurance and Food Stamps," in *The Politics of Social Policy in the United States,* ed.

Having ensured that most southern blacks would remain ineligible for Social Security's social insurance programs, southerners further protected their interests by ensuring that eligibility for means-tested programs remained firmly in local hands. Again, an ostensibly race-blind insistence on states' rights and local autonomy was pressed almost exclusively by southern legislators. And these concerns were reserved, again almost exclusively, for the debate over public assistance programs (which could not be otherwise controlled through occupational exemptions). Fearing "that this measure might serve as an entering wedge for federal interference with the handling of the Negro question in the South," congressional southerners pressed the House Ways and Means Committee to restrain federal oversight of program administration, allow states to impose their eligibility rules, and strike the provision that set pensions at "a reasonable subsistence compatible with decency and health." Though motivated primarily by racial considerations, these concessions also had the effect of leaving most women workers (disproportionately employed in uncovered domestic and agricultural industries), as Suzanne Mettler has argued, "under the provincial, uneven, and generally paternalistic rule of state legislatures" as well. Local administrative discretion invited and accomplished a remarkably uneven and inequitable pattern of provision, reflected in both the regional and racial distribution of benefits and the racially specific enforcement of "suitable home," "man-in-the-house," or "employable mother" provisions. "There will be most likely 48 different interpretations and variations in the effects of these most important social security acts," observed the St. Louis Urban League, "if administered by the states." Or, as the NAACP's Charles Houston put it: "From a Negro's point of view, it looks like a sieve with the holes just big enough for the majority of Negroes to fall through."[23]

Weir, Orloff, and Skocpol, 209–10; Lieberman, *Shifting the Color Line*, 100–2; Key, *Southern Politics in State and Nation*, 315–16; Murray, "Confidential: Unified Democratic Policy Re Health Legislation," Box 89, Decimal 32.22, General Classified Files [GCF] (1944–1950), RG 235, Department of Health, Education, and Welfare [HEW], National Archives.

[23] Quadagno, "Welfare Capitalism and the Social Security Act," 643; (quote) Edwin Witte, *The Development of the Social Security Act* (Madison, Wis., 1963), 142–44; Finegold, "Agriculture and the Politics of U.S. Social Provision," 210; Piven and Cloward, *Regulating the Poor*, 136–41; Lieberman, *Shifting the Color Line*, 52–53, 126–30; Alston and Ferrie, "Labor Costs, Paternalism, and Loyalty," 107–13; Quadagno, "From Old Age Assistance to Supplemental Security Income," 238–39; Katznelson, Geiger, and Kryder, "Limiting Liberalism," 284–86, 289–97; Suzanne Mettler, "Federalism, Gender, and the Fair Labor Standards Act of 1938," *Polity* 26 (1994): 639–40; St. Louis Urban League to Altmeyer (11 Apr. 1935), Box 54, Records of the Committee on Economic Security, SSA Records; Houston quoted in Linder, *Migrant Workers and Minimum Wages*, 147; Robert Lieberman and John Lapinski, "American Federalism, Race, and the Administration of Welfare," *British Journal of Political Science* 31:2 (2001): 303–329.

Local administration of health provision posed a special challenge, because, although conventional public assistance flowed out to recipients, health benefits drew them into doctor's offices, hospitals, and clinics. Health programs, accordingly, were shaped not only by the race of recipients but also by the meager and segregated southern medical system. The Depression saw an infusion of federal funds and federal standards (including Federal Emergency Relief Administration assistance for hospitals and state boards of health, medical education funded by the Works Progress Administration, and medical programs offered by the FSA, the Civilian Conservation Corps, the National Youth Administration, and Social Security's Title IV). But federal agencies, as a practical and political necessity, consistently surrendered control over these programs to state and local administration. States set their own standards for care and eligibility and controlled the pace and scope of federal matching funds. And local political and medical authorities (like voting registrars or sheriffs in other civil rights arenas) wielded considerable informal power and discretion. For these reasons, civil rights activists viewed efforts to include health insurance under or alongside Social Security (as in the Truman and Taft proposals of the late 1940s) with considerable skepticism—at least as long as state and local interests were able to spend federal money in such a way as to reinforce southern race and labor relations rather than challenge them. The NAACP, for its part, was ambivalent about the first Wagner-Murray-Dingell bill because it left basic administration to the states; was more enthusiastic about the 1943 and 1945 versions, which promised stronger federal standards; and, while admiring the universalism of the 1947 and 1948 versions, bemoaned their unwillingness to confront discrimination and their retreat to state administrative control.[24]

The shadow cast by the South over the New Deal was especially apparent in the understanding, expressed by reformers and opponents alike, of the scope of federal health programs. Through 1933–1935, the CES focused much of its attention on underserviced rural settings but also confined its concerns to "the ordinary self-supporting farmer, the poor white farmer." In sharper terms, an AMA official dismissed the universalism suggested by postwar innovations in Saskatchewan: "I do not believe that our Anglo-Saxon people are going to take to the Saskatchewan Plan. The paid doctor before the Civil War in the South was a slave doctor,

---

[24] Michael Grey, *New Deal Medicine: The Rural Health Programs of the Farm Security Administration* (Baltimore, 1999), 7, 40, 59; Beardsley, *History of Neglect,* 156–63; CNH, "Revision of National Health Bills," Box 46, Decimal 011.4, GCF (1944–1950), HEW Records; "Health and Housing" (1945), Part 1, reel 12:0083, NAACP Papers; Dona Cooper Hamilton and Charles V. Hamilton, *The Dual Agenda: Race and Social Welfare Policies of Civil Rights Organizations* (New York, 1997), 73–76.

and then the paid doctor in the South got to be the county physician, and woe to the man in the South who gets to be county physician. . . . He is also the physician to the chain gang." Opponents questioned the very need for health reform on the grounds that dismal indices of the nation's health (including World War II draft statistics) did not make appropriate racial distinctions. In 1948 the Brookings Institution published a book-length assault on health reform in which it based cost estimates on "the ordinary private expenditures of white families," confined comparative mortality rates to the white population on the grounds that higher black mortality was "predominantly the result of economic, cultural and social differences," and concluded that United States was "among the most healthful nations of the world, perhaps the most healthful of the large nations at least with respect to its white population." The AMA seconded the conclusion that rates of non-white mortality or draft deferment reflected "poor sanitation, housing, education, and the lack of ordinary individual and community common sense" rather than inequitable access to care. In arguing that the United States should not be measured against European peers "with purely homogeneous populations," the AMA also followed Brookings by "adjusting" national measures of mortality or life expectancy (in one case using Minnesota instead of national figures) to exclude African Americans and Latinos altogether. Some used such reasoning to argue against the necessity of any federal health programs, others used it to argue for local control: "Different States," Senator Robert Taft put it in 1949, "have different kinds of people and different medical problems for different kinds of people."[25]

Southern anxieties over the confluence of race and social programs emerged again in postwar battles over veteran's rights. The war created an expectation of social provision for veterans and their families, and many opponents of wider health reform championed the VA as a means of distinguishing "deserving" recipients. But for the South, even the VA

[25] Medical Advisory Board, Minutes of Meetings (29 Jan. 1935), pp. 149–50, and "Abstract of a Program for Social Insurance against Illness: Preliminary Draft" (1935), p. 88, both in Box 67, Witte Papers; George Bachman and Lewis Merriam, *The Issue of Compulsory Health Insurance* (Washington, D.C., 1948), 20, 16–17; Chamber of Commerce Proceedings 37 (May 1949), pp. 190–91, Hagley Museum; NPC, "Compulsion: The Key to Collectivism" (1949), p. 37, SHSW Pamphlets; "The Brookings Report," *JAMA* 137:6 (1948): 536; Olin West (AMA) in Official Report of Proceedings before the President's Interdepartmental Committee to Coordinate Health and Welfare Activities (18 July 1938), p. 368, Box 29, Records of the President's Interdepartmental Committee to Coordinate Health and Welfare Activities, Franklin D. Roosevelt Presidential Library [FDRPL], Hyde Park, N.Y.; Frank Dickinson, "An Analysis of the Ewing Report," AMA Bulletin no. 69 (1949), pp. 6–7; Taft in Senate Subcommittee of the Committee on Labor and Public Welfare, *National Health Program, 1949* 81:1 (May 1949), I:119.

crossed the line. "I think it is perfectly silly for a lot of Senators," complained one southerner, "who on account of the fact that they are up for re-election next year, have to get together in the Senate and cry all over each other on account of some nigger who was drafted and forced to tote logs in France." Local and congressional interests besieged veterans' administrator Omar Bradley with demands for segregated facilities. And while both the National Medical Association (NMA) and the NAACP fought the segregation of veterans' care, Bradley rejected "Negro propaganda" and remained "firmly convinced of the necessity of segregated care in the Southern and border States." For Senator Theodore Bilbo of Mississippi, the issue of VA segregation was "just as important as the disposition of the atomic bomb. What difference does it make how our white race and civilization are destroyed? . . . I would prefer to have it destroyed with the atomic bomb rather than to see it destroyed by mongrelizing both races into a brown race."[26]

Civil rights activists and black professionals pressed the New Deal to use the leverage afforded by federal spending. "Our racial plea," stressed the NMA in 1939, "is that, whatever form this National Health Program shall take, that its administration will be minus any discriminatory practices and that this provision will be made one of the federal conditions of the subsidy." Yet as in the larger logic of Social Security, the New Deal had every incentive to placate southern Democrats and little incentive to connect federal social policy to the civil rights struggle. When the FSA returned to the issue in the early war years, it urged reformers to downplay the social impact of national health insurance on the assumption that any public statements to that effect "might possible antagonize others by emphasis on relative advantage to Negroes of liberalization." When war-era reform energies were diverted to hospital construction in 1945–46 (as we shall see), Congress had little trouble including a "separate but equal" provision in the enabling legislation. And while the 1948–49 reform proposals included nondiscrimination language in their discussion of medical care, they did not challenge the practice of segregation in medical education, professional association, or hospitalization.[27]

[26] Williams to McIntyre (9 June 1933), President's Official File [POF] 95d:8, Franklin D. Roosevelt Papers, FDRPL; Louis Wright, "The NAACP in 1946–1947," Part 1, reel 12:0137, NAACP Papers; NMA to HST (30 Mar. 1946), POF 8B, Box 91, Harry S. Truman Papers, HSTPL; Memorandum on Interview with General Bradley (Jan. ? 1946), President's Secretary's File [PSF], Box 140, Truman Papers; Theo. Bilbo to Omar Bradley (19 Nov. 1945), POF 8B, Box 91, Truman Papers; see also I. C. Rayner to John Rankin (22 June 1945), Rankin to Rayner (27 June 1945), H 79A-38.2, RG 233, Records of the House Committee on World War Veterans, National Archives; Rankin memo (6/3/38), POF 95d:9, FDR Papers. My thanks to Roger Horowitz for pointing out the importance of this debate.

[27] Statement of the NMA (1938) in "Resolutions, Statements of Policy, Etc Relative to the National Health Program" (May 1939), Box 10, Decimal 011.4, General Reclassified

190   CHAPTER FIVE

Although health care remained on its margins, the New Deal would
have enormous implications for future patterns of race relations and
health provision. In part this reflected the fundamental irony of the New
Deal welfare state, which was designed to exclude African-Americans but
which, over time, created and promoted a popular and political identifi-
cation of public assistance with a pathologically dependent and primarily
African American "underclass." The very logic of Social Security largely
excluded African Americans from its contributory, social insurance programs and then employed their disproportionate presence on the public
assistance rolls to undermine the legitimacy of those programs. "When
a specific minority group comes to constitute so high a caseload of a
program that is subject to a certain amount of popular disfavor," admitted the National Resources Planning Board as early as 1942, "there is
every likelihood that no great amount of social pressure will be exerted
to improve or even maintain the standards of aid for this group." The
politics of "charitable" assistance (always anxious about malingering and
"disincentives" to work) dovetailed with long-standing stereotypes—routinely voiced in congressional deliberations over Social Security—of African Americans as peculiarly "dependent" or "shiftless." This racialized
welfare state was reinforced by fiscal anxieties, voiced first by congressional Republicans in the 1940s and 1950s and later, in the wake of Vietnam, by Democrats as well.[28]

More important for the immediate future of health care, the New Deal
deferred much of the organization of social provision to private employment. Social Security's core social insurance programs rested on base
employment requirements in covered occupations. In theory, social insurance promised to alleviate discrimination: claims flowed from contributions, and benefits were insulated from local administration. But in
practice, social insurance was doubly discriminatory: it used occupational exemptions to exclude many African Americans and Latinos outright, and then allowed private labor market discrimination to shape the
eligibility of those with a marginal or occasional presence in covered
employment. Tellingly, the reformer Abraham Epstein admitted to the
NAACP in 1935 that his first interest lay in social insurance and that
he "did not see how we can solve the Negro problem through social
insurance." All of this was exaggerated in the case of health insurance.
As a rule, private employment benefits replicated and reinforced existing

Files, (1939–1944), HEW Records; Ivan Asay to Mr. Powell (25 Aug. 1942), Box 2, Decimal
11, Correspondence of the Executive Director, SSA Records; "The President's Message,"
140:1 *JAMA* (1949), 111.
   [28] Lieberman, *Shifting the Color Line*, 6–7, passim; Michael K. Brown, *Race, Money, and the
American Welfare State* (Ithaca, N.Y., 1999), 6–8, 76–86; NRPB, "Security, Work and Relief
Policies" (1942), 224–25, draft in POF 1092:6, FDR Papers.

inequalities. Indeed, as the reform proposals of the 1940s were gradually redrafted around the assumption of employment-based provision, it became increasingly apparent that they would do little to address the health needs of marginal and rural workers. "The benefit rights of Negroes under the WMD bill," one reformer conceded, "will depend primarily upon the employment opportunities available to them."[29]

Those opportunities were decisively shaped by residential and occupational segregation, direct employment discrimination, and the economic fortunes of the postwar city. The formative years of the private welfare state coincided with an era of massive African American migration north in response to the industrial boom of World War II. Yet this boom was at best a mixed blessing and, as Thomas Sugrue has shown for postwar Detroit, also short-lived. The last to benefit from the tight labor markets of the wartime economy, African Americans were the first to bear the costs of economic decline as urban industrial economies suffered a drift of industry and investment to the South and the suburbs in the 1950s and 1960s, and a more general pattern of deindustrialization and political neglect in the 1970s and 1980s. Taken together, postwar employment patterns and the willingness to subsidize private coverage as a surrogate for public policy served, as Michael Brown argues, to "erode blacks' access to permanent, full-time, work, and thus the basis for their integration into the core of the American welfare state."[30]

The mechanization of the cotton South, coupled with the emergence of commercial agriculture in the West and Southwest, gradually shifted the burden of both the New Deal's agricultural exemptions and their reflection in the public and private welfare states. Between 1945 and 1995 labor intensity in southern agriculture collapsed: farmers dropped from over a third of the labor force to barely 2 percent, and the number of farms plummeted by 80 percent. For African-American farmers, the transformation was even more dramatic: the number of black farmers in the South fell from nearly 1.5 million in 1940 to less than 65,000 in 1990—during which time the black share of the southern farm popula-

---

[29] Epstein quoted in Hamilton and Hamilton, *The Dual Agenda*, 30; Lieberman, *Shifting the Color Line*, 7–9, 60, 177–78, 204–6; NRPB, "Security, Work, and Relief Policies" (1942), p. 202 POF 1092:6, FDR Papers; Gwendolyn Mink, "The Lady and the Tramp: Gender, Race, and the Origins of the American Welfare State," in *Women, the State, and Welfare*, ed. Linda Gordon (Madison, Wis., 1990), 112–14; (quote) Falk to Davis (22 May 1944), reel 8, Davis Papers; Jill Quadagno, "How Medicare Promoted Racial Integration in the Health Care System: Explaining Variations in Social Movement Outcomes" (unpublished ms., 1999), 25–26.

[30] Thomas Sugrue, *The Origins of the Urban Crisis: Race and Inequality in Postwar Detroit* (Princeton, N.J., 1996), passim; Brown, *Race, Money, and the American Welfare State*, 192 (quote).

tion fell from over 35 percent to less than 8 percent.[31] At the same time, the agricultural economies of the West and Southwest boomed, thanks largely to the cheap migrant labor provided by a series of "guest worker" programs (most notably the 1951–64 *bracero* program). This transformation is not as easily captured by census data, given the transience and uneven immigration status of the labor force, but it is clear that the booming western agricultural economy relied increasingly on an itinerant Latino workforce.[32] The racial premises of social insurance and Social Security forged by southerners in the 1930s and 1940s were borne increasingly by Latino Americans in the Southwest after 1945. By the late 1990s Hispanic Americans went without health insurance at a much higher rate (33 percent) than either white Americans (14 percent) or black Americans (21 percent). And of the six states with uninsurance rates exceeding 20 percent in 1999, five (New Mexico, Texas, Arizona, Nevada, and California) were in the West and Southwest.[33]

Access to private benefits was further constrained by professional segregation, institutional segregation and discrimination, and discriminatory underwriting conventions. Provider-based insurance plans, such as Blue Cross and Blue Shield, replicated and rarely challenged patterns of professional or institutional segregation. The Blues had a meager presence in the South (as late as the early 1950s, over two-thirds of the Blues' subscribers resided in six northern, urban, industrial states, and plans in some black-belt states had no black enrollees at all).[34] Consumer-based insurance plans (including most of the early group health experiments) were confined by employment-based groups as well and maintained wage thresholds that barred most low-income workers. Private insurers routinely excluded, as one company specified in 1930, "Negroes, Chinese, Japanese, and Mexicans and more than one-fourth blood Indians" as uninsurable risks. And although state laws increasingly disallowed direct racial exclusion, private insurers found other means to "redline" by race and persistently viewed the rural population (as the HIAA put it in 1956) as "beyond the scope of traditional or even possible or proper concern by private insurers."[35]

[31] On changes in southern agriculture, see Orville Burton, "Race Relations in the Rural South since 1945," in *The Rural South since World War II*, ed. R. Douglas Hurt (Baton Rouge, La., 1998), 35–36, 56–58; Wright, *New South, Old South*, 259–74.

[32] See Anne Effland, "Migrant and Seasonal Farm Labor in the Far West," in *The Rural West since 1945*, ed. R. Douglas Hurt (Lawrence, Kans. 1998), 147–54.

[33] Rates of coverage by race and region are calculated from health insurance historical tables at http://www.census.gov/hhes/hlthins/historic, accessed February 2001.

[34] Senate Committee on Labor and Public Welfare, *Health Insurance Plans in the United States*, Report 359:1, 82d/1 (Washington, D.C., 1951), 1–2, 8.

[35] Statement of David Burgess (Georgia CIO), Box 55, Records of the President's Commission on the Health Needs of the Nation [PCHNN], HSTPL; Deborah Stone, "The

Dancing with Jim Crow: Health Care and Civil Rights, 1946–1970

New Deal and Great Society reformers could not contain the contradictions in a liberal tradition shaped equally by southern compromises and universalist pretensions. Indeed, the promise of equity implicit in the profusion of federal programs in the 1930s and 1940s provided the legal and political spark for the modern civil rights movement. In health care, as in education, the principal issue was segregation in facilities built or maintained with federal money. But unlike schools, hospitals were largely private institutions whose relationship to federal funding was fragmented and complex. Civil rights activists found it hard to argue that hospital admission was a right akin to education or voting. Many in federal politics were reluctant to use health spending to leverage civil rights, especially if it meant that hospitals might go unbuilt or patients might go uncovered. And southern interests remained torn between their thirst for federal money and their anxieties about the conditions that might accompany it.[36] For these reasons, the struggle to desegregate southern hospitals proceeded more fitfully, and lasted much longer, than parallel struggles in education, voting, or public accommodation.

At the root of the hospital issue in the South was not only professional and patient segregation but also the ways in which it was countenanced by federal efforts to address the region's dearth of facilities. Federal aid to hospitals, first in 1940 and then under the 1946 Hill-Burton Act, avoided any commitment to maintenance: once built, hospitals would reflect local control and local custom. This reflected a long-standing political strategy of placating reformers by opening the federal purse and placating opponents by relinquishing control to local or private interests. Hill-Burton required its recipients to provide a "reasonable volume" of uncompensated care but also allowed them to do so on a "separate but equal" basis. In part, Hill-Burton applications read: "No person/certain persons (cross out one) in the area will be denied admission . . . because

Struggle for the Soul of Health Insurance," *JHPPL* 18 (1993): 296, 313–14; Cobb, "National Health Program of the NAACP," 334–35; statement by Max Mont, Box 55, PCHNN Records; "Blueprint of Proposed Industry Program" (Oct. 1956), Box 18, Orville Grahame Papers, University of Iowa Special Collections; Joni Hersch and Shelly White Means, "Employer-Sponsored Health and Pension Benefits and the Gender/Race Wage Gap," *Social Science Quarterly* 74:4 (1993): 851, 855; James Shepperd, "Minority Perspective of a National Health Insurance" (paper presented to the Congressional Black Caucus, September 1974), reprinted in *JNMA* 68:4 (1976): 285; USCCR, *Health Insurance: Coverage and Employment Opportunities for Minorities and Women*, 15–38.

[36] See "Alabama" files, File 89A-F13, Box 101, Records of the Senate Committee on Labor and Public Welfare, Subcommittee on Health, RG 46, Records of the Senate, National Archives.

of race creed or color." If the applicant opted for "certain persons," it was required to abide by a provision that "such hospital or addition to a hospital will be made available to all persons residing in the territorial area of the applicant, without discrimination on account of race, creed, or color, but an exception shall be made in cases where separate hospital facilities are provided for separate population, if the plan makes equitable provision."[37]

It is difficult to assess the consequences of Hill-Burton's deference to southern custom. Between 1946 and 1963, only about 1 percent (roughly 70 of 7,000) of applicants invoked the "separate-but-equal" provision. But this did not prevent hospitals from segregating by other means. In order to qualify as "nondiscriminatory," a hospital was required only to grant equal access "to that portion of the facility constructed with federal funds." Applicants routinely juggled their books in order to distinguish one area (typically a "colored" ward or the emergency room) as federally funded. The task of monitoring Hill-Burton compliance was left almost solely to state health agencies—a concession that virtually guaranteed that federal money would do little to challenge local segregation. "By statute and administration," the United States Commission on Civil Rights concluded in 1963, the federal government "supports racial discrimination in the provision of health services."[38]

Hill-Burton's separate-but-equal provision survived legal challenge until 1963, nine years after the 1954 school segregation cases affirmed the principle that "no Federal program may include racial exclusiveness as a permissible standard." While the NAACP's National Health Committee had always placed the issue of federal funding at the center of its litigation strategy, it was not until *Simkins v. Cone* (1963) that the Supreme Court concurred and struck down Hill-Burton's separate-but-equal

---

[37] Arthur J. Altmeyer, *The Formative Years of Social Security* (Madison, Wis., 1966), 117; Kenneth R. Wing and Marilyn G. Rose, "Health Facilities and the Enforcement of Civil Rights," in *Legal Aspects of Health Policy*, ed. Ruth Roemer and George McKray (Westport, Conn., 1980), 243; Kenneth Wing, "The Community Service Obligation of Hill-Burton Health Facilities," *Boston College Law Review* 23 (1982): 591; P. A. Paul-Shaheen and Harry Perlstadt, "Class Action Suits and Social Change: The Organization and Impact of the Hill-Burton Cases," *Indiana Law Journal* 57 (1982): 391; USCCR, *Health Facilities and Services* (Washington, D.C., 1963), 131; Title VI of the Public Health Services Act of 1946, Pub. L. No. 79–725, 622 (f), 60 Stat. 1043; Marilyn Rose, "Federal Regulation of Services to the Poor under the Hill-Burton Act: Realities and Pitfalls," *Northwestern University Law Review* 70 (1975): 171; Brown, *Race, Money, and the American Welfare State*, 102–12, 124–27.

[38] Wing and Rose, "Health Facilities and the Enforcement of Civil Rights," 244; USCCR, *Equal Opportunity in Hospital and Health Facilities: Civil Rights Policies under the Hill-Burton Program* (March 1965), 4–5; Rose, "Federal Regulation of Services to the Poor," 186–87; USCCR, *Health Facilities and Services*, 129–32 (quoted at 129).

clause. The Greensboro, N.C., hospital in question did admit some black patients, but systematically denied admitting privileges to black physicians. This gave the NAACP a legal opening and also won it the support of the NMA (otherwise ambivalent on the issue of patient segregation). Opponents of the ruling included not only southern hospitals and segregationists but also the AMA, which resented the implication that federal funding could transform private institutions into public ones. Although the administration joined the case on the plaintiffs' behalf, HEW continued to hold that grant recipients had the right to segregate patients, that compliance was a state responsibility, and that an assurance of nondiscrimination did not extend to practitioners or beyond a narrow range of "essential" services. Even as the Court completed its deliberations, HEW was overseeing the construction of eight separate-but-equal facilities. In the wake of *Simkins,* HEW redrafted Hill-Burton to ensure equal treatment of patients and providers, require "voluntary nondiscrimination assurances" from current projects, and transform the separate-but-equal clause into a "community service" requirement designed to strengthen the act's original commitment to uncompensated services.[39]

Like other landmark civil rights cases, the symbolic importance of *Simkins* exceeded its immediate impact. In part (as in education and voting rights), this reflected the determination of segregationists to defy the ruling and the federal government's unwillingness to enforce it. In part, this reflected the limited reach of *Simkins,* which did not extend to those hospitals that had received Hill-Burton funds in the past. Because Hill-Burton dispensed one-time construction grants rather than ongoing federal assistance, the *Simkins* decision could not be used or interpreted as a broader mandate to desegregate southern hospitals. For these reasons, attention shifted quickly to Title VI of the 1964 Civil Rights Act, which prohibited discrimination under any program or activity receiving federal financial assistance, and to the institution of Medicare and Medicaid

[39] USCCR, *Health Facilities and Services,* 133–34; Reynolds, "Hospitals and Civil Rights," 898–903; F. L. Blasingame [AMA] to Rep. Oren Harris (6 Mar. 1964), *Simkins v. Cone* file, Box 86, Records of the Senate Subcommittee on Health, RG 46, Records of the Senate; Simkins et al. v. Moses H. Cone Memorial Hospital 376 U.S. 938,84 S.C. 793; Wing, "The Community Service Obligation," 601; Institute of Medicine, *Health Care in a Context of Civil Rights* (Washington, D.C., 1981), 24, 148–53; Rose, "Federal Regulation of Services to the Poor," 171; Kenneth Clement, "Racial Discrimination in Health Services, Facilities, and Programs" (n.d.), in "Health and Welfare," Planning Session Master Book D, Records of the White House Conference on Civil Rights, 1965–1966, *Civil Rights during the Johnson Administration, 1963–1969* (microfilm), Part I, reel 17; USCCR, *Equal Opportunity in Hospital and Health Facilities,* 6–8; Lee White to LBJ (5 Mar. 1964), Part I (WHCF), reel 2:0207, *Civil Rights during the Johnson Administration, 1963–1969;* Celbrezze to Dingell (13 Apr. 1964), Box 291, Secretary's Subject Files [SSF] (1955–1975), HEW Records.

in 1965, which simultaneously presented southern hospitals with an on-going source of federal funds and the conditions (Title VI) that went with it.[40]

Through the gestation of Medicare and Medicaid, southern legislators supported the Kerr-Mills program because it offered unconditional federal funds for state-run health programs. By the same token, civil rights activists saw Kerr-Mills as a throwback to the original southern accommodation of Social Security: states were neither required to participate nor held to any federal standards if they did.[41] As the Medicaid debate continued, however, both the relationship between federal social policy and civil rights, and the southern response, changed dramatically. Agricultural mechanization, black migration north, and the aging of the southern population combined to erode the logic of southern paternalism and soften southern anxieties about federal interference. And a flurry of legislative and legal developments underscored the civil rights implications of federal health spending and girded the efforts of civil rights activists to point out those implications and press the federal government to pursue them.[42]

In health care, the immediate impact of Title VI (which went into effect in January 1965) was simply to affirm and broaden the *Simkins* decision. Although hospitals that had completed Hill-Burton contracts were still untouchable, Title VI did apply to all facilities "which currently receive or will be receiving Hill-Burton funds" and extended its protection to all portions of the facility in question. Medicare and Medicaid, by contrast, raised the prospect of a systematic flow of federal funds into public and private hospitals—all of which would, presumably, come with Title VI attached. Few, however, gave this serious consideration. HEW staff, absorbed with the intricacies of program design and implementation, only belatedly confronted the Title VI implications. The White House viewed health care and civil rights as entirely separate issues (advi-

[40] Institute of Medicine, *Health Care in a Context of Civil Rights*, 141–43; Reynolds, "Hospitals and Civil Rights," 904; Wing and Rose, "Health Facilities and the Enforcement of Civil Rights," 246–47. On patterns of hospital segregation, see Moore and Livingston testimony, USCCR, *Hearings in Memphis* (June 1962), 38–39, 78–82.

[41] Edward Berkowitz, *Mr. Social Security: The Life of Wilbur J. Cohen* (Lawrence, Kans., 1995), 130–31; Rashi Fein, *Medical Care, Medical Costs: The Search for a Health Insurance Policy* (Cambridge, Mass., 1989), 58–60; "Comments on AMA Telecast" (1962), Box 126:7, Wilbur Cohen Papers, SHSW; Smith, *Sick and Tired*, 83, 168.

[42] Wright, *Old South, New South*, 156ff.; Quadagno, "From Old Age Assistance to Supplemental Security Income," 237–63; Young and Burstein, "Federalism and the Decline of Prescriptive Racism," 13–32; Libassi to Cater (18 June 1966), Ball to Califano (21 May 1966), both in WHCF IS 1; Cohen to LBJ (26 Aug. 1966), WHCF IS 2, Lyndon B. Johnson Papers, LBJPL; David McBride, "Black America: From Community Health Care to Crisis Medicine," *JHPPL* 18:2 (1993): 320–22.

sors briefed Johnson for a 1964 meeting with the NMA by urging "that Medicare—*not Civil Rights*—be the focus of the conversation and discussion"). Northern legislators did not press the issue, and southern legislators devoted most of their attention to the preservation of Kerr-Mills. Indeed, it was not until Senator Robert Byrd (D-Va.) asked HEW for an opinion in April 1965 that the administration gave it any serious thought.[43]

The administration viewed Byrd's question as a legislative monkey wrench. It was afraid, on the one hand, that "the liberals will insist on an amendment making this [application of Title VI] clear," and, on the other, that any affirmative stance would be "a signal to some of the Southern supporters of Medicare to reexamine their position." "On balance," HEW counsel Lee White advised, "it seems that we should make every effort to find authority to prevent discrimination without a specific amendment to the Medicare bill—this assumes, of course, that whatever theory is used to support this position can be defended in any court test following enactment." As the fate of the bill hung in the balance, however, the immediate task was to "keep the entire matter as low-keyed as possible." Behind the scenes, the administration worked to avoid the prospect of attaching Title VI to its medical care programs. HEW secretary Anthony Celebrezze's "instinctive reaction" was to argue that "Title VI does not apply on the ground that insurance is expressly excluded from Title VI and that this is an insurance program," and the Justice Department prepared a memorandum to this effect (although the drafters advised that "they could support a theory that the Title does apply if it is desirable to do so"). In the end, the three-layer cake assembled by Congress confounded this strategy: HEW maintained that Title VI did not extend to Medicare's Part B because the voluntary and supplemental medical program was "excluded as a contract of insurance," but that Title VI did apply to both Medicare Part A and Medicaid.[44]

The task of winning the compliance of southern hospitals was immense, unprecedented, and—for most at HEW—unwelcome. "In two decades of debate about government health insurance," Theodore Marmor points out, "almost no-one pressed the issue of racially-segregated medical services. Yet, in the first weeks of the program, the question of certifying southern hospitals under Medicare took up more of the time of HEW's three top health officials than any other feature of

---

[43] USCCR, *Equal Opportunity in Hospital and Health Facilities*, 3, 8; Busby to LBJ (4 Aug. 1964), WHCF HE, Box 1, LBJ Papers; Lee White to LBJ (26 Apr. 1965), Part I (WHCF), reel 13:0320, *Civil Rights during the Johnson Administration, 1963–1969.*

[44] Lee White to the President (26 Apr. 1965), WHCF LE/IS 75, LBJ Papers; Berkowitz, *Mr. Social Security,* 233; USCCR, *Federal Civil Rights Enforcement Effort—1974* (1974), 116–18.

the Medicare program." In late 1965 state health department officials in Alabama estimated that barely 5 percent of the state's 18,600 hospital beds would satisfy Title VI, and throughout the deep South, many communities had no facilities that were either willing or able to comply. "Although there are several problems," concluded one HEW official, "the basic hard-core, tough one is that of bi-racial room occupancy and . . . the predominant use by physicians of certain hospitals for Negro patients and others for white patients." HEW lamented the dilemma posed by "strict enforcement of Title VI of the 1964 Civil Rights Act on the one hand and the necessity for the almost immediate implementation of the Medicare provisions on the other" and remained determined that Title VI not trump the larger task of launching Medicare and Medicaid. On civil rights, as on other issues such as reimbursement, the administration viewed the cooperation of hospitals and doctors as its foremost priority and feared that any "crackdown" might encourage boycotts.[45]

HEW deeply resented both the threat that Title VI posed to a clean takeoff for Medicare and Medicaid and the distraction of enforcing it. For some, Title VI was little more than "a faulty instrument that Congress added to the Civil Rights Act largely to keep Adam Clayton Powell from adding it to every piece of social legislation that came along . . . [it turns HEW] into policeman, judge, and jury." Many at Social Security resented the "interference" of civil rights activists and reacted angrily to their role in training them for surveying compliance in the South. "We were given to understand that anyone who could not, or would not, accept the proposition that the Negro was always in the right, the white administrator always in the wrong—should at once withdraw from the program," complained one trainee. Some felt that the civil rights workshops were little more than "brain washing ceremonies" which "combined an inadequate attempt to furnish trainees with procedures for conducting a Civil Rights compliance hospital survey with use of those trainees as a sounding board upon which to voice the pent-up feelings of certain so-called spokesmen of the Negro community." Others complained of "the feeling I was attending a civil rights rally rather than a government-sponsored workshop" or that HEW was being asked to be a "civil rights agitator" rather than "a calm and forceful Federal Agency." Many were simply unwilling to abandon Social Security's original southern compromise and

---

[45] Theodore Marmor, *The Politics of Medicare* (Chicago, 1970), 88; Robert Ball to the Secretary (19 Nov. 1965), Box 300, Commissioner's Correspondence, 1936–69, SSA Records; (quotes) Murray to Ball (15 Feb. 1966), Box 300, Commissioner's Correspondence, 1936–1969, SSA Records; Libassi to Califano (28 July 1966), Bell to Owen (22 Dec. 1966), both in WHCF HE, Box 17, LBJ Papers; Cater to LBJ (1 Dec. 1966), Box 14, Cater Office Files, LBJPL; Paul Starr, *The Social Transformation of American Medicine* (New York, 1982), 375–76; Judith Feder, *Medicare: The Politics of Federal Hospital Insurance* (Lexington, Mass., 1977).

feared that Title VI enforcement might create the impression that Social Security—"which has so well established its services as a local institution"—"has gone over to the enemy."[46]

Compliance with Title VI was half-hearted and half-heartedly enforced. While some at HEW wanted to certify compliant hospitals before Medicare and Medicaid went into effect, the administration was reluctant to "to move into the compliance program for Title VI before the time comes to pay benefits [or] . . . to extend the scope of our effort beyond the institutions that will be participating in health insurance." SSA officials argued that they should "carry out compliance requirements of Title VI in a manner that will minimize adverse impact on Medicare," beware that Title VI enforcement could constitute "interference with the practice of medicine," and avoid the "severe political repercussions" that might follow a crackdown on southern hospitals. "If our first contact with them . . . is for the Social Security Administration to inspect the hospitals for Title VI compliance," Social Security Commissioner Robert Ball argued, "we will be putting an unnecessary barrier in the way of getting the health insurance program off to a good start."[47] This timidity was reinforced by the fact that HEW did not have the national or regional staff to ensure compliance and relied instead on state health departments or third-party contractors such as Blue Cross and Blue Shield. Before HEW established its Office of Civil Rights in late 1965, Title VI enforcement consisted primarily of mailing compliance forms to hospitals. The role of Title VI in Medicaid was even more ambivalent; as in other programs of public assistance, administrative deference to the states eroded federal (including civil rights) standards.[48]

The early results were disheartening. Through 1965, HEW received numerous reports, both from its own staff and from the NAACP, docu-

[46] Unsigned memorandum (1966), Box 51, Cater Office Files; Blackwell to Murray (26 Apr. 1966), Box 299, Commissioner's Correspondence (1936–1969); Third Meeting of Civil Rights Staff (8 Apr. 1966); Murray to Ball (2 May 1966); Konefsky to Murray (26 Apr. 1966); "Summary of Comments and Reactions by SSA Personnel to Training Sessions" (Apr. 1966); Training and Work Assignment for PHS Equal Opportunity Health Detailees (26 Apr. 1966), all in Box 299, Commissioner's Correspondence, 1936–1969, SSA Records; (quote) Swift to Ball (20 July 1966), Box 298, Commissioner's Correspondence, 1936–1969, SSA Records.

[47] (Quote) Ball to the Secretary (19 Nov. 1965), Box 300; (quote) Gaskill to Swift (13 Apr. 1966), Box 299; (quote) James Murray to Robert Ball (15 Feb. 1966), Box 300; (quote) Richard to Hess (14 Apr. 1966), Box 299; (quote) Robert Ball to the Secretary (19 Nov. 1965), Box 300, all in Commissioner's Correspondence, 1936–1969, SSA Records.

[48] HHH to LBJ (24 Jan. 1966), Part I (WHCF), reel 2:0792, *Civil Rights during the Johnson Administration, 1963–1969*; Robert Ball to the Secretary (19 Nov. 1965), Box 300, Commissioner's Correspondence, 1936–1969, SSA Records; USCCR, *HEW and Title VI* (1970), 8–11; USCCR, *Federal Civil Rights Enforcement Effort—1974*, 130–31, 158.

menting persistent segregation in southern hospitals—including many who had assured HEW of their compliance. Civil rights activists viewed HEW's efforts with disdain: "They do not act on complaints . . . [and] when they do go in they make the mistake of announcing that they are coming and anyone who has dealt with White Southerners knows that this is—I think—way out—because all sorts of shenanigans go on in try- ing to impress the investigator with how desegregated the facilities are." HEW's own staff recorded numerous such cases of hospitals which "delib- erately placed Negro and white patients in the same rooms, closed the Negro dining room, and integrated the nursery for the benefits of the review team—and then promptly shifted everything back to business-as- usual as soon as the review team left the city." Aside from an exchange of paper assurances, HEW's compliance efforts consisted largely of fielding complaints; as the department itself admitted: "We are fumbling . . . we are inundated with complaints. We are ill-equipped to handle them quickly." The NMA and others agreed: "If they are going to pass the money out and then go check on the hospitals and then place the burden on someone really to complain about the way the money is distributed then the law will certainly not work."[49]

And it was not working. As Title VI's first anniversary passed and Medi- care's launch date approached, the Civil Rights Commission found "no discernible pattern of compliance" in two-thirds of the hospitals it sur- veyed. SSA identified nearly a thousand hospitals as "hard-core hold- outs," and even HEW's optimistic assessment (based on self-reporting) found hospitals representing between a third and a half of all hospital beds in Mississippi, Alabama, and Virginia in violation of the law. Nearly a hundred Southern counties (including thirty contiguous counties in western Mississippi) had no participating hospitals and over one hun- dred others were served only by hospitals that had not yet complied. There persisted, as SSA staffers noted, not only a "lack of desire to comply and an expectation of deceit" but the assumption in much of the South that "when a showdown comes they will get in touch with Senator Russell, and Senator Long, and Senator Hill, and the Senators will fix things

[49] Califano to Valenti (19 Feb. 1965), Part I (WHCF), reel 2:0544, *Civil Rights during the Johnson Administration, 1963–1969*; (quote) Planning Session, Panel 4 (Health and Welfare) (17 Nov. 1965), p. 66, Records of the White House Conference on Civil Rights, 1965–1966, Part IV, reel 7:0443, *Civil Rights during the Johnson Administration, 1963–1969*; (quote) James Quigley [HEW], "Hospitals and the Civil Rights Act of 1964" (1 Sept. 1965), in "Health and Welfare," Planning Session Master Book D, Records of the White House Conference on Civil Rights, 1965–1966, Part I, reel 17, *Civil Rights during the Johnson Administration, 1963–1969*; (quotes) Planning Session, Panel 4 (Health and Welfare) (17 Nov. 1965), pp. 69, 101, Records of the White House Conference on Civil Rights, 1965–1966, Part IV, reel 7:0443, *Civil Rights during the Johnson Administration, 1963–1969*.

up." With Medicare scheduled to begin in July 1966, HEW faced uneven compliance and little expectation of improvement. This suggested a number of options—including waiving Title VI for a specified period, cracking down on a few hospitals "as a demonstration that resistance will not be allowed [while], for the moment, ignor[ing] other noncompliance," or cutting off all noncompliant institutions.[50] HEW staked out a middle ground: it would not ignore its Title VI commitments, but it would also not allow them to compromise a smooth launch of Medicare. HEW scrambled to open other "federal beds" (such as those in VA hospitals) where local hospitals had either failed to comply or declined to participate (although, as Wilbur Cohen admitted, "the available beds in Federal facilities are clearly insufficient to make up for civil rights noncompliance"). And it cracked down on some of the more flagrantly segregated hospitals. But the department still lacked the staff, or any clear administrative procedures, to handle Title VI and (by its own admission) could only be "reactive to complaints."[51] Not surprisingly, the push for compliance often came from local activists who were willing to point out the chasm between federal law and local practice.[52]

HEW's interest in Title VI dissipated after the flurry of activity surrounding the implementation of Medicare and Medicaid. By late 1968 HEW celebrated a near 97 percent "commitment" to Title VI while admitting that its field reviews were meager and that "some hospitals and other medical facilities have reinstated some of their discriminatory prac-

---

[50] USCCR, *Title VI . . . One Year After: A Survey of Desegregation of Health and Welfare Services in the South* (1966), 14; (quote) Institute of Medicine, *Health Care in a Context of Civil Rights*, 24; (quote) Third Meeting of Civil Rights Staff (8 Apr. 1966), Box 299, Commissioner's Correspondence, 1936–1969, SSA Records; Swift to Ball (20 July 1966), Box 298, Commissioner's Correspondence, 1936–1969, SSA Records; unsigned memo for the president (29 June 1966), WHCF HE, Box 17, LBJ Papers; Douglas Cater, "Report on Hospital Civil Rights Compliance Efforts in the South" (18 June 1966), Part I (WHCF), reel 2:0902, *Civil Rights during the Johnson Administration, 1963–1969*; (quote) Murray to McKenna (26 Apr. 1966), Box 299, Commissioner's Correspondence (1936–1969), SSA Records; (quote) Confidential Memo for Robert Ball (7 Apr. 1966), Box 299, Commissioner's Correspondence, 1936–1969, SSA Records; (quote) Bryant to LBJ (23 May 1966), WHCF IS, Box 1, LBJ Papers; Bell to Owen (23 Dec. 1966) Box 298, Commissioner's Correspondence, 1936–1969, SSA Records.

[51] Cohen to LBJ (23 June 1966), WHCF IS, Box 1, LBJ Papers; Bell to Califano (18 Aug. 1966), Part I (WHCF), reel 3:0050, *Civil Rights during the Johnson Administration, 1963–1969*; (quote) HHH to LBJ (2 Feb. 1966), Part I (WHCF), reel 2:0792, *Civil Rights during the Johnson Administration, 1963–1969*; "Health Matters" (May 1966), p. 27, Files of the Chairman and Vice-Chairman, Records of the White House Conference on Civil Rights, 1965–1966, Part IV, reel 4:0834, *Civil Rights during the Johnson Administration, 1963–1969*.

[52] Mississippi Freedom Democratic Party Handbill (March 1966); Mississippi Hospital Association to Administrators (18 Mar. 1966), both in Box 299, Commissioner's Correspondence, 1936–1969, SSA Records.

tices." Indeed, HEW routinely fielded testimony to the persistence of "white" and "colored" entrances, separate waiting rooms, and uneven service in hospitals that had assured the department of their compliance. HEW cut its own compliance staff each year and increasingly delegated the task to state agencies. For his part, incoming HEW secretary Wilbur Cohen saw civil rights as only one of many sectional and political considerations and considered HEW's Office of Civil Rights an obstacle to congressional appropriations and program growth. Strict enforcement of Title VI was rare. HEW's first formal hearing regarding a hospital that had agreed to comply but failed to do so came late in 1967, and it was not until 1969 that HEW's Office of Civil Rights issued guidelines for providers and hospitals. In turn, the Office of Civil Rights was chronically understaffed and its field officers rarely "possessed the combination of attributes—program knowledge, investigative skill, commitment to the objectives of Title VI, and an understanding of its legal requirements— which a compliance officer should have to do an adequate job."[53] Not surprisingly, assessments of HEW's record have been uniformly dismal. As a consequence of bureaucratic indifference and meager resources, noted the Commission on Civil Rights in 1970, "Title VI has failed to match the laws' promise." A year later, a follow-up report cited "grossly inadequate performance" and concluded that the deficiencies "were so extensive as virtually to nullify the impact of the important civil rights laws enacted over the last decade and to make a mockery of the efforts of the many men and women who have fought for civil rights."[54]

Race, Health, and Welfare since 1965

Beyond the battle over hospital segregation, Great Society reformers tended to harden or underscore racial inequity even as they attempted to overcome it. This was certainly true of Medicare and Medicaid, which

[53] USCCR, *Federal Civil Rights Enforcement Effort* (1971), 11; Berkowitz, *Mr. Social Security,* 178; USCCR, *HEW and Title VI,* 8–11, 46–47; Wing and Rose, "Health Facilities and the Enforcement of Civil Rights," 247–48; Rose to Bell (23 June 1967), and "Summary of Actions taken by DHEW" (9 June 1967), Part I (WHCF), reel 3:0578, *Civil Rights during the Johnson Administration, 1963–1969;* Institute of Medicine, *Health Care in a Context of Civil Rights,* 141–43; USCCR, *Federal Civil Rights Enforcement Effort—1974,* 206–8; (quote) USCCR, *HEW and Title VI,* 16. For examples of segregation, see testimony of Helen Randle, USCCR, *Hearings in Montgomery, Alabama* (Apr. 1968), 291; USCCR, *Title VI . . . One Year After: A Survey of Desegregation of Health and Welfare Services in the South* (1966), 7–9; USCCR, *Report on New York City: Health Facilities* (May 1964), 11.

[54] USCCR, *The Federal Civil Rights Enforcement Effort* (1970), 805; USCCR, *The Federal Civil Rights Enforcement Effort—One Year Later* (1971), 11, 130; USCCR, *Federal Title VI Enforcement to Ensure Nondiscrimination in Federal Programs* (1996), 13–17.

replicated the New Deal's racially loaded distinction between contributory and charitable programs. In turn, as Michael Brown has shown, the Great Society routinely balanced its fiscal anxieties and its universal pretensions by targeting African Americans directly (through the Civil Rights Act) or indirectly (through urban antipoverty programs). In the absence of either universal social programs or equal access to private social programs, this strategy "put blacks in the position of defending the very programs that allowed white Americans to cultivate the most invidious prejudices . . . and allowed white Americans to sublimate white advantage in the welfare state to black dependence and individual failure." Hemmed in by white racism and budgetary restraint, the Johnson administration increasingly echoed the GOP of the 1940s in its preference for targeted, means-tested programs as a means of protecting both contributory programs and the public purse.[55]

In many respects, the Great Society was over before it began. Having finally fleshed out the skeletal welfare state established in 1935, postwar liberalism almost immediately lost the economic underpinnings, the intellectual momentum, and the political credibility that had made the Johnson administration's innovations in health, welfare, education, and civil rights possible. By 1966 economic and budgetary fallout from the Vietnam War had begun to erode the Great Society's expansionary fiscal logic. By 1968 the administration was in full retreat on both fronts, and the incoming Nixon administration inherited the unbridled optimism of Johnson's domestic and international policies and an economy that could no longer sustain either. The political impact was immediate and devastating. Willfully misinterpreting economic decline as a consequence of high wages and excessive government spending, business interests pushed both Democrats and Republicans to the right and created a new political consensus that turned the logic of growth politics inside out. The politics of decline, rooted in the 1970s and most fully expressed after 1980, focused its efforts on disciplining labor, paring social spending, restraining inflation, and dismantling economic regulation.[56]

With the collapse of the Great Society came a dramatic erosion of the political legitimacy of the welfare state. In part, this reflected a budgetary backlash; a conviction that excessive social spending was both a marker of big government liberalism run amok and a contributor to fiscal woes. Such sentiments were buttressed after 1980 by the intellectual elabora-

[55] Brown, *Race, Money, and the American Welfare State,* 205–34, 260–61, 290–92 (quote at 201–2).

[56] David Gordon, "Chickens Home to Roost: From Prosperity to Stagnation in the Postwar U.S. Economy," in *Understanding American Economic Decline,* ed. Michael Bernstein and David Adler (New York, 1994), 34–76; Joel Rogers and Joshua Cohen, "Reaganism after Reagan," *Socialist Review* (1988): 392–403.

tion of the "white popular wisdom" that welfare spending not only wasted tax dollars but also bred the very poverty and dependency it purported to address. In part this view reflected the persistence of a distinction between contributory and charitable programs. In welfare-reform debates before and after 1980, social insurance programs (Social Security and Medicare) remained sacrosanct while local, state, and federal politicians took aim at welfare programs (AFDC and Medicaid). And in part this view reflected the disproportionate presence of African Americans on the rolls of AFDC and Medicaid. Just as the legitimacy of the early welfare state rested on its exclusion of African Americans, the illegitimacy of the modern welfare state rested on their inclusion. Social programs became more racially inclusive through the 1960s as continued black migration north, the efforts of state and urban politicians to lay claim to federal funds, and a welfare rights movement dramatically narrowed the administrative discretion of state and local officials. But inclusion bred resentment as both welfare programs designed around the needs of white women and their children and poverty programs aimed at the Great Society's "Appalachian poster child" were populated instead by a racial underclass. Even as racial tensions generally seemed to ease, welfare spending became a lightning rod for anxieties about the behavior of that underclass and its claim on public resources.[57]

As federal support for means-tested, grant-based assistance programs waned, so did the enthusiasm of local authorities and providers for participating in them. Southern and urban interests accustomed to controlling public relief began to chafe at federal oversight, leading to a string of local challenges (most famously Louisiana's renewed enforcement of "suitable home" provisions in 1960, and Newburgh, New Jersey's effort to institute work requirements and penalize "welfare mothers"). This local backlash accelerated in the late 1960s, as the promise of federal largesse no longer restrained parochial resentment. Its own budgetary anxieties aside, the Johnson administration saw clear "anti-Negro overtones" in a 1967 congressional freeze on income levels for federal matching of local AFDC and Medicaid spending.[58] Various incarnations of a "new federalism" (invoked by every administration since the late 1960s) moved to cap federal spending and pass responsibility to state and local government. The impact on Medicaid was particularly dramatic as states were squeezed by both federal retreat and health care inflation. As a

---

[57] Gareth Davies, *From Opportunity to Entitlement: The Transformation and Decline of Great Society Liberalism* (Lawrence, Kans., 1996), 46–47, 58–59; Eileen Boris, "The Racialized Gendered State: Constructions of Citizenship in the United States," *Social Politics* (Summer 1995): 164–66; Lieberman, *Shifting the Color Line*, 5.

[58] Gardner to LBJ (11 Dec. 1967), Box 51, Califano Office Files, LBJPL; Lieberman, *Shifting the Color Line*, 150–61, 169.

consequence, states routinely cut services and pinched payments to providers: particularly in poorer states, Medicaid covered less, providers
were less willing to participate, and meaningful health reform was less
likely.[59] The state response to cuts in federal spending and the dismantling of federal standards re-created a welfare system in which regional
variations and local administration reinforce rather than challenge the
intersection of race and class.

Even where federal standards and responsibilities remained un-
changed, federal interests in maintaining them began to slip in the late
1960s and collapsed almost completely after 1980. This was the case, for
example, for Title VI enforcement, a task that was distracted in the mid-
1960s by the higher priority given to a smooth launch for Medicare and
undermined, beginning in the early 1970s, by political and budgetary
pressures. HEW's Health Civil Rights Branch pressed the department to
use Title VI to desegregate southern hospitals but made little headway—
indeed the acting chief of the Civil Rights Branch left in 1969 to help
the National Health Law Program launch a series of class-action suits
against HEW and delinquent hospitals. Legal challenges did press HEW
to clarify its obligations. In the wake of *Cook v. Ochsner* (1972), a case
involving discrimination at a New Orleans hospital, HEW redrafted Hill-
Burton (requiring that hospitals either maintain an "open door" admis-
sions policy or provide uncompensated care at a rate that exceeded 3
percent of their operating costs or 10 percent of federal assistance) and
ultimately replaced it entirely with the National Health Planning Act of
1974—which, for the first time, required federally assisted hospitals to
accept Medicare and Medicaid patients.[60]

Cook v. Ochsner compelled HEW to do what it had proved reluctant to
do since 1965: monitor compliance with Title VI and take remedial action against noncompliant hospitals. Many hospitals entered into negotiations with HEW, but some dug in their heels—and the task of actually
terminating federal funding proved extraordinarily complex (especially

[59] Mettler, *Dividing Citizens*, 223–31; Bruce Vladeck, "The Design of Failure: Health Policy and the Structure of Federalism," *JHPPL* 4:3 (1979): 524–27; Dana Hughes and Zoe
Clayson, "The Debate Is in the States," *Health/PAC Bulletin* (Summer 1990), 5; Wendy Parmet, "Regulation and Federalism: Legal Impediments to State Health Care Reform," *American Journal of Law and Medicine* 29:1 (1993): 121–44; Colleen Grogan, "Hope in Federalism?
What Will the States Do and What Are They Likely To Do?" *JHPPL* 20:2 (1995): 477–83;
Thomas Anton, "New Federalism and Intergovernmental Relationships: The Implications
for Health Policy," *JHPPL* 22:3 (1997): 698.

[60] Paul-Shaheen and Perlstadt, "Class Action Suits and Social Change," 386–99; Cook v.
Ochsner Foundation Hospital, Civ. A No. 70–1969; Institute of Medicine, *Health Care in a
Context of Civil Rights*, 14–15, 148–53; Rose, "Federal Regulation of Services to the Poor,"
168–70; Sara Rosenbaum et al., "Civil Rights in a Changing Health Care System," *HA* 16:1
(1997): 94; Wing, "The Community Service Obligation," 615–16.

as the administrative law judges who heard the cases proved sympathetic to the argument, made routinely by hospitals, that racial imbalances in admission reflected patterns of economic discrimination beyond the hospitals' control). HEW moved again to stiffen its community service provisions in 1979, adopting regulations (challenged by the AHA and the AMA as a threat to freedom of contract) that forbade admission denials based on insurance status, ability to pay, or professional privileges. By the late 1970s, however, the effect of HEW's new standards was almost entirely vitiated by a continued reluctance to enforce them. Both local authorities and HEW tread lightly out of concern for the financial health of the hospitals. And in any case, the resources available for compliance fell steadily through the 1970s (HEW estimated in 1977 that barely 5 percent of its compliance resources went to health care) and all but disappeared after 1980 when HEW split and the new Department of Education claimed what was left of the Civil Rights Branch. The Clinton administration promised to revitalize the Office of Civil Rights, but staffing never reached half of 1981 levels, though complaints increased steadily.[61]

Over time, a combination of black activism, urban and demographic change, and federal programs did nevertheless integrate the nation's hospitals, and in a manner that proved less contentious and violent than parallel efforts in education or public accommodations. Title VI gave the federal government considerable clout, and hospitals considerable incentive, to desegregate. Hospital boards were, for the most part, more insulated from local political pressures than were local politicians or school boards. Steady migration north undermined the conditions that had sustained health segregation. And increased employment of professional and nonprofessional blacks in the modern hospital rendered the logic of segregation less and less tenable. But such progress was muted by the persistence of discrimination in other forms and the persistence of disparate outcomes for black Americans. "The more visible symbols of Jim Crow disappeared quickly," David Barton Smith suggests, "but the underlying structures were more resistant to change." Where Title VI was more difficult to invoke, in nursing homes or private practice, progress was slower.[62] And where Title VI did apply, its enforcement was further

[61] Institute of Medicine, *Health Care in a Context of Civil Rights*, 148–53, 174–84; Wing, "The Community Service Obligation," 581; Mitchell Rice, "Hospital/Health Facilities and the Hill-Burton Obligations: A Secret from the Black Community," *Urban League Review* 9:2 (1985–86): 40; USCCR, *Federal Title VI Enforcement to Ensure Nondiscrimination in Federal Programs* (1996), 611–12; Rose, "Federal Regulation of Services to the Poor," 198–99; Note, "Title VI Challenges by Private Parties to the Location of Health Facilities," *Boston College Law Review* 37:517 (1996); Smith, "Addressing Racial Inequalities in Health Care," 86–89.

[62] McBride, *Integrating the City of Medicine*, 3–5, 171–73; Smith, "Addressing Racial Inequalities in Health Care," 79 (quote), 83–87; Quadagno, "How Medicare Promoted Racial Integration," 32–33.

complicated by the changing nature of segregation and discrimination in the delivery of health services.

By the 1980s the attention of civil rights advocates had shifted from Jim Crow to less-formal patterns of segregation, particularly concerning the impact of closing or moving urban hospitals. Although other elements of civil rights law (including Title VII protection against employment discrimination) covered both intentional and adverse impact discrimination, Title VI remained ambiguous on the latter point. This was especially important in the case of health care, because of the variety of "facially neutral" but effectively discriminatory means of sorting patients by race. Through the late 1970s and early 1980s, civil rights activists lost a series of adverse impact cases—including *Bryan v. Koch* (1980), concerning the closing of a public hospital in New York City, and *NAACP et al. v. Wilmington Medical Center* (1981), concerning the suburbanization of a Wilmington, Delaware, hospital. In health care, as in other arenas of social provision, the accomplishments of the Great Society were blunted or frustrated by the retreat (first fiscal, later ideological) of federal power, the persistence of economic segregation and discrimination, and the accompanying tendency to identify the welfare state less and less with its broader goals and more and more with the race and gender of its beneficiaries.[63]

As secular Reaganism displaced the Great Society, the racial gap in health and health provision began to widen again. Indeed the problems identified in the late 1960s (including the uneven availability of basic services, discrimination in the provision of those services, popular and political suspicions about "welfare medicine," and the fiscal anxieties generated by health inflation) persisted into the 1990s.[64] Part of the problem lay in the economic and spatial discrimination that had always lurked behind the edifice of Jim Crow. The collapse of the postwar American city had enormous implications for the health of those who lived there.

[63] "Title VI Challenges by Private Parties to the Location of Health Facilities," 518–23; Sidney Watson, "Reinvigorating Title VI: Defending Health Care Shouldn't Be So Easy," *Fordham Law Review* 58 (1990): 941–42, 948–54, 966–68, 971–73; Institute of Medicine, *Health Care in a Context of Civil Rights*, 145–48; "The Inner City Hospital Battle," *The Nation* 230 (15 Mar. 1980), 301–2; Bryan v. Koch 627 F. 2d 1980; NAACP v. Wilmington Medical Center 460 U.S. 1052 103 S.C. 1499; Wing and Rose, "Health Facilities and the Enforcement of Civil Rights"; Michael Byrd and Linda Clayton, "The 'Slave Health Deficit': Racism and Health Outcomes," *Health/PAC Bulletin* 21:2 (Summer 1991): 25–26.

[64] McBride, "From Community Health Care to Crisis Medicine," 330–1; "Health" (May 1966): 2–5, Files of the Chairman and Vice-Chairman, Records of the White House Conference on Civil Rights, 1965–1966, Part IV, reel 4:0834, *Civil Rights during the Johnson Administration, 1963–1969*; Nancy McKenzie and Ellen Bilofsky, "Shredding the Safety Net," *Health/PAC Bulletin* 21:2 (Summer 1991): 6, 8; Thomas Brooks, "The Political Agenda of Health Care for African Americans," *Journal of Health Care for the Poor and Underserved* 8:3 (1997): 377–81; USCCR, *Federal Civil Rights Enforcement Effort—1974*, 116–18; "The Emerging Health Apartheid in the United States," *Health/PAC Bulletin* (Summer 1991): 3–4.

Economic decline and white flight contributed not only to high unemployment (and little stable access to private social provision) and declining public services (including health facilities and health professionals)
but to a heightened (and largely unmet) need for basic health services.[65]

This "emerging health apartheid," as one critic dubbed it, was reflected in and reinforced by the institutions of health provision. Medicare and Medicaid mirrored the political and racial distinctions between
Social Security and welfare; in each case, the latter was presumptively
less legitimate and under attack through the 1980s and 1990s.[66] At the
same time Medicaid has proved a remarkably ragged extension of the
welfare system, reaching between one-third and one-half of the poor but
failing altogether where private providers decline to participate. Private
coverage also lagged badly for African Americans and Latinos, especially
as the managed care revolution brought together two actors—private
insurers and private employers—with deep histories of discrimination.
While HMOs and insurers eroded the doctor's freedom to select patients
(and hence to discriminate), they also multiplied the "point of entry"
discrimination (financial barriers, location of facilities, choice of providers) routinely faced by poorer patients.[67]

All of this was accompanied by the new politics of social provision,
which, beginning in the late 1970s and running through the "end of
welfare as we knew it" in 1996, turned the gender assumptions of social
policy inside out (using welfare to press mothers into the labor market
rather than protecting them from it) and hardened a pathological explanation for poverty and dependency. In this political atmosphere, civil
rights were increasingly crowded out by a new ethic of individual responsibility: "Civil Rights have a unique meaning in this country," argued one
of Reagan's civil rights appointees. "People do not have a constitutional
right to health care . . . any more than a farmer has a constitutional right

[65] Gary Orfield, "Race and the Liberal Agenda: The Loss of the Integrationist Dream,
1965–1974," in *The Politics of Social Policy in the United States,* ed. Weir, Orloff, and Skocpol,
315–17; McBride, "From Community Health Care to Crisis Medicine," 330; Chamber of
Commerce, "Improving Our Nation's Health Care System: Proposals for the 1970s" (1971),
Box II:27, Chamber of Commerce Papers, Hagley Museum; testimony of Dr. Nobel Guthrie
(Shelby County Health Department) in USCCR, *Hearings in Memphis* (June 1962), 23.

[66] Helen Slessarev, "Racial Tensions and Institutional Support: Social Programs during
a Period of Retrenchment," in *The Politics of Social Policy in the United States,* ed. Weir, Orloff,
and Skocpol, 258.

[67] Sara Rosenbaum et al., "Civil Rights in a Changing Health Care System," *HA* 16:1
(1997): 97–100; Hersch and Means, "Employer-Sponsored Health and Pension Benefits,"
851–55; McKenzie and Bilofsky, "Shredding the Safety Net," 6–7; McBride, "From Community Health Care to Crisis Medicine," 326–28; Mitchell Rice and Woodrow Jones, "Black
Health Care in an Era of Retrenchment Politics," in *Contemporary Public Policy Perspectives
and Black Americans,* ed. Rice and Jones (Westport, Conn., 1984), 157.

to a tobacco subsidy or Chrysler to a bailout." Racially disparate measures of public health were increasingly understood in cultural terms: Clinton-era reformers noted the widening racial gap in mortality, but argued that "one should look toward the patient population as the source of the problem." And the consequences of a history of economic injustice and uneven social provision were increasingly held up as arguments against public solutions: "When you compare our country to Canada," the AMA's James Todd reasoned in 1992, "we have a very different demography. We have more violence. We have more drugs. We have more poverty . . . because we don't have a homogenous population, you would intuitively expect our health care expenditures to be greater."[68]

The discrimination that runs through the history of health provision in twentieth-century America is important and telling. It offers a compelling case study of the interaction of race and region in U.S. social policy. In this respect, American health provision has been both ordinary and exceptional. Like other facets of social policy, health care in the twentieth century was shaped by a combination of direct and indirect discrimination, southern recalcitrance and local administration, the uneasy intersection of public and private (job-based) benefits, and the sharp political distinctions routinely drawn between contributory and charitable programs. Unlike other facets of social policy, health care was also shaped by a tangle of private interests—hospitals, insurers, doctors, medical societies—who were both directly responsible for the delivery of services and marked by their own distinct relationships to Jim Crow and its aftermath. All of this offers at least a partial explanation for the failure of national health insurance in the United States. Health provision always sat uncomfortably against the employment basis of public and private provision—indeed, the most compelling public health issue during the formative years of the American welfare state was the dismal status of rural (and especially southern) services. Because the logic of health insurance was necessarily more universal, and because health care was delivered in institutional settings, it also posed a more direct threat to the southern racial order. Accordingly, southern interests rebuffed the expansion of federal health programs and forced reformers to retreat to meager and deeply racialized alternatives: job-based private insurance, locally administered subsidies for hospital construction, and penurious charitable programs for those left behind.

<hr/>

[68] Morris Abrams quoted in Charles V. Hamilton, "Social Policy and the Welfare Rights of Black Americans," *Political Science Quarterly* 101:2 (1986): 247; John Feibel to Ira Magaziner (1 Feb. 1993), Box 600, Records of the Clinton Health Care Task Force, National Archives College Park, Md.; Todd testimony in House Committee on Ways and Means, *Hearings: President's Proposals on Health Care Reform* 102:2 (Mar. 1992), 419.

6

Private Interests and Public Policy: Health Care's Corporate Compromise

DEMOCRATIC capitalism sets capitalist boundaries around democratic rule (and vice versa). This logic is exaggerated in its American setting, which invites economic influence and organizes political competition around investments in parties and candidates. The absence of a social democratic tradition and the weakness of state institutions both reflect this pattern of economic influence and contribute to it. The federal system exaggerates the clout of economic interests, which are able to play political jurisdictions off against one another. Over time, the political status of economic interests has yielded considerable cultural clout as well. All of this has had a direct political effect: powerful economic interests throttle popular reform efforts that might otherwise threaten them. It has had a chilling effect: legislators narrow debate to ensure that important patrons are not displeased. And it has had an administrative effect: economic interests capture public policy in order to minimize the costs of state intervention or turn it to their advantage.[1]

Health interests have employed a variety of strategies in the long, episodic debate over national health insurance. Most commonly and crassly, they have simply outspent reformers. The AMA emerged as one of the first powerful political lobbies and has persistently led the pack in direct and indirect political spending. Because medical societies controlled licensing, consulting, and admitting privileges, they not only maintained a stable dues-paying membership but were also able to chill provider participation in group practice experiments.[2] Other interests emerged

[1] Charles Lindblom, "The Market as a Prison," *Journal of Politics* 44 (1982): 324–36; Thomas Ferguson, *Golden Rule: The Investment Theory of Party Competition and the Logic of Money-Driven Political Systems* (Chicago, 1995), 3–110, 17–172; Sanford Jacoby, "American Exceptionalism Revisited: The Importance of Management," in *Masters to Managers: Historical and Comparative Perspectives on American Employers*, ed. Sanford Jacoby (New York, 1991), 173–87; Colin Gordon, "Why No Corporatism in the United States? Business Disorganization and Its Consequences," *Business and Economic History* 27:1 (1998): 29–46.

[2] Oliver Garceau, *The Political Life of the American Medical Association* (Hamden, Conn., 1961), 103–11; Michael Davis, "Restrictions on Free Enterprise in Medicine" (Apr. 1949), Box 43 (0.11.4), Office of the Administrator, General Classified Files [GCF], 1944–1950, Federal Security Agency, Records of the Department of Health, Education, and Welfare [HEW], RG 235, National Archives, College Park, Md.; Frank Kennedy, "The American Medical Association: Power, Purpose, and Politics in Organized Medicine," *Yale Law Journal*

as their stakes in the health system grew. Hospitals became increasingly important as changes in medical practice magnified the importance of the institutional provision of health care, and as hospitalization insurance or capital funding emerged as an alternative to national health insurance. Hospitals often joined the AMA in defense of private provision, but their economic fate (and political activity) was much more intertwined with that of private insurers, the nonprofit Blues, employers, and (especially after 1965) government. The commercial insurance industry emerged as an influential political actor once it began offering group health plans in the 1930s and 1940s. For their part, some employers supported the emergence of employment-based insurance (although they increasingly resented its costs), after which health politics were shaped by their relationship with unions, hospitals, and insurers.

In a polity in which economic interests enjoy profound political advantages, innovations in social policy have always been difficult—and often succeeded only when they promised to even out competitive disparities, ensure social stability, or socialize private costs. American health politics offers a telling glimpse of these patterns of economic influence, but this story is not one in which private interests merely dig in against public solutions. Unlike other facets of social policy, health care has been controlled by a vast and complex private industry. Public policy has confronted a tangle of interests whose shared distrust of the state veiled considerable disagreement over the virtues of private health care and the promise of political solutions. The result, as observers of the modern health debate have noted, has been an uneasy "corporate compromise" among employers, insurers, doctors, and hospitals.[3]

Medical Politics before the New Deal: Interests versus Reform, 1910–1932

The 1914–1920 AALL debate sparked an uncertain response, largely because doctors were initially divided over the issue of public health insurance and employers and insurers were not yet involved in health provision in any serious way. The AMA initially hoped that the AALL plan would buttress doctors' incomes, but drifted into opposition when it became apparent that it might cap those incomes.[4] Before 1920 local medi-

---

63 (1954): 939–50; Memoranda on Attitudes of the AMA (10 Feb. 1944), Box 45:284, Series II, Isidore Falk Papers, Sterling Library, Yale University, New Haven, Conn.

[3] David Himmelstein and Steffie Woolhander, "The Corporate Compromise: A Marxist View of Health Policy," *Monthly Review* (May 1990): 14, 20–22.

[4] "Recommendations on Health Insurance" (n.d.), Box 4 (Mss 400), Arthur J. Altmeyer Papers, State Historical Society of Wisconsin [SHSW], Madison, Wis.; Ronald Num-

cal societies still wielded most of the political clout in the AMA, and the national organization had not yet emerged (as AMA officials projected hopefully) as a "compact organism, whose power to influence public sentiment will be almost unlimited, and whose requests for desirable legislation will everywhere be met with that respect which the politician always has for organized votes." While AMA leadership flirted with the idea of reform, state and local medical societies staked out what would become the profession's stock positions, including a deep distrust of "contract" practice and resistance to the intrusion of any third party in the patient-physician relationship.[5]

Employers were also ambivalent. Some were attracted by the Progressive promise of tying health care to industrial efficiency. Some argued that if health insurance was to be considered, "such insurance cannot be made general in its application without some form of compulsion"; that "to be equitable and reasonable and effective, health insurance should be national in scope: it should be compulsory." But most argued that the AALL bill tied health care too closely to employment, placing "the burden on the employer of things which are not his fault." In this sense, the AALL's business supporters demanded that the costs of coverage be spread among all firms, while its business opponents argued for a broader public health program and scored the limited coverage of employment-based benefits.[6]

The decisive influence through 1915–1920 was wielded by the insurance industry. Although the AALL posed no direct threat to commercial health insurance, its draft bill did threaten to shut insurers out of the lucrative market for burial insurance. Insurers feared the precedent of compulsory state programs and the socialization of other lines of cover-

---

bers,"The Specter of Socialized Medicine," in *Compulsory Health Insurance: The Continuing American Debate*, ed. Ronald Numbers (Westport, Conn., 1982), 5–8, 12–14; "The Doctor's Future in Relation to National Medical Insurance" *JAMA* (11 Jan. 1913): 153.

[5] James G. Burrow, *AMA: Voice of American Medicine* (Baltimore, 1963), 139–51; Donald Madison, "Preserving Individualism in the Organizational Society: 'Cooperation' and American Medical Practice, 1900–1920," *BHM* 70:3 (1996): 455–56 (AMA quote at 450); David Moss, *Socializing Security: Progressive-Era Economists and the Origins of American Social Policy* (Cambridge, Mass., 1996), 144–45; "Memorandum re Doctors" (1918), reel 63, American Association for Labor Legislation [AALL] Papers (microfilm); notes on informal joint meeting (1916), reel 62, AALL Papers; Margarett Hobbs, "History of the Health Insurance Movement in America" (1919), reel 63, AALL Papers.

[6] "Recent American Opinion in Favor of Health Insurance," *ALLR* 6 (1916): 345–52; Margaret Stecker, "A Critical Analysis of the Standard Bill for Compulsory Health Insurance" (1920?), untitled testimony (Mar. 1919), Box V:9; Seventh Meeting of the National Industrial Conference Board [NICB] (21 Dec. 1916), all in NICB Papers, Hagley Museum and Library, Wilmington, Del.; "European Employers Find that Health Insurance Pays" (1911), reel 62; "Memorandum on the Action of the Manufacturers' Associations" (1916), and "Notes on Hearings on Mills Health Insurance Bill" (1917), reel 62, AALL Papers.

age. The AALL bills, as one New York office warned its agents, "would mean an end to all insurance companies and agents and to you personally the complete wrecking of the business and connections you have spent a lifetime in building and the loss of your bread and butter." Major insurers (led by Prudential and Metropolitan) established the Insurance Economics Society (IES) in 1917, and the IES, in turn, financed state and local anti-AALL coalitions. The opposition, as one reformer put it, was simply "better organized and financed." State health commissions invariably approached the problem as one of appealing to the demands and anxieties of those with the time and resources to dominate hearings—a process by which "commercial opposition," one critic noted, always won out. The IES outflanked and outspent the AALL in a brief pamphlet war. Insurers convinced employers that the AALL plan was actuarially unsound, used their clout in the National Civic Federation to silence liberal employers, and pressed the AMA to consider the professional implications of state medicine.[7]

After 1920, health interests hardened their positions. Scattered experiments in company medical care aside, employers saw health insurance as neither a pressing issue nor a viable aspect of welfare capitalism. Insurers remained leery of federal intervention, while continuing to consider health care an uninsurable moral hazard. Organized medicine dug in against public programs, refining its methods for defeating them, and, by decade's end, emerged as a much more powerful and active political force. At the top of the AMA's agenda was the pursuit, as Robyn Muncy puts it, of an "uncompromisingly exclusive, profit-seeking, elitist, professional code." This was starkly apparent, for example, in the AMA's opposition to Sheppard-Towner. At the program's passage in 1921, the AMA was relatively inactive while state health officers and the AMA's own pediatrics section supported the law. As the 1920s wore on, however, the political emergence of the AMA and the experience of private physicians under Sheppard-Towner solidified the AMA's fears. AMA delegates voted to oppose Sheppard-Towner in 1922 and, in a deeply gendered cam-

[7] Moss, *Socializing Security*, 138–39, 148–50, 55 (insurer quoted at 146, reformer at 150); Daniel Rodgers, *Atlantic Crossings: Social Politics in a Progressive Age* (Cambridge, Mass., 1998), 261–65; Lee Frankel, "Some Fundamental Considerations in Health Insurance," in U.S. Department of Labor, *Proceedings of the Conference on Social Insurance*, Bureau of Labor Statistics Bulletin 212 (Washington, D.C., 1917), 599–601; Hobbs, "History of the Health Insurance Movement"; John Lapp, "The Findings of Official Health Insurance Commissions," *ALLR* 10 (1920): 27–31; Forrest Walker, "Compulsory Health Insurance: 'The Next Great Step in Social Legislation,' " *JAH* 56 (1969): 302; (quote) New York State League of Women Voters, "Report and Protest . . . New York League for Americanism, Box 209, Edwin Witte Papers, SHSW; Memorandum for Dr. Lambert (1919), reel 63, AALL Papers; Frederick Hoffman, *Facts and Fallacies of Compulsory Health Insurance* (Newark, N.J., 1917), 7–12.

paign of local noncooperation and legislative opposition, pressed the Senate to kill the program outright in 1929.[8]

The AMA also took aim at others (unions, rural cooperatives, hospitals) who threatened to displace fee-for-service care with "contract medicine." In these campaigns, organized medicine drew cynically on a variety of conflicting notions: at times defending physicians as professionals facing the commercialism of contract practice; at times defending physicians as entrepreneurs facing the "unfair competition" of mass-production medicine. Over the course of the 1920s the AMA retreated from its rigid defense of fee-for-service care, by separating the issue of group payment from the thornier issue of group practice. Doctors were willing to countenance schemes that prepaid or insured fee-for-service care, but dug in against "fee splitting" (paying more than one doctor on the same bill) or capitation plans (providing care for an annual fee). State medical societies continued to penalize those who participated in contract plans—expelling maverick doctors, denying admitting privileges, and in one case, dissolving the county medical society entirely in order to reincorporate without the offending physicians.[9]

The final issue to galvanize medical politics before the New Deal was the 1932 report of the Committee on the Costs of Medical Care. While the report was not accompanied by any legislative proposals, it served as a lightning rod for organized medicine and provoked a dramatic display of the AMA's power. The private doctors on the CCMC drafted a blistering minority report, condemning the majority's cautious interest in group insurance and suggesting that "government care of the indigent be expanded with the ultimate objective of relieving the medical profession of this burden." The AMA also took aim at the foundations that had funded the CCMC. In a stark indication of organized medicine's economic clout, the AMA attacked the Milbank Fund by boycotting Borden products (fund president Albert Milbank was chair of the Borden

[8] Starr, *The Social Transformation of American Medicine* (New York, 1982), 260–72; Madison, "Preserving Individualism," 458–60; Burrow, *AMA: Voice of American Medicine,* 157–58, 160–64; Robyn Muncy, *Creating a Female Dominion in American Reform, 1890–1935* (New York, 1991), 135–42 (quote at 136); Douglas Parks, "Expert Inquiry and Health Care Reform in New Era America: Herbert Hoover, Ray Lyman Wilbur, and the Travails of the Disinterested Experts" (Ph.D. diss., University of Iowa, 1994), 104–8; Theda Skocpol, *Protecting Soldiers and Mothers: The Political Origins of American Social Policy* (Cambridge, Mass., 1992), 501–2; Molly Ladd-Taylor, *Mother-Work: Women, Child-Welfare, and the State, 1890–1930* (Urbana, Ill., 1994), 170–75, 184–86; "Federalization of Health and Hygiene through Sheppard Towner-ism," *JAMA* 98:5 (1932): 404–5.

[9] "Excerpts from CCMC Minority Report" (31 Oct. 1932), Box 4 (Mss 400), Altmeyer Papers; William Burns, "The Michigan Enabling Act for Non-Profit Medical Care Plans," *Law and Contemporary Problems* 6:4 (Winter 1931), 559–63; Starr, *Transformation of American Medicine,* 200–25, 272; "Cooperative Hospital," *The Nation* 174 (2 Feb. 1928): 12.

board of directors, and nearly half of the fund's income came from Borden stock). This pressure both diluted the CCMC's final report (although not enough to assuage the AMA) and led to the abrupt dismissal of Milbank's executive secretary, John Kingsbury.[10]

The Limits of the New Deal: Interests versus Reform, 1932–1940

Through the 1920s and early 1930s, organized medicine emerged as the most important and influential opponent of both public health insurance proposals and private experiments in group medicine. The Depression dramatically raised these stakes, both by exacerbating uneven access to health care and by raising the specter of new federal health programs. For the AMA, the economic crisis brought with it the prospect of both popular demands for public health insurance and a "sort of mental panic" among "physicians . . . willing to embrace almost any scheme which holds out promises of a more definite financial return."[11]

Although its political power would not fully emerge until the 1940s, the AMA and its affiliates exercised political and economic influence in a number of ways. Medical societies continued to act as trade associations with real teeth, willing and able to revoke the privileges of members who participated in group practice experiments. Such tactics were so widespread they caught the attention of the Justice Department and led to a series of antitrust prosecutions in the late 1930s and early 1940s.[12] At the same time the AMA retreated from its opposition to any form of

[10] Frank Dickinson, "A Brief History of the Attitude of the American Medical Association toward Voluntary Health Insurance," *AMA Bulletin*, no. 70 (1952), 8–13; CCMC, *Medical Care for the American People* (Chicago, 1932), 172 (quote); Falk to Kingsbury (2 Apr. 1932), Box 38:120, Series II, Falk Papers; Starr, *Transformation of American Medicine*, 272; notes on conversation with Falk (12 Aug. 1935), Box 208, Witte Papers; Falk memo of phone conversation with Milbank (26 Sept. 1934), Box 39:132, Series II, Falk Papers; James Rorty, "The Case of John A. Kingsbury," *The Nation* 142 (24 June 1936): 801–2.

[11] AMA Bureau of Medical Economics, "Some Phases of Contract Practice" (1934), 27.

[12] James Rorty, "The Attack on Group Medicine," *The Nation* 143 (4 July 1936): 15; Rorty, "'Organized Medicine' Sees Red," *The Nation* 145 (6 Nov. 1937): 500–501; Kennedy, "The American Medical Association," 947–53, 988–90; Andrew and Hannah Biemiller, "Medical Rift in Milwaukee," *Survey Graphic* (Aug. 1938); Oliver Garceau, "Organized Medicine Enforces Its Party Line," *Public Opinion Quarterly* 4:3 (1940): 419–25; Department of Justice press release (1 Aug. 1938), Box 208, Witte Papers; Patricia Ward, "United States versus American Medical Association et al.: The Medical Antitrust Case of 1938–1943," *American Studies* 30:2 (1989): 123–53; Benjamin Raub, "The Antitrust Prosecution against the American Medical Association," *Law and Contemporary Problems* 6:4 (1939): 595–605; "Medicine and the Antitrust Act" (1941), Box J7:5, and "Presentation of the Government's Evidence" (n.d.), Box J11:4, Walton Hamilton Papers, Rare Books and Manuscripts, Tarlton Law Library, University of Texas, Austin, Tex.

group practice and pressed the passage of "Blue Shield" laws in most states that ensured that group practice would remain firmly under the control of the profession. "No measure opposed by the medical societies," one state legislator conceded, "had a chance of passage."[13] Organized medicine's clout rested on both the coercive character of the medical societies and the community of interest that the AMA established with advertisers (especially pharmaceutical companies) in its *Journal of the American Medical Association (JAMA)*. By the mid-1930s, *JAMA* pumped nearly a million dollars a year into the AMA's coffers. The AMA also began levying special fee assessments for the support of political lobbying and publicity. At a cost of about $700,000 a year, the AMA maintained a Bureau of Health Education, a Bureau of Legal Medicine and Legislation, and a Bureau of Medical Economics.[14]

The AMA's clout led the New Deal's Committee on Economic Security—which initially assumed that health insurance was the most promising of the proposed Social Security titles—to conclude glumly "that the design of a system of health insurance has limitations which are not inherent in the design of other systems of social insurance." The CES still clung to the "possibility that a program for health insurance reasonably acceptable to the medical profession might be worked out," but medical interests ensured that the committee would do little more than promise further study, encourage the development of private plans, and defer to the AMA and its allies.[15] The AMA objected to the staffing of the CES and its authority to even consider health insurance, and besieged the administration and Congress with "a barrage of letters and telegrams

[13] Burrow, *AMA: Voice of American Medicine*, 230–43; CNH, "Record of the American Medical Association" (May 1949), Box 209, Witte Papers; Dorothy Pearson, "The AMA Hedges," *The Nation* 148 (11 Feb. 1939), 171; New York legislator in *The Nation* 145 (18 Dec. 1937): 675.

[14] James Rorty, "Whose Medicine?" *The Nation* 143 (11 July 1936): 42–44; J. Mitchell Mores, "Medicine and Politics," *The Nation* 158 (10 June 1944): 677; "Minutes of the Special Session of the House of Delegates, Sept. 16–17, 1938," *JAMA* 111:13 (1938): 1200–1201; Kennedy, "The American Medical Association," 953–55; "The American Medical Association," *Fortune* 18:5 (Nov. 1938): 150; Daniel Hirshfield, *The Lost Reform: The Campaign for Compulsory Health Insurance in the United States from 1932 to 1943* (Cambridge, Mass., 1970), 33–35, 44–59; notes on conversations with Falk (12 Aug. 1935), Box 208, Witte Papers; Plumley Memorandum Re: NPC (23 Sept. 1943), Box 60:524, Series II, Falk Papers; Falk memo of phone conversation with Milbank (26 September 1934), Box 39:132, Series II, Falk Papers.

[15] (Quote) CES, Preliminary Report of the Staff of the CES (Sept. 1934), Box 70, Witte Papers; Appendix A, CES, "Final Report on Risks to Economic Security Arising out of Illness" (1935), Box 67, Witte Papers; Edwin Witte, *The Development of the Social Security Act* (Madison, Wis., 1963) quoted at 180; Medical Advisory Board to Witte (22 May 1935), Box 2, Altmeyer Papers; Proceedings of the Meeting of the Medical Advisory Board (29–30 Jan. 1935), p. 5, 215–17, Box 42:236, Series II, Falk Papers; Medical Advisory Board, Minutes of Meetings (29 Jan. 1935), p. 16, Box 67, Witte Papers.

from state and county medical societies." The White House complained that "telegraphic protests poured in upon the President . . . generally in batches from a particular section of the country and identical in wording." As the CES retreated, staffers noted that that "the kicks from the state medical societies appear to be dying down; at least we do not have to answer so many telegrams daily," although the mere mention of health insurance in the committee's final report was enough to "once more bring down the wrath of the opposition." As the CES was fine-tuning its final reports in mid-1935, health insurance was a dead letter. "We can't go up against the State Medical Societies," Roosevelt concluded. "We just can't do it."[16]

Some on the CES hoped that "the opposition of organized medicine groups, which may be significant when functioning as a whispering campaign, [would] dwindle in effectiveness when drawn into the open forum of legislative hearings and public discussion." But the AMA chilled debate before it ever reached that stage. With the CCMC experience in mind, CES members anticipated the AMA's reaction, sought to avoid confrontation from the outset, and assured doctors of their support for "the basic principle that the private practice of medicine . . . should be conserved and strengthened." Such deference made it difficult to envision any alternative to private practice and ultimately became an excuse for shelving the health title entirely. The administration even used its timidity in 1935 to assure the profession that the "Administration contemplates no action detrimental to their interests. . . . The action taken in the field of health as shown by the provisions of the splendid Social Security Act recently enacted is clear."[17]

[16] Summary Memoranda (n.d.), President's Official File [POF] 1086, Franklin Roosevelt Papers, Franklin D. Roosevelt Presidential Library [FDRPL], Hyde Park, N.Y.; "The Administration Studies Social Insurance," *JAMA* 103:8 (1934): 609–10; "The Conference on Economic Security," *JAMA* 103:21 (1934): 1624; (quote) Witte to West (21 Dec. 1934), Box 40, CES Records, RG 47, Social Security Administration [SSA], National Archives; Witte, *Development of the Social Security Act*, 174–88 (quotes at 174, 182); (quote) Memo for Altmeyer (29 Oct. 1934), Box 54, CES Records; Medical Advisory Board Minutes (29 Jan. 1935), pp. 20–31, Box 67, Witte Papers; Bureau of Research and Statistics, "Memorandum on Health Insurance" (1937), pp. 44–47, Box 34, Decimal 056, Chairman's File, Commissioners' Records, SSA Records; FDR quoted in Starr, *Transformation of American Medicine*, 279.

[17] (Quote) Michael Davis, "Some Relations between Health and Economic Security" (9 Oct. 1934), Box 18, CES Records, SSA Records; Witte, *Development of the Social Security Act*, 173–75, 188–89; Falk to Altmeyer (22 May 1935), Box 54, CES Records; CES, "Final Report on Risks to Economic Security Arising out of Illness" (1935), pp. 3, 32–36; Medical Advisory Board Minutes (30 Jan. 1935), 220; Abstract of a Program for Social Insurance against Illness" (1935), p. 21; Medical Advisory Board, Interim Report (Jan. 1935), all in Box 67, Witte Papers; (quote) FDR Address at Jersey City Medical Center (2 Oct. 1936), POF 511a; Memoranda in POF 1710:2, FDR Papers.

For the rest of the 1930s, the New Deal deferred to the AMA on the administration of health programs and the boundaries of prospective policy. New Dealers conceded that it was "unlikely (and probably unwise) that anything can be done along these lines without very considerable support from the medical profession." When the Interdepartmental Committee on Health and Welfare convened in 1938, the AMA lobbied successfully to strip serious consideration of health insurance from its deliberations. "Faced with the bitter opposition of organized vested interests—the medical and allied professions and the insurance companies," Abraham Epstein noted bitterly, "the aims of health insurance are today less known and less popular than they were twenty years ago." Some held out the hope that doctors might "eventually be led to demand compulsory health insurance in order to get away from the evils of voluntary arrangements not under government [or medical] control."[18] But at least through the 1930s, such arrangements were not widespread enough to encourage anyone to think seriously about socializing them, and doctors were able to police their "evils" through professional rather than political intervention. This was true, for example, of organized medicine's cooperation with the Farm Security Administration's health programs, which crept under the AMA's radar largely because they were so solicitous of local medical societies and because they addressed the impoverishment of rural practitioners alongside the needs of rural citizens. Other economic interests expressed little interest in the health insurance battle. Although some employers supported federal unemployment and pension law as a means of spreading the costs of private and state-level plans, there was little parallel incentive to socialize health insurance. Because, as *Business Week* noted, "the direct cost of medical care which [business] bears is not appreciable," business generally supported the AMA in its antitrust battles.[19] Commercial insurers, not yet extensively involved in health provision, remained on the sidelines.[20]

[18] AMA, "Report of the Reference Committee, Special Session House of Delegates" (16 Feb. 1935), Box 209, Witte Papers; (quote) Harris to Altmeyer (28 May 135), Box 54, CES Records; (quote) Witte, "Suggestions for Consideration to the Advisory Council" (1935), pp. 13–14, Box 65, Witte Papers; Minutes of the Interdepartmental Committee and Technical Subcommittee on Medical Care (19 Dec. 1939), Box 45, Interdepartmental Committee to Coordinate Health and Welfare Activities [ICHWA], FDRPL; Abraham Epstein, "Health Insurance—the Next Step," *New Republic* (17 Feb. 1937): 35; (quote) Bureau of Research and Statistics, "A Memorandum on Health Insurance" (1937), p. 17, Box 34, Decimal 056, Chairman's File, Commissioners' Records, SSA Records.

[19] Folsom to Altmeyer (26 Mar. 1935), Box 55, CES Records; *BW* (6 Aug. 1938), 36; Michael Grey, *New Deal Medicine: The Rural Health Programs of the Farm Security Administration* (Baltimore, 1999), 59–68, 99–103, 125–44.

[20] (Quote) "What Is Socialized Medicine?" (1938), Box 8, ICHWA; Starr, *Social Transformation of American Medicine*, 309; Robert Cunningham III and Robert M. Cunningham, Jr., *The Blues: A History of the Blue Cross and Blue Shield System* (De Kalb, 1997), 20, 34–55, 308–9.

Public Defeats and Private Alternatives: Interests versus Reform, 1941–1950

The emergence of health insurance as a workplace benefit transformed health care's corporate compromise. Employment-based insurance enabled insurers to leap the moral hazard of individual enrollment and expand a line of coverage they had long avoided. Employers suddenly had a stake not only in public health policy but also in their relationship with workers, providers, and insurers. And the nation's hospitals were the beneficiary of both a dramatic increase in private insurance and a windfall of public spending as legislators routinely fell back on hospital construction as an alternative to public insurance. For employers and insurers, the issue of public health insurance was secondary to the emerging contours of a private welfare state. Although employers preferred the prewar pattern of sporadic provision and managerial discretion, they increasingly faced the argument that only the rapid spread of private provision could stem the greater evil of national health insurance. "As long as we can keep a fluid advancing front on our medical plans," noted General Electric's director of employee benefits, "then we can keep government intervention as only a threat."[21] These fears were cultivated by doctors and insurers, whose stake in private health care was more pressing, and who persistently reminded employers of the larger implications of state intervention or competition.

Insurers had an immense stake in the emerging system of employment provision. Commercial insurers wanted to protect a new and promising line of insurance from public alternatives and federal regulation. Periodic efforts by the Federal Trade Commission (FTC) to oversee advertising by multistate carriers had sown legal confusion and prompted Congress (at the industry's behest) to reconfirm state regulation of insurance in 1945. The prospect of national health insurance threatened that compromise. In turn, insurers wanted not only the freedom to offer a range of risk-based rates (as nonprofits, the Blues were required to offer uniform "community" rates) but also assurance that the Blues would not be privileged as intermediaries in any public plans.[22]

[21] "American Beveridge Plan and American Business" (1943), POF 1710:3, FDR Papers; Control of Employee Benefit Plans during World War II, Box IV:109, National Association of Manufacturers [NAM] Papers, Hagley Museum; NICB Proceedings, "The Insurance Drive: What's Ahead at the Bargaining Table" (May 1950), 81, Box I:33, NICB Papers; Alexander Sachs, "Notes on the Coal Agreement," (7 June 1946), Box 123, Alexander Sachs Papers, FDRPL; E. S. Willis (GE) in NICB Proceedings, "Getting the Most for Your Insurance Dollar" (Jan. 1953), 130, Box I:43, NICB Papers.

[22] Wendy Parmet, "Regulation and Federalism: Legal Impediments to State Health Care Reform," *American Journal of Law and Medicine* 19 (1993): 126–27; Grahame to Elliott (10

As employers and insurers struggled with the implications of private provision, doctors again took the lead in opposing public programs. The AMA worked closely on Republican alternatives to the Truman-era proposals and took the initiative in establishing a Joint Informational Committee that acted as a clearinghouse for business and insurance opinion.[23] At the same time, however, AMA leadership raised some tensions as various interests accompanied their opposition to the WMD bill with contingency plans for its passage. Insurers worked behind the scenes to get a "contracting-out" provision (which would have allowed employers using private insurers to opt out), an effort the AMA agreed to support as long as the insurers pledged their "help in amending the administrative set-up so as to give large control to the medical societies." And some business interests feared that, by blindly following the AMA, employers were not only "shirking a plain duty" to shape the emerging health system but inviting both future state intervention and spiraling health costs: in this respect, the AMA's blanket opposition, as *Fortune* concluded, was nostalgic and "obviously mendacious."[24]

Organized medicine opposed any extension of state-funded health insurance, although it increasingly conceded support for voluntary forms of group insurance. "The sword of federal control through compulsory sickness insurance," the New Jersey Medical Society argued in late 1948, "will hang over the profession until the physicians of this country develop these [private] Plans."[25] And the AMA supported federal expenditures on health as long as they did not displace private practice or threaten professional control.[26] The task of getting the AMA's message across (and coordinating the influence of other health interests) required a sophisti-

---

Oct. 1946), Box 17, Orville Grahame Papers, University of Iowa Special Collections, Iowa City, Iowa; Falk, "Notes on Meeting of October 15, 1946," Box 63:579, Series II, Falk Papers.

[23] Miller to Willcox (7 Nov. 1944), Box 42, Decimal 011.1, GCF (1944–1950), HEW Records; Geraldine Sartain, "California's Health Insurance Drama," *Survey Graphic* 34:11 (Nov. 1945): 44; Wagner to Dingell (3 May 1945), Box 60:525, Series II, Falk Papers; CNH, "Legislative Memorandum" (Aug. 1947), Box 210, Witte Papers; Elmer Henderson, Report on NEC (8 Sept. 1950), Box 60, Caroline Ware Papers, FDRPL.

[24] AFL Committee on Social Security Meeting (6 Jan. 1949), Box 16, Nelson Cruikshank Papers, SHSW; Elizabeth Wilson, "Hazards of Compulsory Health Insurance," *Barron's* (8 Apr. 1946); "U.S. Medicine in Transition," *Fortune* (Dec. 1944): 158–59, 186.

[25] NJMS quoted in Alan Siegel, *Caring for New Jersey: A History of Blue Shield of New Jersey, 1942–1986* (Montclair, N.J., 1986), 47; Transcript of Panel on Group Practice (1948), Box 1, Records of the President's Commission on the Health Needs of the Nation, Harry S. Truman Library [HSTPL], Independence, Mo.; Dickinson, "Brief History of the Attitude of the AMA," 16–23.

[26] "National Health Program" (1948) in AMA Kit on Health Insurance, Box 43, Decimal 011.4, GCF (1944–1950), HEW Records; "Program of the AMA for the Advancement of Medicine" (1949), Box 209, Witte Papers; "National Health Program," *JAMA* 130:10 (1946): 641.

cated and expensive political effort. The Chicago-based AMA opened a Washington, D.C., office in 1944 and began to employ outside expertise in public relations and political lobbying in 1946. Prohibited (as a non-profit) from direct political activity, the AMA formed the National Physicians Committee for the Extension of Medical Care and charged it with stemming "political control of medicine," guarding "the independence of the profession," and selling the American people "on the incomparable advantages of the American Way of Life." The NPC, which began as an anti–New Deal effort backed by the Gannett newspaper chain, was by 1946 widely recognized as "a blind through which the reactionary elements of organized medicine can pursue obstructive tactics and propaganda without legally involving the American Medical Association." To maintain its arm's length relationship with the NPC, the AMA tapped a reliable source—the drug companies who advertised in *JAMA*—to pay for it. The NPC spent $208,000 in 1946, $389,000 in 1947, and $592,000 in 1948—most of which went to political advertising, printing, and postage (including the distribution of over twenty-five million pamphlets).[27]

Through the NPC and on its own, the AMA became increasingly active in legislative and electoral politics. Doctors and medical societies (the AMA made an effort after 1945 "to locate the personal physician of every Congressman and every U.S. Senator") routinely assumed that they controlled the votes, at least on legislation in which the AMA expressed an interest, of their congressional delegations. Organized medicine could "win any fight in Congress . . .[and] defeat the Wagner Bill at any time," the AMA boasted, simply by "flashing the word [from] Chicago." The AMA buried legislators with boilerplate mailings from medical societies, chambers of commerce, and local women's clubs—all of which reiterated a familiar defense of medical practice, free enterprise, and family privacy.[28] Beginning with the 1948 elections, the AMA organized local

[27] Burrow, *AMA: Voice of American Medicine*, 334–35; NPC quoted in "Analysis of 'Abolishing Private Medical Practice' " (1945?), Box 210, Witte Papers; "Behind the Wagner Bill," *Medical Care* 3:3 (1943): 258 (quote); (quote) Peters to Galbraith (5 Dec. 1941), Box 2:41, Series I, Peters Papers; Oscar Ewing OH, pp. 185–86, HSTPL; Richard Polenberg, *Reorganizing Roosevelt's Government: The Controversy over Executive Reorganization, 1936–1939* (Cambridge, Mass., 1966), 55–78; "Dirty Work by the Doctors," *New Republic* (30 Aug. 1943): 272; Confidential RNC study of Pennsylvania District 26 and New York Senate Races, POF 103, Box 575 and Summary of RNC document in POF 103G, Box 177, Harry S. Truman Papers, HSTPL; NPC Statement of Income and Expenditures (9 Jan. 1948) and Margaret Stein memo (27 Oct. 1948), both in Box 45:288, Series II, Falk Papers; NPC Statement of Income and Expenditures (Jan. 1949), reel 8, and "Contributions by Large Drug Companies to the NPC" (1948), reel 7, Michael Davis Papers, HSTPL; Sartain, "Who Fights Health Insurance?" 691–92.

[28] (Quote) CNH Release (5 Jan. 1950), Box 60, Ware Papers; (quote) "Discussion," *JAMA* 113:27 (1939): 2429; (quote) handwritten notes (1955?), AMA Administration file, Box

"healing arts committees" that bombarded doctors with political appeals, distributed pamphlets extolling the evils of socialized medicine, and flooded the airwaves with spot announcements and canned "news" briefs. In New York in 1948, AMA-Republican healing arts committees generated over two million doctor-to-patient letters, 32 pages of newspaper ads, 218 radio spots, and 18 longer radio programs. The AMA devoted considerable resources to defeating those who had supported the WMD bill in 1948 and 1949 and, in the wake of the 1950 elections, claimed to have forced many candidates to renounce their support of health insurance and to have defeated "90 percent" of those who would not be swayed, including Frank Graham (D-N.C.), Claude Pepper (D-Fla.), and Andrew Biemiller (D-Wi.).[29]

Perhaps the starkest illustration of the AMA's economic and political clout came in the National Education Campaign (NEC) of 1950. By 1949 the NPC's stridency had begun to wear thin: a craven effort to solicit anti-WMD political cartoons and the NPC's redistribution of a far-right religious newsletter attacking the Truman reforms were the last straws. In response, the AMA disbanded the NPC and retained the public relations firm Whitaker and Baxter (which had come to its attention by helping to defeat a state health plan in California in 1945).[30] Whitaker and Baxter's NEC targeted politicians and public opinion, illustrating the political importance of money and the limits of a free press beholden to large advertising accounts. The AMA financed the NEC with a special $25 assessment on members—generating a war chest of over $3.5 million, most of which the NEC spent on newspaper, radio, and magazine advertising and the distribution of between fifty and eight million pamphlets. The NEC had a staff of almost forty and supported a dramatic

---

52, Frank Kuehl Papers, SHSW; File 81A-H7.2, Boxes 182 and 183, Records of the House Committee on Foreign and Interstate Commerce, RG 233, Records of the House of Representatives, National Archives; Delaware Senate Resolution 20 (1949), Mississippi Senate Resolution 16 (1950), File 81A-H7.2, Box 182, Records of the House Committee on Foreign and Interstate Commerce, Records of the House of Representatives.

[29] Republican National Committee (RNC) study of Pennsylvania District 26 and New York Senate races, POF 103, Box 575, and Summary of RNC document in POF 103G, Box 177, Truman Papers; NPC Statement of Income and Expenditures (9 Jan.1948) and Margaret Stein memo (27 Oct. 1948), Box 45:288, Series II, Falk Papers; Physicians Forum to Truman (16 Dec. 1949) Box 45, Decimal 011.4, FSA, Office of the Administrator (GCF, 1944–1950), HEW Records; Numbers, "Specter of Socialized Medicine," 9–10; *Medical Economics* (Jan. 1951); George Smathers OH (Senate Historical Office, 1989), 92.

[30] *Congressional Record* 95:4 (1949): 4589–90; Kennedy, "The American Medical Association," 1013–14; "Dan Gilbert's Washington Letter" (Dec. 1948), reel 7, Davis Papers; "The National Physicians Committee," *JAMA* 139:40 (1949): 924; Fred Stein to Davis (28 Sept. 1945), and NPC clippings, reel 7, Davis Papers; Chamber of Commerce, "Business Support of Private Enterprise" (1950), Box, II:18, Chamber of Commerce Papers, Hagley Museum; Henderson, "Report on NEC"; Burrow, *AMA: Voice of American Medicine*, 361.

expansion of the political presence of the AMA—which registered fifteen new lobbyists in 1949 and 1950.[31]

The NEC's genius lay less in its pamphlet blitz than in its management of the press. "It is vital," Whitaker and Baxter argued, "that much of this flow of words should reach the public through normal newspaper and magazine channels, rather than through direct publicity releases," adding that "we intend to work with the great newspapers and the national magazines to get them to do special jobs." The AMA outflanked reformers and the administration—indeed columnists and editorialists routinely based their assessments not on the WMD bill itself but on a widely distributed AMA digest of it. In radio as well, the AMA was conscious of its considerable resource advantage: "We do not believe it is a sound campaign practice to sponsor too many debates," counseled Whitaker and Baxter. "They make a forum for the opposition which would be difficult for them to secure otherwise."[32] The AMA exploited the fact that "newspapers largely followed the interests of the advertisers" and bought full-page ads in virtually every daily in the country. "There will be some duplication of circulation," conceded Whitaker, "but the added impact of that duplication is desired so that medicine's story can be hammered home by repetition." The AMA provided advertising copy for adoption by local doctors, druggists, used-car lots, and grocery stores; each tied the virtues of small enterprise to the doctor's fight and ended with the slug line: "The voluntary way is the American Way." As the campaign progressed, AMA officials crowed that the newspapers "are wonderfully enthusiastic about medicine's advertising program and are planning to build support for it from their local advertisers which probably will far surpass our expectations." And newspapers praised the AMA and the infusion of advertising dollars: "AMA ad copy best we have seen in years," cabled the advertising director of the *New York Post*. "Tie-in advertising program excellent and one of the most complete ever sent to our office." Little wonder that reformers lamented the gap between public support and a hostile press. "Would I be undermining the 'freedom of the press,'" asked George Addes of the United Auto Workers bitterly, "if I were to infer that some relationship might possibly exist between the fact that these three groups [doctors, employers, drug companies] control

[31] Kennedy, "The American Medical Association," 1013–14; *NYT* (3 Dec. 1948); "AMA Advertising Program," *JAMA* 143:8 (1950): 744; "The President's Page," *JAMA* 144:9 (1950): 767; "The AMA Lobby," Box 43, Decimal 011.4, FSA, Office of the Administrator (GCF, 1944–1950), HEW Records.

[32] Whitaker and Baxter quoted in "What Will We Do with the Doctor's $25.00?" *Dallas Medical Journal* clipping in Box 43, Decimal 011.4, FSA, Office of the Administrator (GCF, 1944–1950), HEW Records; "Analysis of 'Abolishing Private Medical Practice' . . ." (1945?), Box 210, Witte Papers; *Detroit News* (27 Jan. 1944).

most of the newspaper and magazine advertising in the nation and that practically every newspaper in America either gives the Bill silent treatment or actively opposes it?"[33]

The political and legislative consequences were dramatic. As early as 1942, when Social Security staff began toying with health insurance in response to both abortive prewar reforms and the elaboration of the British Beveridge Plan, reform was framed by fear of medical opposition and deference to fee-for-service care. Any health plan, as then vice president Henry Wallace stressed in 1943, needed to be drafted in such terms that "it may be possible to put it over without opposition from Fishbein and the American Medical Association."[34] Dancing around the opposition of health interests proved as unproductive as confronting them. The administration persistently failed to overcome the opposition and the resources wielded by organized medicine, private insurers, and employers. The problem was one of "health, money, and politics," the Committee for the Nation's Health observed, while lamenting that "the first of this trio is the third."[35]

Health Care and Growth Politics: Interests versus Reform, 1950–1960

After the defeat of the Truman proposals, health care's corporate compromise and the political activities of its constituent interests shifted once again. With national health insurance off the table and reformers devoting their attention to fragments of Social Security–based coverage, organized medicine and others retreated from the apocalyptic politics of the late 1940s. And with the expansion of employment-based insurance increasingly trumping public proposals, employers and commercial insurers emerged as more important and distinct political actors.

After its successes of the late 1940s, the AMA moved to entrench its political influence. The Washington office was expanded and reorga-

[33] (Quote) Sartain, "California's Health Insurance Drama," 44; Whitaker quoted in CNH Release (28 Aug. 1950); Henderson, "Report on NEC"; CNH Release (25 Sept. 1950); "To Newspaper Advertising Directors . . . , " all in Box 60, Ware Papers; *Editor and Publisher* (Sept. 1950) clippings, Box 209, Witte Papers; George Addes, "The Plot against the W-M-D Bill" (17 Feb. 1944), Box 60:519, Series II, Falk Papers.

[34] Altmeyer Memorandum (29 Dec. 1942), President's Secretary's File 165, FDR Papers; "Proposed Expanded Social Security System Compared with the Beveridge Plan" (15 Dec. 1942); Altmeyer Memorandum to the President (29 Dec. 1942), both in Box 3 (Mss WP), Altmeyer Papers; Wallace to FDR (4 Feb. 1943), POF 4351:2, FDR Papers.

[35] Willcox to Rosenfeld (24 Oct. 1947); Crabtree to Parran (29 Oct. 1947); and "Informal Conference on National Health Insurance" (6 Nov. 1947), all in Box 46, Decimal 011.4,

nized in order to ensure a " 'grass-roots to Congressional hall' chain of influence." This reorganization (under the direction of Wisconsin lawyer Frank Kuehl) included the establishment of a "Legislative Key Man" system (charged with building "personal contacts with national legislators") in 1946, a Committee on Legislation (charged with prepping congressional witnesses) in 1950, and field offices (charged with building grass-roots support) in 1958. The goal, as Kuehl saw it, was to build an organization with the "ability to strike quickly." The AMA generally supported Republicans (spinning off a National Professional Committee for Eisenhower and Nixon in 1952) but was also careful to employ Democrats in its Washington office in order to keep all channels to Congress open.[36] For the AMA, the keystone of its political influence was its ability to exploit the "inherently close relationship between physicians and Senators and Representatives that is enjoyed by no other group in the country." This relationship reflected both the doctors' local and professional stature and the resources the national office devoted to nurturing it: "a closely knit nationwide organization of doctors should be formed and maintained even at heavy cost, an organization willing to keep in touch with *all* Senators and Representatives. This is within our capabilities, both organizationally and financially." The AMA also cultivated contacts with liberal legislators "who are generally on the opposite side from us on most issues," reasoning "while we know they won't be with us on most of the big issues, until we and our friends can knock them out of Congress we should be able to reach them with our arguments; our efforts may bring them to our side on some issues and may dilute their opposition on the major issues."[37]

All of this depended upon a substantial resource base. The AMA continued to lean heavily on *JAMA* revenues and member dues and maintained, for a time, the $25 "special assessment." In the wake of 1949–50, spending slowed: the NEC spent $500,000 in 1951, $250,000 in 1952, and was disbanded in 1953. But resources still poured into the Washing-

---

FSA, Office of the Administrator (GCF, 1944–1950), HEW Records; (quote) CNH, "Considerations for 1948," reel 1, Davis Papers.

[36] "Reorganization of Washington Office," Box 52, Kuehl Papers; Lull to Stettler (30 Dec. 1955), AMA Committee on Legislation file, Box 52, Kuehl Papers; Kennedy, "The American Medical Association," 1017; CNH Release (26 Sept. 1952), Box 60, Ware Papers; Kuehl to Fister (13 Aug. 1958), Box 52, Kuehl Papers.

[37] (Quote) Confidential memo (1957?), and Senate Committee to Investigate Lobbying file, both in Box 57; "The Washington Scene" (16 Sept. 1955); (quote) Minutes of AMA [Washington Office] Staff Conference (8 Nov. 1955), Staff Meetings file, Box 52; Alphin to Lull (29 Dec. 1955), AMA Committee on Legislation file, Box 52; "Memorandum to Board of Trustees" (Dec. 1953), Correspondence files, Box 54; handwritten notes (1955?), AMA Administration and Personnel file, Box 52; Kuehl to Fister (13 Aug. 1958), Box 52, all in Kuehl Papers.

ton office and the AMA was quick to respond to threats. It remained active on the electoral front: "Those of us with deep convictions must do more than vote," observed the AMA's James Foristel in 1956; "we must financially support the high costs of present-day electioneering." The AMA not only continued the healing arts committees that had worked so effectively for Republicans in 1950 and 1952, but also pioneered the management of "soft money" contributions to the Republican and Democratic national committees.[38] The results were impressive. The AMA was "the only organization in the country," the *Washington Post* noted in 1952, "that could marshal 140 votes in Congress between sundown Friday Night and noon on Monday." The AMA proved adept at both shaping debate and engineering "grass-roots" (telegrams, letters, phone calls) interest. By the late 1950s, the AMA gloated that it been able to "extend its influence from the purely legislative fields to the agencies where it has been able to shape bills before their introduction and to help direct regulations after passage of laws." As federal programs expanded, AMA lobbyists increasingly appreciated the importance of capturing their administration. "Once laws are passed, whether we approve of them or not," Foristel argued, "[we should] get in on the ground floor of regulation-writing. If ordinary discretion were observed at the outset, it is likely that the agencies would welcome, or at least tolerate, the help of the medical profession . . . the importance of this activity cannot be overemphasized; a bad law can be minimized in the proper regulations."[39]

While organized medicine consolidated its position, health insurers established a political presence virtually from scratch. Commercial health insurance had only just emerged as an important line of business, and given the industry's history of state regulation, political activity had been largely behind the scenes of state insurance commissions. But after 1945 commercial insurers recognized the political implications of their increasingly complex relationship with employers, doctors, and hospitals. The IES remained the most the most active industry group in the early 1950s, but it was leery of expanding membership to include either "the giants who might attempt to dictate policy" or "companies not com-

[38] Kuehl to Fister (13 Aug. 1958), Box 52, Kuehl Papers; Theodore Marmor, *The Politics of Medicare* (Chicago, 1970), 31; Foristel in AMA Law Department, "Conference of Legal Counsels for Medical Societies" (Apr. 1956), p. 269, Box 53, Kuehl Papers.

[39] (Quote) "AMA Is Potent Force" *Washington Post* (15 June 1952), E7; Drew Pearson, "How Doctors' Lobby Operates," *Washington Post* (22 June 1952); Kuehl to Fister (13 Aug. 1958), Box 52; Foristel in confidential memo (1952?), Senate Committee to Investigate Lobbying file, Box 57; Staff Meeting, AMA DC Office (19 Sept. 1955), Box 52, all in Kuehl Papers.

pletely in accord with our aims and purposes."[40] Insurers increasingly saw the need for the "establishment of one major trade association with an affirmative public relations approach" that could distinguish health insurers from the industry's umbrella life and accident trade association and look beyond the political horizons of the IES. Toward this end, leading health insurers organized first under the auspices of the Health and Accident Underwriters Conference, and then used HAUC to create, in 1956, the Health Insurance Association of America. HIAA established a base annual budget of $850,000, financed by dues set as a percentage of each firm's premiums. "I would hope that we could join with organized medicine, the U.S. Chamber of Commerce, and other private insurers' organizations," a founding member argued, "to do something of the same kind of job that [the] American Medical Association did in 1948 when Whitaker and Baxter spearheaded a national education program that resulted in the defeat of the Wagner, Murray, Dingell Legislation."[41]

For the HIAA, three issues were of immediate and lasting political concern. The first was the scope and stability of private health insurance. Although the HIAA felt that freedom to cancel coverage or deny renewal was a basic contractual right, it acknowledged that cancellation was also a matter of "public and legislative relations" and that while there was "nothing legally wrong with cancellation . . . the important consideration . . . [is] the extent of unfavorable public reaction, which in turn has transmitted into a political question." This issue captured the politics of private insurance before Medicare, as the HIAA struggled to champion private coverage against growing evidence of its limits. "We have witnessed a series of inquiries into the effectiveness of voluntary health insurance" since 1950, one insurer warned, to which the industry had responded "without adequate organized representation, with a dearth of statistical data [and] with no satisfactory answer to the problems of the aged or to

[40] O'Connor to Skutt (15 Oct. 1954), Box 28, Grahame Papers; Tentative 1952 Budget, Insurance Economic Society, IES Financial Report (1954), Tentative Budget (1959), O'Connor to Powell (1 May 1956), O'Connor to Grahame (13 Oct. 1954), IES Minutes (1952–1954), Grahame to O'Connor (20 Oct. 1955), all in Box 28; Washington Representation correspondence (1954), Box 29, Grahame Papers.

[41] Executive Committee Meeting, Health and Accident Underwriters Conference (8 May 1955), Box 17; HIAA correspondence files, Box 19; (quote) HAUC Memo (9 Mar. 1956); memo for Grahame (16 Mar. 1955), Box 17; Report of Task Force for Jan. 16, 1955 Meeting of the Joint Committee on Health Insurance, Box 17; Joint Committee on Health Insurance, Report of Finance Committee (Oct. 1955); HIAA, Projected Budget 1957–1958 (Jan. 1957), Box 19; "Outline of Proposal to Establish the Health Insurance Association of America" (Oct. 1955), Box 19; (quote) Faulkner to Miller (6 Aug. 1958), Box 18, all in Grahame Papers.

the problems of nonrenewal or cancellation."[42] This anxiety echoed that of many employers: could private insurance expand "fast enough to avert legislation"? "I believe the time has come—now," one insurer stressed in 1958, "for the HIAA to ask its members . . . whether, by their conduct of the business, they are casting a vote for voluntary health insurance or whether, by their inaction and adherence to traditional ways, they are voting for compulsory governmental administration of hospital and medical facilities." As legislators begin toying with coverage for the aged, the HIAA worried that such efforts might create "enormous pressures for a complete compulsory health insurance plan" and warned its members "we have only months in which to prove the capacity of private health insurance to provide adequately for the aged."[43]

The HIAA's second concern was its ongoing tug-of-war with the non-profit Blues for the group insurance market. The Blues had signed up many employers before commercial insurers had given health insurance a serious look, forged strong ties to the labor movement, and maintained natural advantages in their relationships with hospitals and doctors. As a condition of their nonprofit status, however, the Blues were also required to offer a community rate to group clients. Commercials, by contrast, could "cherry pick" group risks by offering experience rates based on "occupation, educational and skill levels, income levels, size of family, stability of home, [and] characteristics with respect to spending, savings, budgeting." As commercials picked off the good risks, community rates rose and exposed the Blues even further. As medical costs rose, the gap between community and experience rates widened and, by the mid-1950s, the Blues began to retreat from community rating. Commercial insurers were also able to offer national employers "one-stop shopping" for all their plants and for other lines of group coverage. Although the Blues offered more expansive benefits, commercials introduced "major medical coverage" in the mid-1950s as a means of offering the same "peace of mind" without the inflationary pressures that they feared would accompany a full service plan.[44]

[42] "Individual Health and Accident Insurance" (n.d.); (quote) "Confidential Memorandum Concerning Cancellation" (Mar. 1958); Minutes of the HIAA Special Committee on Cancellation (17 Apr. 1958); (quote) Miller to Wallace (1 Aug. 1958), all in Box 18, Grahame Papers.

[43] (Quote) Miller to Wallace (1 Aug. 1958); "Blueprint of Proposed Industry Program" (Oct. 1956), both in Box 18, Grahame Papers; (quote) Ardell Everett, "The March to Utopia," *Weekly Underwriter* (2 Jan. 1960); (quote) Faulkner to Miller (Aug. 6, 1958), Box 18, Grahame Papers; "Meeting with Consultant on Health Insurance" (20 Nov. 1959), Box 225, Decimal 900.1, Secretary's Subject Files [SSF] (1955–1975), HEW Records.

[44] Report to [HIAA] Board (28 Oct. 1958), Box 18, Grahame Papers.

Finally, insurers fretted about the threat federal policy posed to a carefully nurtured system of state regulation. Members insisted that the HIAA "go all out in its attack on FTC intrusion and in its support of a state system of regulation," and many saw even the Eisenhower administration's tepid reinsurance proposals as the top of a slippery slope.[45] At the same time, large insurers grew leery of the administrative hassle and competitive disadvantage that came with fragmented state regulation: "I judge you have more confidence in your domicilary state than I have in mine," one HIAA executive wrote in 1956. "If we should get an incompetent or vengeful insurance commissioner or legislature or governor, we could be in a rough spot if such party or parties attempted to control us throughout the Country on all aspects of our business." And some worried that the "race to the bottom" encouraged by state regulation might actually invite the federal presence it was intended to thwart: "On the issue of the effectiveness of state regulation we will all sink or swim together, whether we like it or not," a Travelers official argued. "If we cannot agree among ourselves on this subject then we not only invite, but in effect require, the establishment of a federal regulatory body."[46]

While doctors and insurers developed clear political positions (and the means of fighting for them) through the 1950s, employers remained ambivalent and divided. As unions increasingly won service benefits, employer financing, and dependent coverage, many employers began to fall back on the argument that health care was not a consequence or cost of industrial employment. Such anxieties also reflected the pace of health care inflation—which, by the mid-1950s, employers blamed on hospital mismanagement, union corruption, and the perverse logic of third-party billing. Because the scope of private insurance remained quite meager, employers faced constant pressure for more expansive plans. But as health costs (and the employers' share) rose, employers also sought efficiency and economy. Employers were torn between abandoning health commitments and spreading their costs more broadly. Most were leery of new commitments (such as retiree plans) but open to public policies (such as the 1954–55 reinsurance proposals) that promised to prop up the existing system. And some (resenting the fact

[45] "Motion for Leave to File Brief" (14 Nov. 1956); Hubbard to Grahame (2 Nov. 1956), both in Box 26, Grahame Papers; see also files of the Subcommittee on FTC Jurisdiction (1956–1961), Boxes 26–27, Grahame Papers; "Suggested Modifications to Reinsurance Bill" (28 May 1954), Box 235, Decimal 901, GCF (1951–1955), HEW Records; Memo for Grahame (16 Mar. 1955), Box 17; Minutes of the Joint ALC-LIAA Social Security Committee (12 Apr. 1960), Box 20, both in Grahame Papers; *BW* (7 Apr. 1956): 117.

[46] Grahame to Hubbard (26 Nov. 1956); Hubbard to Grahame (22 Apr. 1959), both in Box 26; Legislative Committee Minutes, Boxes 21–23, Grahame Papers.

that private insurance had transformed employers into the health care system's only dependable cash cow) were willing to consider public solutions—especially, as Benson Ford noted, "while we have an administration sympathetic to private enterprise principles."[47]

Doctors, insurers, and employers shared class interests and political status, but also confronted each other in private bargaining and policy debates. Unions, providers, employers, and insurers battled over the cost of private health provision. And each approached politics with the often-contradictory goals of staving of state intervention and gaining political advantage over others. Organized medicine's anxiety about third parties was apparent in its continued battles with group and union health plans—and increasingly in its dealings with employers as well, especially when the latter ventured any input on benefits, utilization, or reimbursement. Unions and employers routinely accused doctors of gouging union health and welfare funds or employment-based insurance plans.[48] Hospitals were much more dependent upon patterns of public and private insurance and, accordingly, proved much less predictable. The American Hospital Association worked closely with the Eisenhower administration on its reinsurance proposals and, along with Blue Cross, devoted considerable effort in the late 1950s to drafting a preliminary version of Medicare. The AMA and AHA had drifted apart through the decade as the latter proved willing to consider anything that would subsidize its capital costs or deliver more patients.[49] In turn, unions, doctors, and employers maintained an often-tense relationship with insurers. Most unions cultivated close ties to Blue Cross and Blue Shield and resented their move away from full-service benefits and community rating. Doctors worked closely with insurers on many issues, but also resented

[47] Bureau of National Affairs, "Administration of Health and Welfare Plans" (1954), Box 849:1, Pennsylvania Railroad [PRR] Papers; Edwin Grace, "Keep Your Employees Out of the Hospital" *HBR* 37:5 (Sept./Oct. 1959): 119–26; "Lunch with A. L. Kirkpatrick" (2 Dec. 1958), Box 124, Decimal 900.1, SSF (1955–1975), HEW Records; (quote) Benson Ford, "A Businessman Looks at Health" (1955), Box 208, Witte Papers; Sanford Jacoby, *Modern Manors: Welfare Capitalism since the New Deal* (Princeton, N.J., 1997), 216–20.

[48] Preliminary Draft of Proceedings, Association of Labor Health Administrators (28 Mar. 1957), Box 37:212, Series II, Lorin Kerr Papers, Sterling Library; "History of Local 119 Health Fund of the Male Apparel Industry of Allentown" (1957), Box 37:212, Series II, Kerr Papers; Henry Kaiser to Charles Wilson [GM] (21 Mar. 1952), Box 92, Edgar Kaiser Papers, Bancroft Library, University of California, Berkeley; "Dr. Jekyll and the AMA," *The Nation* 184 (22 June 1957): 539–40; George Baehr,"The Attitude of Medical Societies to Prepaid Group Practice," *NEJM* 247:17 (23 Oct. 1952): 625–27; *BW* (14 June 1958), 30; E. Trefethen, "Organization and Business Management of Medical Care Operations in Southern California" (1956), Box 272, Henry J. Kaiser Papers, Bancroft Library.

[49] "Report of Meeting with Representatives of Hospital Associations" (22 Dec. 1954), Box 8, Decimal 011, GCF (1951–1955), HEW Records; Cunningham and Cunningham, *The Blues,* 124; Michael O'Neill, "Siege Tactics of the AMA," *The Reporter* 26:8, 29.

insurers' efforts to control costs through benefit or fee schedules, and insurers blamed doctors for rising costs. Finally, while employers enjoyed natural ideological and economic alliances with doctors and insurers, they also blamed them for health inflation and the headache of managing employment-based plans.[50]

These tensions aside, health interests enjoyed uncommon political influence through the 1950s. This reflected not only the effort they put into political organizing but also the Eisenhower administration's natural deference. Reformers routinely accused the Eisenhower-era HEW of coddling the AMA, the insurance industry, and the Chamber of Commerce—a trio dubbed the Hobby Lobby for its access to Eisenhower's first HEW secretary, Ovetta Culp Hobby. In crafting its reinsurance proposals, the administration "work[ed] assiduously to meet the objections" of insurers, relied on them for background data and cost estimates, and deferred to them on most of the details. As Medicare gained momentum in 1959 and 1960, Eisenhower's Bureau of the Budget directed HEW to work something out with the industry.[51] The influence of the AMA was even starker, and HIAA officials recognized that the administration would defer to organized medicine whenever the interests of doctors and insurers were at odds. HEW adopted the AMA's "12-Point Program" of 1949 as a blueprint for federal policy, worked closely with the AMA's Legislative Liaison Committee, and strove to keep "the latest thinking of the AMA" at the forefront.[52] This deference also reflected the AMA's

[50] Subcommittee on Claims Cost Control (8 Apr. 1955), Box 17; "To Members of the Planning and Finance Committee" (22 July 1958), Box 28, both in Grahame Papers; George Wheatley, "Voluntary Health Insurance—Progress and Problems," NEJM 257:3 (18 July 1957): 117–18; "The Doctor's Dilemma," *NEJM* 257:26 (26 Dec. 1957), 1293; P. C. Irwin, "Economic Tolerance," *JAMA* 165:12 (1957): 1574–75; "Comprehensive or 'Single Plan Major Medical' Insurance," *JAMA* 166:5 (1958): 472; "Health Insurance for the Aged," *JAMA* 170:6 (1959): 689–91; Ford, "A Businessman Looks at Health"; Confidential Memoranda, Box 57, Kuehl Papers.

[51] "Hobby Lobby" quote in Rockefeller to Sen. Smith (2 June 1954), Box 235, Decimal 901, GCF (1951–1955); "Meeting with Insurance Representatives" (5 Nov. 1956), Box 125, Decimal 900.1, SSF (1955–1975); "Agenda for Conference with Insurance Executives" (26 Jan. 1954), Box 235, Decimal 901, GCF (1951–1955); Thore to Rockefeller (26 Oct. 1954), Box 235, Decimal 901, FSA, Office of the Administrator (GCF, 1951–1955); "Cost estimates" (27 Apr. 1960), Box 225, Decimal 900.1, Secretary's Subject Correspondence [SSC] (1956–1974); "Luncheon Meeting" (25 Apr. 1960), "Meetings with Outside Groups" (6 Apr. 1960), Box 225, Decimal 900.1, SSC (1956–1974); "Recent Questions and Discussions Re Health Insurance" (29 Jan. 1960), Box 225, Decimal 900.1, SSC (1956–1974); "Notes for Monday Luncheon with Insurance Executives" (14 May 1954), Box 235, Decimal 901, GCF (1951–1955); Pond to Flemming (17 Mar. 1960), Box 225, Decimal 900.1, SSC (1956–1974); Skutt to Flemming (8 Mar. 1960), Box 225, Decimal 900.1, SSF (1955–1975), all in HEW Records.

[52] Pond to Flemming (16 Mar. 1960), Box 225, Decimal 900.1, SSC (1956–1974); "Discussion with Dr. Elmer Hess" (26 Oct. 1954), Box 235, Decimal 901, FSA, Office of the Admin-

close ties to Congress, where even the "introduction of legislation offered little difficulty," one lobbyist boasted, and "committee and floor amendments could be added whereupon the original legislation would be radically altered." The AMA applauded the administration, noting typically (in response to the president's 1956 Health Message) that it was "pleased to know the extent to which our previous recommendations have been incorporated in the new program." The AMA took it upon itself to draft the health platform for the Republican National Committee in 1956, which it privately summarized as one in which "the Republican party would want to pledge itself to leave the whole subject of medicine in the hands of the medical profession, but stand ready to cooperate with the medical profession, at any time, and in such manner that the medical profession might request."[53]

The political clout of health interests was evident in the administration's reinsurance proposals in 1954–55, the expansion of Social Security to cover permanent disability in 1956, and the first rounds of the Medicare fight after 1958. The AMA, which viewed any legislative solution with trepidation, instinctively opposed reinsurance—fearing it would "provide a vehicle which can be amended and can then lead to compulsory health insurance and socialized medicine." But the administration was able to bring the doctors around by playing off its broader alliance with the AMA.[54] The HIAA opposed reinsurance and major employers were lukewarm, seeing considerable danger in passing a health insurance measure that promised new coverage but was unlikely to deliver it.[55] The administration tried to allay these fears by inviting doctors and insurers to "put what you might call the finishing touches" on the pro-

istrator (GCF, 1951–1955); Foristel to Perkins (27 Oct. 1954), Box 235, Decimal 901, "Outline for Discussion with Liaison Committee of the AMA" (28 Oct. 1954), Box 235, Decimal 901, FSA, Office of the Administrator (GCF, 1951–1955), "Meeting with AMA Representatives" (11 Feb. 1958), Box 73, Decimal 056.1, Cruikshank to Rockefeller (3 Dec. 1954), and (quote) "Next Meeting with AMA Liaison Committee" (26 Nov. 1954), Box 235, Decimal 901, all in FSA, Office of the Administrator (GCF, 1951–1955) HEW Records; (quote) Chad Calhoun to Henry Kaiser (18 Mar. 1953), Box 77, Henry Kaiser Papers; (quote) Pond to Flemming (11 Dec. 1959), Box 51, Decimal 011, SSF (1955–1975), HEW Records.

[53] (Quotes) Committee on Legislation to Board of Trustees (10 Feb. 1956), Correspondence files, Box 54, Kuehl Papers; Avery to Shephard (9 July 1959), Box 225, Decimal 900.1, SSF (1955–1975), HEW Records; (quote) Kuehl to Alphin (15 June 1956), RNC file, Box 59, Kuehl Papers.

[54] (Quote) Conversation with Dr. Martin of the AMA (16 Nov. 1954), Tenney to Eisenhower (7 Dec. 1954); (quote) "Meeting with AMA Liaison Committee" (7 Dec. 1954); "Meeting with AMA and Insurance Executives" (9 July 1954), all in Box 235, Decimal 901, FSA, Office of the Administrator (GCF, 1951–1955), HEW Records.

[55] AMA News Release (28 Nov. 1954); "Tax Exemptions" (9 Apr. 1954); discussion with E. S. Willis (26 Nov. 1954), all in Box 235, Decimal 901, FSA, Office of the Administrator (GCF, 1951–1955) HEW Records.

posal themselves, but was left with a bill that satisfied no one; still, it concluded that congressional Republicans would "stay with the AMA on any showdown."[56] The debate over disability played out quite differently, as the AMA overestimated its political clout on an issue peripheral to medical politics and closely identified with the popular Social Security program. When the issue first arose in 1952, organized medicine telegrammed every member of Congress in a day and buried the bill. When the issue came before Congress again in 1955, doctors lost the fight, but their response underscored a distinct understanding of the role of interest groups in the legislative process. "The AMA's *important job*," one lobbyist put it, "is to sleep with legislative leaders in both houses right now to determine who will be conferees and to *indoctrinate the entire membership* on the hazards, if not evils, of [the disability bill]."[57]

When an early version of Medicare was first proposed in 1957, the AMA and the HIAA opposed the idea and congratulated the administration for doing the same—lauding HEW secretary Arthur Flemming for "the firm and courageous stand you have taken on the Forand Bill" and promising that "the AMA will mobilize its entire resources to assist you." But health interests and the administration struggled to come up with a credible alternative. The AMA's "Medicredit" plan struck HEW as little more than "a totally Federally-financed blank check to the insurance carriers," but the administration's own ideas were not much better. To complicate matters, the AMA and others wanted to avoid floating alternatives until they were sure that Forand was a real threat. "If we were to introduce the measure early in the next session of Congress as the administration's firm proposal in the field, we could not count on the support of the insurance industry, Blue Cross—Blue Shield, the hospital organizations, or organized medicine," one HEW official noted in late 1959. "However, . . . if it was evident that the Forand Bill was likely to move out of Committee, we at that time could anticipate the support of many of the above-mentioned groups on the grounds that our proposal would represent the lesser of two evils." Many in Congress urged the doctors to consider alternatives (hospital construction, insurance subsidies, means

---

[56] Kuehl to State Medical Society of Wisconsin (17 Nov. 1954), Box 54; "Health Service Reinsurance," Box 54; notes on Civil Service Commission Meeting (16 Nov. 1954); Irons to Wilson (26 Jan. 1955), Box 55, Kuehl Papers; "Gaps in Provision for Economic Security" (1 June 1955), Committee on Social Security Correspondence, Box 16, Nelson Cruikshank Papers; (quote) Counihan to Folsom (16 July 1954), Box 235, Decimal 901, GCF (1951–1955), HEW Records.

[57] Memo: Social Security Amendments of 1955, Correspondence files, Box 54, Kuehl Papers; "AMA Is Potent Force," E7; (quotes) Kuehl to Alphin (23 Nov. 1955), Box 57, Kuehl Papers; (quote) Staff Meeting, AMA DC Office (19 Sept. 1955), Box 52, Kuehl Papers; Edward Berkowitz, *America's Welfare State* (Baltimore, 1991), 164–66.

testing) as the only way of slowing Forand's momentum. Although the AMA prevailed in 1960, its stance had the effect of "waking a sleeping dog," one congressional staffer saw it. "Many folks wouldn't have known what the Forand bill was if it hadn't been for the crusading or publicity given it by doctors."[58]

Making Medicare: Interests versus Reform, 1960–1965

After the 1960 elections, most conceded that even the AMA was unlikely to keep the issue of health care for the aged at bay. But Medicare and Medicaid were not unambiguous victories over entrenched interests. The 1965 reforms were possible, in large part, because reformers had retreated to a fragment of coverage (hospitalization for the elderly) that was least likely to threaten commercial insurers or private providers. "Some of our friends on the Hill are asking us if this is not a good 'substitute' for compulsory health insurance," worried the AMA, "[but] when we tell them that it is essentially the same as compulsory health insurance, they seem confused with our rationale, insisting that this would be free enterprise health insurance." While organized medicine flatly opposed Medicare, other health interests saw some promise in it: hospitals welcomed the prospect of stable third-party insurance for elderly patients; the Blues positioned themselves as the intermediary for a vast flow of federal funds; and insurers and employers were intrigued by a program that would relieve the private welfare state of its worst risks. Indeed, Medicare ceded so much ground to private providers that "the result will not be so much the subsidizing of needy people," one cynic observed, "as the subsidizing of an industry."[59]

The AMA's response drew on long-standing arguments about the dangers of state intervention, the incompatibility of health care and social insurance, the costs of public coverage, and the unrealized promise of private insurance. The AMA continued to rely on member fees and *JAMA* revenues and, by the early 1960s, also made nearly $1 million annually selling its subscriber list to direct mail firms. In 1962 the AMA collapsed its healing arts committees into a formal political action committee

[58] Orr to Flemming (3 Aug. 1959), Box 51, Decimal 0.11, SSF (1955–1975); Blasingame to Flemming (5 Feb. 1960), Box 225, Decimal 900.1, SSF (1955–1975); "Meeting on Health Insurance" (1959); (quote) Merriam to Flemming (19 Sept. 1960); (quote) "Meeting with Consultant on Health Insurance" (20 Nov. 1959), all in Box 225, Decimal 900.1, SSC (1956–1974), HEW Records; Foristel to Alphin (2 Jan. 1958), Box 57, Kuehl Papers; congressional staffer quoted in Kuehl to Alphin (7 Mar. 1958), Box 57, Kuehl Papers.

[59] Kuehl to Fister (13 Aug 1958), Box 52, Kuehl Papers; "Cold Eye on Johnson," *The Nation* 202 (3 Jan. 1966), 5.

(AMPAC) that was able to both engage in direct political and electoral work and solicit money from non-AMA members. AMPAC disbursed about $250,000 in direct political contributions in the 1962 election cycle, although another $1.3 million was raised and spent locally and the budget for AMPAC's public relations work ran close to $8 million. The AMA's Operation Hometown furnished doctors, medical societies, and the press with posters, pamphlets, canned editorials, and speech and debate kits. In 1964 the AMA devoted nearly $2 million to a campaign that featured quarter-page ads in seven thousand dailies, full-page ads in every major metropolitan daily, ads in most major weeklies, thirty national one-minute TV spots, and hundreds more local TV spots. In 1965 the AMA spent more than the next nine national political lobbies combined, and its expenditures in the first quarter alone approached the benchmark it had set in 1949 and 1950.[60] The Kennedy and Johnson administrations distanced themselves from the AMA, but also admitted (as a Kaiser official recalled) to being "scared to death" of it. And administration officials found that many legislators made no bones about being "committed to the AMA"; the first step in any congressional contact was to establish, as Wilbur Cohen put it, "whether he is beholden to the AMA or independent of them."[61]

At the same time, organized medicine did not claim the same political clout it had enjoyed in the late 1940s. Its apocalyptic arguments were increasingly out of step with the cold war liberalism of the 1960s. Its support of Goldwater in 1964 backfired badly, and (in an era in which doctors' incomes and health costs were both rising) Democrats saw some promise in confronting the AMA. "Have you ever fed chickens? . . . chickens are real dumb," Lyndon Johnson confided to AFL-CIO president George Meany. "They eat and eat and eat and they never stop. Why they start shitting at the same time they're eating, and before you know it, they're knee deep in their own shit. Well, the AMA's the same. They've been eating and eating nonstop and now they're knee deep in their own

[60] Richard Harris, "Annals of Legislation: Medicare," *New Yorker* (16 July 1966), 49–50, 65; Edward Annis, "Government Health Care: First the Aged, Then Everyone," *Current History* (Aug. 1963): 105–6; Marmor, *Politics of Medicare*, 49–50, 63; "MDs Organize to Fight," *WSJ* (24 July 1962); "Facts about Fedicare" (1964), Box 2, Donovan Ward Papers, University of Iowa Special Collections; AMA News (22. Feb. 1960), clipping Box 206, Witte Papers; "Drug Firms Provide Millions" clipping (Apr. 1961), Box 2; AMPAC clippings, Box 10; DNC Report on AMPAC (22 Mar. 1963), Box 1; "AMA Crusades clipping (May 1961), Box 2, *Congressional Quarterly* clipping (Aug. 1966), Box 9; "AMA Lobby" clipping (July 1965), Box 9, all in Democratic National Committee [DNC] Records, Lyndon Baines Johnson Presidential Library [LBJPL], Austin, Tex.

[61] Kaiser official quoted in Rickey Hendricks, *A Model For National Health Care: The History of Kaiser Permanente* (New Brunswick, N.J., 1993), 107; (quote) Manatos to O'Brien (25 July 1964), Box 9, Manatos Office Files, LBJPL; (quote) Cohen OH [72–26], p. 1:19, LBJPL.

shit and everybody knows it. They won't be able to stop anything." While doctors continued to shape radio and newspaper coverage, they were less successful with television—indeed the major networks declined AMA ads in 1964, citing a policy against selling time on controversial issues. In turn, the AMA claimed a shrinking share of the profession as many doctors and other professional groups (including the American Nurses Association and the American Public Health Association) fell out of step and endorsed Medicare. All of this was reflected in Medicare politics: for the first time, the AMA accompanied its opposition with a serious alternative, conceding that the question was not whether Medicare would pass but what form it would take.[62]

The politics of Medicare proved complex, in different ways, for insurers. The HIAA dug in against Medicare on the grounds that any regulation or displacement of private coverage would be "an undesirable and objectionable move," and that there was no need for "a permanent program to take care of what is essentially a temporary situation [the slow growth of retiree coverage]." At the same time, many insurers saw little danger in federal programs that simply picked off the poorest risks.[63] For insurers, the choice between fighting federal programs and shaping them to their advantage also rested on a calculation of their political standing vis-à-vis consumer, labor, and elderly lobbies on the one hand and other health interests on the other. Like the AMA, the HIAA had devoted much of the 1950s to cementing its political influence and capacity. Member dues brought the HIAA an annual income of about $1.5 million, of which about a third went to salaries, a third to general operating expenses, and a third to a public relations arm, the Health Insurance Institute.[64] The HIAA stayed in close touch with "sympathetic con-

[62] "AMA in Disarray" clipping (July 1965), Box 9, DNC Records, LBJPL; Nestingen Address (13 Mar. 1965), Box 346, SSF (1955–1975), Decimal 900.1, SSF (1955–1975), both in HEW Records; Mrs. Charles Peck to House of Representatives (15 Sept. 1964), Box 1, Medicare Correspondence, Records of the House Committee on Ways and Means, 88th Congress, RG 233, Records of the House of Representatives; Johnson quoted in Robert Dallek, *Flawed Giant: Lyndon Johnson and His Times* (New York, 1998), 209–10; Anne Somers and Herman Somers, "Health Insurance: Are Cost and Quality Controls Necessary," *ILRR* 13:4 (1960): 584; O'Neill, "Siege Tactics of the AMA," 29–31; Wilbur Cohen, "Reflections on the Enactment of Medicare and Medicaid," *Health Care Financing Review,* supp. (1985): 6.

[63] Confidential Report of the Subcommittee to Review Regulatory Policy (Feb. 1964), Box 24; HIAA Statement to the Mass. Joint Legislative Committee (8 Feb. 1960), Box 21; (quote) HIAA Annual Report of the General Manager (1964/1965), Box 20, all in Grahame Papers; Singletary to Ribicoff (6 Jan. 1961), Box 225, Decimal 900.1, SSF (1955–1975), HEW Records.

[64] Hellgren to Grahame (11 Aug. 1961), Box 28; Andersen to HIAA Board (1 May 1962), Box 20; Statement of Income and Expenses, March 1965, Box 20; Statement of Income and Expenses, March 1964, Box 24; Health Insurance Institute, Proposed Budget (5 Feb.

gressional contacts," and worked diligently not only to elect conservatives but to "learn to live persuasively with any Congressman." And it was able to shape press coverage through both its information services and the industry's status as a major advertiser: when CBS began work on a health insurance documentary in 1963, for example, HIAA officials observed that "in view of the fact that [the industry] is spending over a million and a half dollars with CBS on football games in the fall, someone from one of our organizations should be in a strong position to obtain information from the network as to what they are planning."[65]

At the same time, the industry remained divided between mutual and stock companies, between national and regional firms, and by the disparate interests of companies selling different lines of insurance. HIAA officials routinely lamented that "the internal politics of the health insurance business was such as to make a suggested compromise from the insurance business as a whole virtually impossible to come by." This organizational weakness reflected the industry's history of state regulation, which gave its members less contact with national legislators and mired them in the arcane politics of state insurance commissions. And it reflected the uncertain political atmosphere of the early 1960s, in which other health interests were also scrambling to shape federal legislation and congressional deference could no longer be taken for granted. HIAA leaders bemoaned the "gradual loss of our conservative friends in Congress" and the fact that "that coalition between the Republicans and the Southern Democrats which had helped preserve free enterprise, was now ineffective because of the integration question."[66]

Under these circumstances, the industry remained ambivalent. On the one hand, the HIAA doubted "that any type of federal program involving private insurers could be developed without intolerable interference and regulation by the Federal Government [and] . . . the likelihood of future expansion of the Federal program to younger ages or to other areas of benefits." Because it was so leery about "partnering up" with the federal government, the HIAA even opposed an option that would have allowed

---

1965), Box 25; Annual Report of the General Manager (1964/1965), Box 20, all in Grahame Papers.

[65] HIAA Legislative Committee Minutes (25 Apr. 1962), Box 22; Graham memo (13 Oct. 1965), Box 20; (quote) Minutes of the Meeting of the ALC-HIAA-LIAA "Medicare Task Force" (5 Apr. 1965), Box 14; (quote) Thore Memo (22 Jan. 1960), Box 20; (quote) Beebe to Neal (6 Sept. 1963), Box 23, all in Grahame Papers.

[66] Martha Derthick, *Policymaking for Social Security* (Washington, D.C., 1979), 136–42; Cox to Grahame (23 Apr. 1959), Box 26; (quote) Minutes, Joint Committee on Social Security (1 Dec. 1964), Box 21; (quote) Grahame to Neal (8 Aug. 1965), Box 20; Washington Reports, Box 14; To the Members of the Joint Committee on Social Security (25 July 1962), Box 21; (quote) Harrington to Grahame (19 Sept. 1958), Box 26, all in Grahame Papers.

retirees to opt out of Medicare and use their "accounts" to buy private insurance (although the HIAA did toy with the idea of using tax deductions—a subsidy without regulatory strings—for the same purpose).[67] On the other hand, many HIAA members argued that the industry should back Medicare and position itself to administer it—admitting privately that the industry was unlikely to make much progress in over-65 coverage and that public coverage might actually "strengthen Blue Cross and commercial health insurance" by picking off the market's poorest risks. "Our position with respect to coverage below age 65 would be somewhat stronger," one HIAA official reasoned, "if any legislation in this field is within the scope of the OASI system," adding that "the viewpoint that the OASI system is a safer refuge is shared by most Conservative Congressmen and Senators."[68]

Employers too were torn. While trumpeting the virtues of private coverage, most resented any hint of their responsibility for postretirement care. Some offered retiree plans or continuation of group coverage, but most saw care of the elderly as a personal or public responsibility. Indeed, most employers rejected the "toe in the door" reasoning of the AMA and argued "if the most pressing need—institutional services for aged persons— is met, the pressure for more sweeping governmental action will be greatly reduced."[69] The employers' stance reflected their anxieties concerning health costs and their lack of enthusiasm for committing either general revenue or payroll taxes to meeting the escalating demands of patients and providers. Although umbrella organizations such as NAM worked closely with the HIAA to "counteract the flood of favorable publicity," employers' active involvement in the debate was slight. Different firms and industries had divergent stakes in reform, and because most employers continued to see health interests as important political allies, they were not yet prepared to confront them over health costs.[70]

[67] (Quote) Confidential Report of the ALC-HIAA-LIAA Task Force (8 Jan. 1965), Box 25; Financing Medical Care for the Aged (May 1961), Box 21; Minutes of the Meeting of the ALC-LIAA Joint Committee on Social Security and Health Care (8 June 1961), Box 21, all in Grahame Papers.

[68] Minutes of the Meeting of the ALC-HIAA-LIAA Medicare Task Force (5 Apr. 1965), Box 14; To the Members of the Joint Committee on Social Security (25 July 1962), Box 21; Minutes, Joint Committee on Social Security (1 Dec. 1964), Box 21; (quote) Minutes of the Meeting of the ALC-LIAA Joint Committee on Social Security and Health Care (8 June 1961), Box 21, all in Grahame Papers; (quote) Report of the 1964 Task Force on Health (Nov. 1964), Box 1, Task Force Reports, LBJPL; (quote) Thore to Grahame (20 Apr. 1960), Box 20, Grahame Papers; Marion Folsom, "How to Pay the Hospital," *Atlantic* (June 1963): 79–83.

[69] (Quote) Flemming to Keene (24 July 1961), Box 366, Edgar Kaiser Papers; Confidential Report of the ALC-HIAA-LIAA Task Force on Medicare (8 Jan. 1965), Box 25, Grahame Papers; Gaston Rimlinger, "Health Care of the Aged: Who Pays the Bill?" *HBR* 38:1 (Jan.–Feb. 1960): 110–11.

[70] Leo Wade, "Needed: A Closer Look at Industrial Medical Programs," *HBR* 34:2 (Mar.–Apr. 1956), 82; Scott Flemming to Clifford Keene (5 July 1961), Box 366; Edgar Kaiser to

Hospitals strayed even further from the AMA line. The AHA was composed of at least three factions: a small group "convinced that massive government financing is necessary to enable the voluntary general hospital to carry the care of the aged," a slightly larger group that was "ready to accept the S[ocial] S[ecurity] principle because they see no other way to get the needed money," and a slim majority of conservative hospital boards and administrators "heavily infected with the AMA virus." As the debate wore on the AHA warmed up to Medicare, especially as it became clear that Blue Cross would serve as the principal intermediary. The fact that the AHA and the national Blue Cross Association (BCA) supported Medicare, however, did not mean that all their constituents agreed. Many private, parochial, and southern hospitals remained uneasy about the implications of federal spending. Larger Blue Cross plans were "convinced that the future of Blue Cross is at stake in the present issue, that Social Security financing is the only way the necessary money can be had," and hoped that Medicare would solidify their relationship with organized labor and defend community rating against the inroads of the commercials. But many of the smaller state and regional Blue Cross plans "have the point of view of insurance companies," one reformer complained; they feared that support of Medicare would be seen as "giving aid and comfort to the enemy."[71]

Medicare was shaped more by divisions among health interests than by their direct influence. Insurers balked at supporting means-tested alternatives, which they viewed as cynical and meager: the "AMA plan would lead to onerous governmental regulation and would be subject to the central deficiency of the Kerr-Mills program," an industry task force concluded, "namely, that some states will either refuse to participate or will enter the program in a sufficiently minimal basis as to leave a major portion of the need unsatisfied." Insurers and doctors jockeyed for position by blaming each other for health inflation. The doctors are "favorably disposed toward our cause [but] labor under many erroneous assumptions," observed an HIAA official in 1963, " . . . [they] are fully persuaded that that the insurance companies are making a large profit in the health insurance business." The AMA dug in against any role for insurers in policing "reasonable charges." Through 1965 this tension was exacerbated by the insurers' willingness to surrender the elderly to

---

Kuchel (6 Oct. 1964), Box 387, both in Edgar Kaiser Papers; (quote) "To Members of Health and Benefits Committee" (7 May 1962), Box I:23, National Association of Manufacturers [NAM] Papers, Hagley Museum.

[71] (Quotes) "Memorandum re Blue Cross–American Hospital Association" (27 Dec. 1961); "Health Areas for Discussion" (22 Sept. 1965), Box 120:3; "American Hospital Insurance" File, Box 126:6, Wilbur Cohen Papers, SHSW; "Criteria for a Good Bill," *The Nation* 194 (17 Feb. 1962): 136; Cohen to Cater (3 Sept. 1965), WHCF HE, Box 1, LBJ Papers, LBJPL; Cunningham and Cunningham, *The Blues*, 127–34.

public coverage. Many HIAA members argued that supporting Medicare might build legislative goodwill "for use in opposing proposals to provide Federal health benefits for those below 65" but also feared "the danger of being shot at from all sides . . . certainly the AMA and other groups vigorously opposing HR 4222 [the House version of the Medicare bill] would feel they had been deserted." Insurers were torn between the actuarial logic of supporting Medicare and the political danger of breaking with the AMA: "It is possible that [the] Forand or Kennedy approach [of] leaving before age 65 to us and Blues would better preserve private insurance in the long run," reasoned the HIAA's Orville Grahame, "[but] we would naturally prefer not to abandon [the] American Medical Association . . . [and] may be required on account of our friends to stay in opposition to all proposals." Behind all of this lay the admission that "few politicians will want to take on the doctors, but this same restraint will not apply in the case of large insurance corporations. If we fight legislation within the framework of the OASI system to the last ditch . . . we can foresee some serious long range damage to the insurance industry."[72]

Hospitals also broke with the AMA, a split reflected in Medicare's legislative history and in its decision to separate hospitalization and medical insurance. And employers confronted insurers and doctors over both the rising costs of health care and the relationship between Medicare and job-based coverage. Insurers, for example, lobbied for separate payroll taxes to finance Parts A and B (hoping that, under such an arrangement "the public will be more aware of the cost of hospital type benefits and, hence, will be less likely to press for future liberalization"), while employers either pressed for a simpler payroll tax system or fought the imposition of new payroll taxes altogether. And while many employers fought to ensure that Medicare would accommodate cost-conscious benefit and reimbursement procedures, the AMA continued to block any third-party intrusions.[73]

Faced with such divergent stakes and influences, the debate revolved less and less around the principle of a Medicare program and more and more around its details. Many "have accepted the Bill," a Kaiser official noted in late 1964, and were "merely tr[ying] to protect [their] special

[72] (Quote) Confidential Report of the ALC-HIAA-LIAA Task Force on Medicare (8 Jan. 1965), Box 25; (quote) Memo on Medical Relations (20 May 1963), Box 24; (quote) Alternative Policy Positions (20 Mar. 1961), Box 20; (quote) telegram, Grahame to Thore (13 Apr. 1960), Box 20; (quote) Thore to Grahame (20 Apr. 1960), Box 20, all in Grahame Papers; Cohen to Cater (19 July 1966), WHCF IS, Box 1, LBJ Papers.

[73] Confidential Report of the ALC-HIAA-LIAA Task Force on Medicare (8 Jan. 1965), Box 25; Occidental Life to All Agents (12 May 1965), Box 14, both in Grahame Papers; Weissman to Keene (10 Dec. 1964), Box 387, Edgar Kaiser Papers.

interests." The AMA and AHA continued their private lobbying, but also established a presence on advisory committees within the fledgling Medicare structure. "Special pleading, pressure, and negotiations now moved into a new arena," Herman and Anne Somers note, "circumscribed by the law but just as intensive."[74] The hospitals and Blue Cross, which had years of experience with the problems now confronting the federal government, took the lead in the politics of implementation. "Our course has not been . . . . to romance political parties," the BCA's Walter McNerney noted, "but rather . . .through a process of continual negotiations [to] get close to people who are making the decisions." Until passage was a certainty, insurers tried to play it both ways, opposing aspects of the program while simultaneously offering to administer them. By early 1965, the HIAA thought it prudent to drop its opposition altogether and work for "amendments to the bill in order to provide the best legislation it can under the circumstances."[75] Organized medicine remained aloof but, fearing a provider boycott, the administration reached out to the AMA, promising that "you fellows can be on the inside looking out if you want." The AMA agreed privately that it "must *actively participate* in the development of the rules and regulations, . . . [in] the actual *implementation* of the legislation," and "develop a strong, vigorous, and convincing program to *contain* the law."[76]

After the bill's passage, attention shifted to arcane battles over the choice of intermediaries, the establishment of "reasonable costs," and mechanisms for reimbursement or utilization review. In these respects, the new law was a bonanza for private interests. It relieved private employers and commercial insurers of their most troublesome risks and, in doing so, buttressed the politics of employment-based private insurance. For hospitals and doctors, virtually all of whom scrambled to participate in the new programs, it promised to transform underinsured and underserviced populations into a stable pool of patient-consumers. The tone of the debate, as one UAW official noted, seemed to be: "We are opposed to H.R.

---

[74] (Quote) "Discussion of Proposed Amendments" (Dec. 1964), Box 387, Edgar Kaiser Papers; Herman Somers and Anne Somers, *Medicare and the Hospitals: Issues and Prospects* (Washington, D.C., 1967), 35–40 (quote at 35).

[75] McNerney quoted in Cunningham and Cunningham, *The Blues*, 141–42; Minutes, Joint Committee on Social Security (15 Apr. 1965), Box 21; (quote) Legislative Committee Minutes (24 Feb. 1965), Box 23, both in Grahame Papers.

[76] Morris to Mills (29 May 1964), Box 32, Medicare Correspondence, Records of the House Committee on Ways and Means, 88th Congress, Records of the House of Representatives; Cohen OH [72–26], p. 2:13, LBJPL; (quote) Cater to LBJ (17 Sept. 1965), Box 14, Cater Office Files, LBJPL; Cater to LBJ (28 July 1965), Cohen to Cater (26 July 1965), Cohen to Cater (16 July 1965), and Gardner memorandum for the President (13 Dec. 1965), all in WHCF IS, Box 1, LBJ Papers; (quote) "We the People of the United States: Are We Sheep?" *JAMA* 193:1 (1965): 117.

6675 [Medicare] but as long as it is going to pass we wish to make as much money as possible from it." Or as a congressional opponent observed, "we are confronted with a bill that has been so drafted that quite a bit of honey has been placed under the beehive to attract the bees."[77]

In its final form, Medicare/Medicaid testified to providers' political clout and the administration's anxieties. The 1965 reforms made the now-routine distinction between charitable public assistance (Medicaid) and contributory social insurance (Medicare), but also, driven by the divergent interests of hospitals and doctors, distinguished hospitalization insurance from medical coverage.[78] Both programs deferred administration to private carriers and the choice of the appropriate "intermediary" to the hospitals ("the voluntary hospital system and the federal government started going steady last month," Wilbur Cohen observed, "and they both seem pleased with the whole thing, if a little nervous at times"). While insurers worked to "contain and modify" Medicare in such a way that they could "step forward and undertake the administration," the hospitals turned to Blue Cross—designated intermediary for thirty-one states and nearly 90 percent of the hospital beds covered by Medicare. Blue Shield captured about 60 percent of Part B, with commercials picking up the rest.[79] Finally, HEW abandoned any pretense of fee schedules in favor of a system (pioneered by Blue Cross) by which providers could bill "usual, customary, and reasonable" charges and hospitals could roll depreciation and other costs into a "cost-plus" reimbursement formula. HEW was convinced that any regulation or monitoring of charges would "get us into the touchy doctor area" and that deferring this task to private insurers and the Blues was "the only way to get the bill passed."[80]

[77] Somers and Somers, *Medicare and the Hospitals*, 41; *BW* (6 Dec. 1964), 103–4; Report of the Comprehensive Coverage Subcommittee (24 Jan. 1966), Box 23; Grahame to Myers (21 Apr. 1965), Box 14, both in Grahame Papers; *BW* (16 Jan. 1965), 132; "Optometry's Position with Respect to H.R. 6675" (May 1965); Cohen to Byrd (1 June 1965), both in Box 291, SSF (1955–1975), HEW Records; Cunningham and Cunningham, *The Blues*, 157; (quote) Glasser to Roy Reuther (6 May 1965), Box 3, Part I, Series I, Records of the UAW Social Security Department, Archives of Labor History and Urban Affairs, Wayne State University, Detroit, Mich.; (quote) *Congressional Record* 111:12 (1965), 16071.

[78] HEW Administrative History, Box 9, Part 18, pp. 82–84, LBJPL; Elizabeth Wickenden Goldschmidt OH, 2:20, LBJPL; Blasingame to Gardner (7 July 1966), WHCF WE 15, LBJPL; Cohen to O'Brien (29 July 1965), WHCF IS, Box 1, LBJPL.

[79] Cunningham and Cunningham, *The Blues*, 145–70 (Cohen quoted at 147); (quote) Occidental Life to All Agents (12 May 1965), Box 14, Grahame Papers; Group Health Mutual to Cohen (4 June 1965), Box 291, Commissioner's Correspondence (1936–1969), HEW Records; Somers and Somers, *Medicare and the Hospitals*, 33–35; Robert Ball, "Report on Implementation of the Health Insurance Program" (26 Feb. 1966), Box 287, Commissioner's Correspondence (1936–1969), SSA Records; "Memorandum re Blue Cross–American Hospital Association" (27 Dec. 1961), Box 120:3, Cohen Papers.

[80] Cunningham and Cunningham, *The Blues*, 151–53; "Raid on Medicare," *The Nation* 203 (11 July 1966): 36; Theodore Marmor, "Coping with a Creeping Crisis: Medicare at

The Corporate Compromise in Crisis: Interests versus Reform, 1966–1992

Medicare and Medicaid were designed to protect the fiscal integrity of Social Security and the political legitimacy of private provision. The AMA felt that the 1965 reforms marked the outer boundaries of public responsibility and redoubled its efforts to defend "a constantly advancing health care system in America—a system based on incentives and freedom of choice." The HIAA thought it "increasingly important" after 1965 "for the insurance carriers to develop an effective public relations story that will demonstrate to the non-indigent segment of the population why they are better off with private insurance than under a governmental program." For their part, reformers lamented that 1965 could be considered little more than "a manageable beginning . . . within boundaries of cost derived mainly by political considerations," I. S. Falk concluded, adding that "its *insurance* design was dictated largely by its *insurance opponents* . . . [and] its *medical service* design was dictated largely by its *professional opponents*."[81] More important, both public insurance and private insurance were immediately in trouble. An explosion of demand for health services and the new programs' reimbursement policies created a lasting fiscal crisis. In turn, the argument that Medicare and Medicaid would allow private group coverage to thrive collapsed. Employers responded to health care inflation in an increasingly uncertain competitive environment by questioning the terms and premises of managerial responsibility.

The most striking characteristic of the new corporate compromise was its cost-consciousness. After 1965, health politics revolved less around the willingness of private or public plans to expand coverage and more around their ability to slow health inflation. This set health interests against each other, as providers sought to shift the blame for rising costs, private and public interests refashioned a long-standing debate about what form of provision sustained the appropriate medical and market

---

Twenty," in *Social Security: Beyond the Rhetoric of Crisis*, ed. Theodore Marmor and Jerry Mashaw (Princeton, N.J., 1988), 184–85; Hughes to Moyers (18 May 1965), WHCF LE/IS 75, LBJ Papers; (quote) Wilbur Cohen, "Random Reflections on the Great Society's Politics and Health Care Programs after Twenty Years," in *The Great Society and Its Legacy: Twenty Years of U.S. Social Policy*, ed. Marshal Kaplan and Peggy Cuciti (Durham, N.C., 1986), 118; John Robson, "Possible Actions Re Medical Costs" (n.d.), Box 13, Robson-Ross Office Files, LBJPL.

[81] "Analysis of Communications of the AMA" (Mar. 1969), Box 1:5, Philip Lesly Papers, SHSW; Report of the Comprehensive Coverage Subcommittee (24 Jan. 1966), Box 23, Grahame Papers; Isidore Falk, "Beyond Medicare" (Nov. 1968), p. 4, Box 4 (Mss 400), Altmeyer Papers.

incentives, and payers (especially employers) confronted providers with a litany of administrative waste, medical excess, and high costs. Doctors, insurers, and employers devoted renewed energy and resources to health care issues, but found it harder and harder to establish any common political ground.

Employers emerged as the leading advocates of reform. As the politics of growth unraveled, managers and politicians blamed slow productivity, stagnant profits, and competitive pressures on a combination of high wages and excessive social spending. In this setting, health care was especially vulnerable. Health inflation preceded the "stagflationary" crisis of the 1970s, ran well ahead of even the double-digit rates of the mid-1970s, and persisted in the leaner deflationary politics of the 1980s and 1990s. Although American social spending remained meager by international standards, health programs (especially Medicaid) were targeted as budget-busting outliers. Business anxieties were magnified by the fact that health inflation continued even as firms pared back wages and other benefits; by the fact that many American firms did not provide health benefits; and by the fact that health care was not a business cost in competing nations. Employers and politicians identified the health care market as a textbook example of American sloth and inefficiency, blasting doctors and hospitals as "an army of pushcart vendors in an age of supermarkets." "If our national health system is to escape the fat layers of administrative expense and the inevitable abuses that accompany greater federal control," argued a W. R. Grace executive, "business organizations must provide these three 'wonder drugs': (1) real management, (2) a meaningful system of incentives and disincentives, and (3) the opportunity for each consumer to choose the basic medical services he feels he can afford." In this sense, business echoed the reformers' long-standing lament about fragmentation and administrative waste, but toward competitive efficiency rather than redistributive ends.[82]

One measure of business anxiety was the explosion of coalitions and task forces charged with tackling the health care crisis. In part, this re-

[82] Ford, "A Businessman Looks at Health"; Minutes of the Employee Health and Benefits Committee (30 Nov. 1962), Box IV:109, NAM Papers; Draft Memo to President's Advisory Committee (15 Aug. 1966), Box 21, Edgar Kaiser Papers; *BW* (16 May 1977): 127; (quote) "It's Time to Operate," *Fortune* 81:1 (Jan. 1970): 79; "Better Care at Less Cost with No Miracles," *Fortune* 81:1 (Jan. 1970): 80–83, 126–30; "Hospitals Need Management Even More than Money," *Fortune* 81:1 (Jan. 1970), 96–99, 150–51; Linda Bergthold, *Purchasing Power in Health: Business, the State, and Health Care Politics* (New Brunswick, N.J., 1990), 22–27; Chamber testimony in House Committee on Ways and Means, *Hearings: National Health Insurance Proposals: Part 11* 92:1 (Oct.–Nov. 1971), 2500–2501, 2524–28; Chamber of Commerce, "Improving Our Nation's Health Care System: Proposals for the 1970s" (1971), Box II:27, Chamber of Commerce Papers.

flected a broader trend in business organization and representation through the 1970s and 1980s. In response to the ongoing economic crisis and a more inviting political climate after 1980, the resources devoted to business organization multiplied. Between 1961 and 1979, the number of firms with registered lobbyists grew from 130 to 650, nearly half of which boasted full-time Washington staffs. And between 1974 and 1982 the number of corporate political action committees grew almost twentyfold, from 89 to over 1,500. Again health care was a uniquely urgent focus of attention. The proliferation of health care coalitions and commissions included special task forces created by the Chamber of Commerce, the Business Roundtable, and the Washington Business Group on Health (WBGH) for the express purpose of establishing corporate leadership in health reform. The WBGH relied on a combination of member dues and foundation support and by the mid-1980s claimed a membership of nearly two hundred firms and a full-time staff of over twenty-five.[83]

This flurry of organization again altered the terms of the corporate compromise. Business pulled even with, even surpassed, the political stature of organized medicine. Although the AMA claimed an established political presence, it could not claim the natural clout of major employers. "The AMA will send car loads of lobbyists up the Hill on an issue," the WBGH's Willis Goldbleck gloated, "and we only have to write one note."[84] But such advantages were not accompanied by any lasting consensus as to solutions. Most agreed that health costs were spiraling out of control and believed that business bore a disproportionate share of the burden. But beyond this, business opinion was fragmented by firm size, industry, competitive horizons, and experience with private insurance. A political solution that controlled costs or eased the burden for some firms, after all, was likely to do so by imposing those costs and burdens on others. Business interests matched their new prominence in the health care debate with a fundamental confusion as to whether they should expand the private welfare state or abandon it.

For providers, business anxieties represented a direct challenge to their economic interests and their political clout. Organized medicine remained a formidable political force. The AMA bumped up its dues in the late 1960s and early 1970s, a move that yielded an extra $4 million "to put its views across" and an annual budget of nearly $30 million. By the early 1970s, AMPAC claimed over 60,000 members and an annual war chest of about $3.5 million, and remained "one of the best operations in

---

[83] David Vogel, *Kindred Strangers: The Uneasy Relationship between Business and Politics in the United States* (Princeton, N.J., 1996), 132; Bergthold, *Purchasing Power in Health*, 3–6, 35–58, 141–45.

[84] Goldbleck quoted in Bergthold, *Purchasing Power in Health*, 46–47.

the country from the standpoint of gathering political intelligence." At the same time, the AMA was losing ground to other interest groups and losing stature within the profession. Beginning in the mid-1960s, some state medical societies dropped national membership and dues as requirements for membership. New doctors joined at a tepid rate (barely 20 percent) and some of the conservative specialist groups quit in response to the AMA's flirtation with reform in the early 1970s. By 1971 national membership had tumbled to just over 150,000—representing, for the first time since the 1920s, less than half of the nation's doctors. In a struggling economy, efforts to protect professional autonomy and privileges seemed increasingly reactionary and selfish. The AMA's reputation, as one doctor observed in a letter of resignation, "wouldn't be envied by the Teamsters."[85]

As employers pressed doctors to streamline provision, doctors dug in against intrusion on their professional turf. "Passengers who insist on flying the aircraft," said AMA president Russell Roth in 1976, "are called hijackers." Organized medicine objected especially to the profusion of business groups interested in health reform—a development that the Colorado Medical Society dismissed as the equivalent of "putting together physicians to discuss how to manufacture automobiles." Insurers, and especially Blue Cross, were caught in the cross fire. When the Blue Cross Association (at the urging of employers) endorsed experimentation with health maintenance organizations in the late 1960s, the AMA and the National Association of Blue Shield Plans (NABSP) reacted angrily—the former going so far as to formally censure BCA chair McNerney. At the same time, organized medicine and business struggled to maintain the common ground that had girded earlier joint efforts against state medicine. The WBGH worked closely with the AMA; the latter established a corporate liaison program in the mid-1970s. And the AMA and the Business Roundtable joined the AHA, the Blues, the HIAA, and labor representatives on the Dunlop Group of Six, a short-lived effort to bring leading health care interests together to discuss their common problems.[86] In all, however, the relationship between providers and employers was drifting from a compromise centered on employment-based insurance to a confrontation over costs and political solutions.

As the new politics of health made it difficult for health interests to reconcile their competing stakes, it also made it difficult for politicians

---

[85] "Doctors Told to Resist" clipping (July 1966) and "AMA Busy" clipping (June 1966), both in Box 1, DNC Records; *BW* (24 June 1972): 108–9 (quote at 109); (quote) *WSJ* (7 Feb. 1969), 1.

[86] Roth quoted in Starr, *Social Transformation of American Medicine*, 402; Bergthold, *Purchasing Power in Health*, 47–51, CMS quoted at 54.

to accommodate them. The Nixon administration boasted close ties to the AMA (1974 AMA president Malcolm Todd traveled with the Nixon campaign in 1952 and 1960 and chaired Physicians for the President in 1972).[87] Nixon staffers argued for an "overall interest-group strategy" in which accommodation of powerful interests could be accompanied by at least the illusion of "a major health initiative." "We must be careful not to alienate any more of our natural friends," cautioned one official. "Attention must be given to doctors, nurses, hospital administrators, insurance companies, state medical authorities, drug manufacturers, etc." This proved an impossible task. The AMA and AMPAC felt the administration was slow to pay attention to health care and unreliably deferential when it did. And the administration had to keep in mind its own stake as an institutional consumer of health services. It grew increasingly frustrated with the penchant of health interests to rail against federal intervention in one breath only to demand a greater share of federal programs with the next—a pattern of lobbying that prompted one staffer to lament that the AMA and others were "too stupid to know [they] can't have it both ways."[88]

The administration's "potpourri of efforts" in the early 1970s was shaped by a shortsighted desire to please providers and insurers and employers simultaneously. The AMA's "Medicredit" proposal earned organized medicine few points for compromise and considerable grief from its more conservative members. The AHA's "Ameriplan" proposal fell flat, as both Blue Cross and the AMA lined up against it.[89] Business interests, less interested in expanded coverage than in cost controls, grew increasingly leery as attention shifted to the prospect of mandated employment-based care. Although some supported a mandate accompa-

[87] Cavanaugh to Chapin (21 Mar. 1972), Box IS:2; "Meeting with AMA" (4 Feb. 1974), Box IS:3; Malek to Cole (14 Mar. 1972), Box HE:2; Cavanaugh to Cole (29 June 1972), Box IS:2, all in White House Special File (Confidential Files) [WHSF], Richard M. Nixon Papers, National Archives.

[88] (Quote) Morgan to Chapin (12 June 1970), Box HE:1, WHCF; (quote) Moore to Cole (3 Feb. 1972), Box IS:1,WHSF; Cavanaugh to Cole (29 June 1972), Box IS:2, WHSF; (quote) Timmons to Cole (29 Jan. 1974), Box IS:3, WHCF; "Proposed Health Game Plan" (12 Mar. 1971), Box IS:1, WHSF; Duffy to MacGregor (26 May 1971), Box IS:2, WHSF; Henry Hyde to Chapin (20 Oct. 1969), Box HE:1,WHCF; Dent to Harlow (12 May 1970), Box HE:1, WHCF; (quote) Cole to Cavanaugh (8 June 1971), Box IS:1, WHSF, all in Nixon Papers.

[89] (Quote) Theodore Marmor, "The Struggle over National Health Insurance" (1972), in Box 23, George Wiley Papers, SHSW; Moore to Cole (3 Feb. 1972), Box IS:1; Cole to Cavanaugh (5 Mar. 1971), Box IS:3, both in WHSF, Nixon Papers; House Committee on Ways and Means, *Hearings: National Health Insurance Proposals: Part 11* 92:1 (Oct.–Nov. 1971), 2626–27; *JAMA* 216:8 (1971): 1264; Cunningham and Cunningham, *The Blues*, 187–89.

nied by cost controls, most employers and leading business organizations opposed the baggage that came with it.[90] Commercial insurers, meanwhile, were able to negotiate the reform flurry fairly effectively. Through 1969 and 1970, the industry publicly opposed reform while privately preparing to administer new federal benefits and offer supplemental coverage. In the 1972 round, Congress offered an even more expansive role for insurers and, by 1974, the leading reform proposal was little more than a vast federal subsidy shaped, as the *New York Times* observed, by "the recognition of that industry's power to kill any legislation it considers unacceptable."[91]

In the end, the 1971–74 reforms collapsed in much the same way, and for much the same reasons, that the Clinton plan would collapse twenty years later. While Nixon's HEW worked closely with organized medicine, insurers, and business interests, each had quite divergent motives and stakes. As the administration reworked its proposal—appeasing providers by paring back the basic benefit package, appeasing business by offering to phase in or subsidize mandates, and appeasing insurers by accomodating commercial coverage—these contradictory goals made moving ahead both futile and politically dangerous. It proved impossible, in short, to assure employers that controlling costs was worth the risk of mandating coverage, while assuring providers and insurers that a vastly expanded market was worth the risk of cost controls.[92]

As the prospect for reform evaporated, attention turned to the promise of the health maintenance organization (HMO). The HMO strategy reflected a desire to steal the thunder of congressional Democrats, restrain domestic spending, and focus on supply-side market reforms. More important, the 1973 HMO Act allowed the administration and Congress to negotiate, for the moment, the shifting politics of the corporate compromise. The HMO represented both employers' insistence that federal policy facilitate cost savings and market discipline (goals, not inci-

[90] Chamber of Commerce, "Improving Our Nation's Health Care System: Proposals for the 1970s" (1971), Box II:27, Chamber of Commerce Papers; *BW* (30 Oct. 1971): 104; NAM, "Proposed Policy Recommendation" (Dec. 1970), Box I:103, NAM Papers; House Committee on Ways and Means, *Hearings: National Health Insurance: Part 4* 93:2 (Apr.–July 1974), 1780–88; Cole to Cavanaugh (8 June 1971), Box IS:1, WHSF; Cook to Altman (21 Dec. 1973), Box IS:3, WHCF, both in Nixon Papers.

[91] "Draft of the Minutes of the Technical Advisory Group of CNHI" (18 Nov. 1969), Box 3 (Mss 400), Altmeyer Papers; Minutes of the Meeting of the CNHI Technical Committee (5 July 1972 and 31 Aug. 1972), Box 3, Altmeyer add.; Draft: The Problem of Extending Health Coverage to the Uninsured (22 Jan. 1966), Box 23; McDougal to Grahame (10 June 1966), Box 24, both in Grahame Papers; *NYT* cited in Vicente Navarro, *The Politics of Health Policy: The U.S. Reforms, 1980–1994* (Cambridge, Mass., 1994), 203.

[92] "Proposed Health Game Plan" (12 Mar. 1971), Box IS:1, WHSF; Weinberger to Nixon (11 Jan. 1974), Box IS:3, WHCF, Nixon Papers.

dentally, shared by the federal government) and insurers' interest in sustaining private coverage and restraining health inflation—even at the price of some federal preemption of state regulation. Providers proved less enthusiastic. Hospitals welcomed the prospect of HMO's delivering new covered groups to their doors while resenting the restraints proposed on hospitalization and hospital charges. And doctors dug in against another third-party threat—a stance that dragged out the HMO debate but could not block the passage of the bill in 1973.[93]

After the mid-1970s, health care politics settled into an anxious pattern by which health interests sought to shuffle the burden of (and blame for) rising costs. Employers pressed policymakers and private providers alike, reminding the latter of their clout as health consumers and the former of their role as a surrogate for public provision. Providers fended off pressure from health consumers to control costs. Insurers worked to convince employers and providers of their willingness and ability to rein in inflation. And state and federal politicians scrambled to trim their own health spending and facilitate "competitive" solutions. The governing political assumption, expressed repeatedly by the Carter administration after 1976, was that health costs had to be controlled before any consideration was given to broader coverage. The administration rebuffed those who hoped that a Democratic president might revisit Edward Kennedy's proposals of the early 1970s. To the reformers' dismay, the administration insisted on keeping any new health programs off the federal budget and on maintaining a place for private insurers—a stance that prompted I. S. Falk to reflect: "I have never been confident [that we] could wholly exclude the insurance industry, but I have thought that we should go down fighting."[94]

These interests and anxieties were captured by the administration's efforts at hospital cost containment. Eager to do something about health inflation, the administration targeted hospitals in order to avoid confronting the AMA. The proposal to cap hospital spending was shaped largely by business demands, but the administration also sought the advice of "groups representing the widest possible range of interested parties"—an approach one critic saw as "a formula for building fortifications around the status quo" because "most of the 'interested parties,' with just a few quibbles here and there, are quite pleased with the extravagant

---

[93] "Sensible Surgery," *Fortune* 87:4 (Apr. 1973): 110; NAM, "Policy Recommendation" (Dec. 1970), Box I:103, NAM Records; Congressional Quarterly, *Health Policy: The Legislative Agenda* (Washington, D.C., 1980), 68–69; Himmelstein and Woolhander, "The Corporate Compromise," 20–26.

[94] CNHI Executive Committee (20 Mar. 1978) and Corman (D-Calif.) to Fraser (17 May 1978), both in Box 146:2131; Falk to Willcox (1 Mar. 1977), Box 147:2142, Series III, Falk Papers.

nature of American medicine, and when they are not, their discontent derives from self-perceived failure to get their share." Only insurers (who had to both pay hospital bills and pass on the inflationary bad news to employers) went along. Employers saw little distinction between the promise of hospital cost containment and the peril of broader price controls. Organized medicine dug in against the indirect threat of federal intervention. And hospitals, not surprisingly, went nuts. The bill made it no further than the House Commerce Committee, where "the hospitals and the AMA were just throwing money at the Committee as fast as they could," Representative Toby Moffett (D-Conn.) recalled. "It was coming in in wheelbarrows."[95]

The election of Ronald Reagan in 1980 gave political and ideological direction to what was already a well-established, if haphazard, response to economic decline. For health interests, Reagan offered nothing new: business pressed for relief from spiraling costs and spent the decade herding employees into HMOs, forcing employees to bear more of the costs, and paring back coverage. Providers remained leery of both "market" reforms and cuts in state and federal health spending. The AMA, which saw the administration as an ideological ally, nevertheless remained on the defensive and spent close to $12 million between 1981 and 1991 on congressional campaigns. The dilemma, for employers and providers, was that the administration remained fundamentally ambivalent about supply-side solutions and proved willing to adopt coercive measures as long as they cut federal spending.[96] Behind broad ideological agreement that "restoring" competition in health was a good idea, the administration was torn between leading a retreat from government health spending and using its clout as a health consumer to coerce

[95] Congressional Quarterly, *Health Policy: The Legislative Agenda*, 24–25, 28; (quote) Daniel Greenberg, "Cost Containment: Another Crusade Begins," *NEJM* 296:12 (24 Mar. 1977): 699; WBGH, "Statement of Concern about National Health Insurance" (Oct. 1977), Box 489, Edgar Kaiser Papers; Joseph Onek, "President Carter's Principle for Health Care Cost Containment and National Health Insurance," in *Industry's Voice in Health Policy*, ed. Richard Egdahl and Diane Walsh (New York, 1979), 20–21; Philip Stern, *The Best Congress Money Can Buy* (New York, 1988), 7, 22, 141–42 (quote at 102–3).

[96] Thomas Bodenheimer and Kip Sullivan, "How Large Employers Are Shaping the Health Care Marketplace," *NEJM* 338:14 (1998): 1003–5; Vicki Kemper and Vivieca Novak, "What's Blocking Health Care Reform?" *IJHS* 23:1 (1993): 71; Common Cause, "Why the United States Does Not Have a National Health Program: The Medical Industrial Complex and Its PAC Contributions to Congressional Candidates, January 1, 1981 through June 30, 1991," *IJHS* 22:4 (1992): 621–44; Bergthold, *Purchasing Power in Health*, 36–37; Robert Evans, "Finding the Levers, Finding the Courage: Lessons from Cost Containment in North America," *JHPPL* 11 (1986): 589, 596; Alain Enthoven, "How Interested Groups Have Responded to a Proposal for Economic Competition in Health Services," *American Economic Review* 70 (May 1980): 143, 146.

change. Efforts to restrain health consumers invariably set the market's deference to private interests against an older antistatist standard—the autonomy of private providers. The riddle, for an administration eager to champion private markets and private medicine, was that doctors objected to both the third-party threat posed by state intervention and the third-party threat posed by consumers and insurers.[97]

The Fifth Time as Farce: Interests versus Reform in the 1990s

The Democrats took over the White House in 1992 with a willingness to tackle health reform, but without any inclination to confront either the logic of the corporate compromise or the clout of its constituent interests. In the twenty years since national health insurance had last been considered, health interests were more entrenched, and more divided, than ever. Some reformers argued that such disarray, against a backdrop of health inflation and tenuous private coverage, was a real political opportunity. But the administration's Health Care Task Force devoted much of its energy to meeting with interests and tailoring the plan-in-progress to accommodate their quite contradictory goals. Overtures to reform interests were more sporadic and more cynical—and revolved largely around the task of persuading organized labor, single-payer advocates, and others that they could do no better than the administration's plan. The Clinton health plan was more a catalogue of concessions than a solution, a legislative tack (as one critic noted) "close to handing blank paper to special interest lobbyists and saying, Hey, you do it."[98]

While the CHP was inspired by business anxieties, the business community remained ambivalent. Any firm's stand on health reform was a reflection of what it was paying, what it was liable to pay in the future, and what its competitors were paying. Those with a greater burden of current and retiree benefits were more interested in socializing that burden. Many firms remained unsure whether they should confront the

[97] John Iglehart, "The Administration's Assault on Domestic Spending and the Threat to Health Care Programs," *NEJM* 312:8 (21 Feb. 1985): 526–27; Bergthold, *Purchasing Power in Health*, 67–68, 126–27; David Young and Richard Saltman, "Preventive Medicine for Hospital Costs," *HBR* 61:1 (Jan.–Feb. 1983): 129.

[98] Jacob Hacker, "National Health Care Reform: An Idea Whose Time Came and Went," *JHPPL* 21:4 (1996): 67–671; "Meetings with Outside Groups" (14 Mar. 1993) and Starr to Magaziner (16 Dec. 1992), both in Box 3305, Records of the Clinton Health Care Task Force [CHTF], National Archives; "Lobbyists of Every Stripe on Health Care," *NYT* (24 Sept. 1993): A1, A12; "Surprise! Health Care's Fever May Have Finally Broken," *BW* (26 Apr. 1993); "Health Care Plan Moves to Center of Political Stage," *NYT* (9 Aug. 1993): A1, A8; (quote) David Corn in *The Nation* (20 Sept. 1993): 271.

health industry as its principal consumer or abandon that role by forcing workers to bear more of the costs or by dumping coverage altogether. The administration strove to appeal to every shade of business opinion, but it could not, as the drafting process dragged on, skirt the reality that reform was an exercise in "picking winners and losers within and among industries" (as a General Mills executive put it) in such a way as to impose new costs on small and service sector firms while offering "sizable, guaranteed, government hand-outs" to large unionized firms with poor records of cost containment.[99]

For many large firms, reform had real appeal: "some of us who today are free market advocates," conceded GE vice president Art Puccini, "[may have] to reexamine our thinking and positions with respect to government sponsored national health insurance." Or as one benefits consultant mimicked his corporate clients: "They say, 'What do we do now?' and I smile and say, 'Write your congressman and ask for national health insurance.' " For such firms, as the American Automobile Manufacturers Association (AAMA) noted, an employer mandate "leveled the playing field between firms and eliminated unfair competitive advantages based on health care costs." Or as a Baltimore construction firm testified: "We would be willing to accept an incremental increase in our costs [alongside mandated coverage] for very selfish reasons. A lot of our competitors don't provide any insurance at all and that puts us at a competitive disadvantage." In turn, the CHP would allow large employers to escape the indirect burden (taxes and insurance premiums) of caring for the uninsured. "Right now, big companies pay all of the health costs of small companies that are not providing insurance," argued WBGH chair Willis Goldbleck. "It's just another form of tax." Chrysler chair Robert Eaton, claiming that 28 percent of his industry's health care costs went to the uninsured, characterized the current system as "Robin Hood medicine."[100] Nowhere was this competitive disparity more glaring than

[99] "Cynthia Sullivan et al., "Employer-Sponsored Health Insurance in 1991," *HA* 11:4 (Winter 1992): 172–85; Lawrence Brown, "Dogmatic Slumbers: American Business and Health Policy," *JHPPL* 18:2 (1993): 340–52; "Clinton's Health Care Sell-A-Thon," *BW* (24 May 1993): 30–32; "Employees Face Shift in Benefits," *NYT* (14 Sept. 1991): A18; Beth Mintz, "Business Participation in Health Care Policy Reform: Factors Contributing to Collective Action within the Business Community," *Social Problems* 42:3 (1995): 411; Michael Peel (General Mills) quoted in testimony in Senate Committee on Labor and Human Resources, *Hearings: Health Security Act of 1993: Part I* 103:1 (Oct.–Nov., 1993), 328–30.

[100] Puccini quoted in *Washington Post National Weekly Edition* (11–17 Sept. 1989): 10–11; consultant quoted in *National Journal* (9 Sept. 1989): 2201–05; (quotes) AAMA testimony in Senate Committee on Labor and Human Resources, *Hearings: Health Security Act of 1993: Part IV* 103:2 (Jan.–Mar., 1994), 498; Baltimore construction in House Committee on Ways and Means, *Hearing: Private Health Insurance Reform* 102:2 (Mar. 1992), 229; (quote) "The Battle for Health Insurance," *Fortune* 118:7 (26 Sept. 1988), 148; *BW* (25 May 1987), 62;

over the provision of health benefits to retirees—a cost borne disproportionately by unionized mass-production firms for whom the ravages of
economic decline and health inflation were also particularly acute. Such
firms, as *Business Week* concluded, "will stick with almost any reform that
promises to cut the costs of caring for aging, unionized workers." After
a 1993 adjustment in federal accounting standards compelled firms to
record their health care liabilities as they accrued rather than as they
were paid out, many moved to shake commitments to retirees at the
bargaining table and in the courts.[101]

The administration appreciated these anxieties and designed its
health plan accordingly. "Most businesses now insuring employees will
pay less and their fears of ongoing cost increases should be abated," the
task force reasoned, adding that "large businesses will benefit from a
reduction in cost-shifting and will have the option to continue managing
their own health benefits plans." But large employers remained uncertain whether mandating employment-based care was preferable to escaping such responsibilities altogether. Many who were sympathetic to the
idea of spreading health costs across all employment nevertheless worried that the "basic" coverage floated by the administration was too generous and that the employers' share (80 percent) of premiums was too
high. One of the ironies of business's health care politics, in this respect,
was that those firms who were most interested in socializing their health
care costs were also the most reluctant to join the public insurance pools
that might have made that possible. Large firms already providing health
insurance had no interest in forgoing the fruits of experience rating and
insisted on the freedom to opt out of regional health alliances.[102] For the
same reasons large employers were drawn to the CHP, small and service
sector employers dug in against it. Opposition was led by the National
Federation of Independent Business (NFIB), "a political force, particularly in the South," one observer noted, "second only to the Elvis Presley

---

"Companies' Costs: How Much Is Fair?" *NYT* (7 Jan. 1992): C2; "Excerpts from Clinton's
Conference," *NYT,* (15 Dec. 1992): A14; "Movement to Sell Basic Health Plan Is Found
Faltering," *NYT* (10 Dec. 1991): A1; Eaton quoted in *NYT* (23 Aug. 1993): A9; *BW* (29 Mar.
1993): 66; memo from Ford, Chrysler and GM for Magaziner (16 Mar. 1993), Box 3305,
CHTF Records.

[101] (Quote) *BW* (25 July 1994): 32–33; "GM Orders Staff to Pay Part of Health Care Cost,"
NYT (26 Aug. 1992): C3; "Utilities Want to Raise Rates to Meet Future Health Costs," *NYT*
(7 Jan. 1992): A1; "Navistar May Sell Stock," *WSJ* (9 Dec. 1992): B6; *BW* (10 Aug. 92): 32;
"Breaking Promises to Retirees," *NYT* (15 Sept. 1991); (quote) "Ford to Cut 7.7 Billion,"
NYT (17 Dec. 92): C1; "Witco Sees Charges" *WSJ* (9 Dec.1992): B6.

[102] (Quote) Garamendi to Clinton (4 Dec. 1992), Box 4001; Zelman memo (14 Dec.
1992), Box 3279, both in CHTF Records; Chamber of Commerce testimony in Senate,
Health Security Act of 1993: Part I, 349–50; Sullivan testimony in Senate, *Health Security Act of
1993: Part II,* 46–47.

Fan Club in its pressure that can be brought to bear on Members of Congress." Eager to dampen dissent, the task force ducked the logic of an employer mandate (which imposed the costs of new coverage on laggard firms) and offered to subsidize subscription in the new health alliances. This became an intensely political issue—not only over which firms would qualify for federal subsidies but over the budgetary implications of using public money to pay for private coverage. The White House, under pressure from large low-wage firms (including Arkansas's Tyson Chicken), pressed the task force to juggle the employer mandate in such a way as to accommodate such firms and "alleviate one major source of opposition."[103]

Business disarray was reflected in the politics of business organization. Early on, the Chamber of Commerce, the Business Roundtable, the National Leadership Coalition, and the WBGH were cautious proponents of the CHP. But as the debate wore on, divergent stakes forced peak associations (like the chamber) to retreat and single-issue groups (like the leadership coalition) to narrow their membership to a like-minded few. The chamber faced pressure from both small business members and congressional ideologues (who reminded the chamber that it was its "duty to categorically oppose everything Clinton was in favor of") and executed an about-face in early 1994—firing its chief congressional lobbyist and joining the opposition. The Business Roundtable split into at least four factions: some large employers favored a mandate, large service-sector employers (including PepsiCo, Marriott, and Sears) opposed a mandate, insurers and drug companies opposed the entire plan, and many resented the very idea of such a massive new program. Even groups formed specifically to facilitate business influence over health policy, including the WBGH, found it impossible to establish any meaningful political stance without risking the defection of those who felt they had gone too far or not far enough. Small business, disenchanted with the willingness of national business groups to toy with the employer mandate, threw their lot in with the insurance industry in coalitions such as the Health Care Equity Action League or the Health Care Leadership Council.[104]

[103] Cathie Jo Martin, "Together Again: Business, Government, and the Quest for Cost Control," *JHPPL* 18:2 (1993): 380; Jennifer Edwards et al., "Small Business and the National Health Reform Debate," *HA* (Spring 1992): 169–70; (quote) Eamonn McGeady testimony in House Committee on Ways and Means, *Hearing: Private Health Insurance Reform* 102:2 (Mar. 1992), 230; "Subsidies" (21 Feb. 1993), Box 672; Starr to Magaziner (5 Sept. 1993), Box 3210, both in CHTF Records.

[104] John Judis, "Abandoned Surgery: Business and the Failure of Health Care Reform," *American Prospect* (Spring 1995): 68–69; "Call It the Tortured Chamber of Commerce," *BW* (25 Apr. 1994), 32; "Chamber of Commerce Splits Again," *WSJ* (17 Feb. 1994), 3; Martin,

Business support evaporated as the task force strove to accommodate all these anxieties. Those with heavy health care liabilities saw little hope of spreading that burden or ending cost shifting as long as small business would be exempted from mandated coverage or subsidized for their compliance. Although eager to spread costs, large employers were also leery of surrendering managerial discretion or preferential insurance ratings. The attraction of mandates faded with the administration's retreat on cost controls: while many liked the idea of forcing small firms and competitors to pay for care, few were willing to bind themselves to an inflationary insurance system. When cost controls reemerged in the form of taxes on premium health plans, large employers argued that reform would press them to gut the care they were currently providing. "Big Business," noted *Business Week* in July 1994, "is shifting from passive acceptance of broad reform to sullen resistance." Business interest in health reform was gradually displaced by hopeful claims that cost control efforts were paying off, that the crisis had "fixed itself."[105]

For doctors, health care reform was a threat from the state, insurers, or both. While proponents of managed competition and public health alliances battled for the administration's attention, both wanted those who paid for care to exercise a greater say in its provision. This scrambled the doctors' response and their influence. Pleas for protection of professional autonomy were aimed less at the threat of political intrusion than they were at managed care, preferred providers, and HMOs. Some doctors resigned themselves to this managerial *putsch*; some feared that reform would sanction and accelerate it; and some hoped that a different political agenda might retrieve the patient-provider relationship. Organized medicine was hard pressed to offer a meaningful response to efforts that, as one observer noted, were "being most aggressively promoted (and paid for) by American corporations, the ideological brethren of most practitioners on the dangers of centralized government." In the end, doctors' doubts contributed to a general unease about political interference but did little to question the direction of reform.

"Together Again," 383; Colin Gordon, "Cosmetic Surgery: Health Care the Corporate Way," *The Nation* 252:11 (1991): 377–78; "Big Business' Health Plan Isn't Feeling So Hot," *BW* (18 Nov. 1991): 48.

[105] (Quote) *BW* (25 July 1994): 32–33; *NYT* (19 Aug. 1994); *NYT* (7 Aug. 1994); NAM letter to Gephardt cited in *Washington Post,* National Weekly Edition (8–14 Aug. 1994), 14; Cathie Jo Martin, "Stuck in Neutral: Big Business and the Politics of National Health Reform," *JHPPL* 20:2 (1995): 431–33; Martin, "Together Again," 361; Martin, "Mandating Social Change: The Business Struggle over National Health Reform," *Governance* 10:4 (1997): 403–14; "Surprise! Health Care's Fever May Have Finally Broken," *BW* (26 Apr. 1993); "Radical Surgery for Medicine: Hold That Scalpel," *BW* (12 July 1993); Alain Enthoven and Sara Singer, "Health Care Is Healing Itself," *NYT* (17 Aug. 1993): A11.

The AMA's time-worn political reflex obscured the broader anxieties of doctors—many of whom attacked the CHP from the left, embracing the "Canadian" single-payer solution as the only guarantor of professional autonomy.[106]

Commercial insurers worried about the shape and scope of reform and the precedent of federal policy. Even large companies, who persistently complained about the administrative burden of operating in "51 states with 51 different laws," were reluctant to cede regulatory authority to Washington in exchange for uniform or national standards of coverage.[107] While generally in agreement on regulatory politics, however, large and small insurers split over virtually every other aspect of the CHP. The industry's Gang of Five (Prudential, Met Life, Aetna, CIGNA, and John Hancock) broke with the HIAA and put themselves forward as the logical managers of managed care. A Prudential executive put it bluntly: "The best case scenario for reform—preferable even to the status quo—would be enactment of the managed care proposal." Leading insurers were willing to accept community rating, and even some regulation of plans and premiums, in exchange for political support of managed care. Given its fascination with managed care and its desperation for private sector allies, the administration courted insurers and incorporated many of their suggestions—a tack that led one wag to dub the bill in progress "The Health Insurance Industry Preservation Act." As the debate wore on, deference to leading insurers both magnified the anxieties of small insurers and made it harder to address the cost controls demanded by employers. By late 1993 insurers had largely lost interest and turned their attention to private strategies of managed care and market consolidation.[108]

For small insurers, the CHP posed a more direct threat. Most HIAA members were not large enough to erect managed care networks or ab-

---

[106] "Doctors Softening Stand," *NYT* (4 Mar. 1993): A1, A10; "AMA Rebuffed," *NYT* (5 Mar. 1993): A1, A8; AMA "Dear Colleague" circular (24 Sept. 1993); (quote); Iglehart reply to letters, *NEJM* (17 Apr. 1995): 1174; AHA testimony in Senate, *Health Security Act of 1993: Part I*, 113; "AMA Opposes Clinton Plan," *NYT* (9 Dec. 1992): A14; Lonnie Bristow, "The View from Organized Medicine," in *Social Insurance Issues for the Nineties* (proceedings of the Third Conference of the National Academy of Social Insurance), ed. Paul Van de Water (Dubuque, Iowa, 1992), 49–52; AMA testimony in Senate, *Health Security Act of 1993: Part I*, 146–48; David Andleman, "Prescription for a Powerful Lobby," *Management Review* (Feb. 1997): 30.

[107] Insurer quoted in Daniel Fox and Daniel Schaffer, "Health Policy and ERISA," *JHPPL* 14 (1989): 241–43, 247; testimony of Helms in House, *Private Health Insurance Reform Legislation*, 198; "Reforming the Health Insurance Market," *NEJM* 326:8 (1992): 565–69.

[108] "Whose New Health Plan Is This Anyway?" *NYT* (15 Nov. 1992): E5; Prudential executive quoted in Navarro, *The Politics of Health Policy*, 207–8; Thomas Bodenheimer in *The Nation* (22 Mar. 1993): 375; Howard Paster to Magaziner (7 Mar. 1993), Box 3308; Allen Schaeffer to Arnold Epstein, Box 3207, CHTF Records; Martin, "Together Again," 377–78.

sorb the costs of running them. "The big companies are saying 'You've got to go along with this community rating stuff. We've got to throw them a bone,' " complained one small insurer, "but the bone they're throwing puts our business in jeopardy if it doesn't put us out of business." Smaller concerns and the HIAA attacked the CHP as an unwarranted federal intrusion on both private consumption and state regulation. The HIAA's political clout (like that of small employers) proved extraordinarily effective—in part because the administration found it difficult to convince anyone that its tortuously complex plan would not do more harm than good, in part because the larger insurers and employers were tentative and ambivalent and in part because opponents claimed virtually unlimited resources in the battle for congressional attention and public opinion.[109]

Throughout the debate, health interests stepped up their political spending. Medical and insurance political action committees more than doubled their annual spending between 1989–90 ($11 million) and 1990–91 ($23 million). Through the 1992 election cycle, health and insurance interests increased their contributions by over 20 percent, with the AMA leading the pack. Most of this attention was lavished on incumbents occupying key committee or leadership positions. Even leading health and pharmaceutical firms—all traditionally Republican—did an about-face when Clinton's victory was evident and squeezed over $500,000 in soft money into the late days of the campaign. After the election legislators continued to have their coffers filled, although much of the money began drifting from the potential architects of reform to its opponents.[110] Echoing the AMA's campaigns of the late 1940s, a little

---

[109] "Leading Health Insurers into a New Age," *NYT* (6 Dec. 1992): A11; "Suddenly, Momentum for Health," *NYT* (10 Dec. 1992): A22; *BW* (27 Sept. 1993): 42; *BW* (12 July 1993): 134; John Grummere [Phoenix Home and Life] quoted in "Health Care Lobbies" *WSJ* (27 Nov. 1992): 34; Thomas Oliver, "Health Care Market Reform in Congress," *Political Science Quarterly* 106:2 (1991): 467–68; Sheila Sinler, "AHA Struggles to Reach Consensus," *Modern Healthcare* 14 (Mar. 1982): 28–29; Mark Peterson, "The Politics of Health Policy," in *The Social Divide: Political Parties and the Future of Activist Government*, ed. Margaret Weir (New York, 1998), 184; "Landmines" (n.d.), Box 670, CHTF Records.

[110] Nicholas Lehman, *A Lost Cause: Bill Clinton's Campaign for National Health Insurance* (Westport, Conn., 1996), 45–56; Common Cause, "Why the United States Does Not Have a National Health Program," 619–44; Michael Podhorzer et al., "Unhealthy Money: The Growth in Health PACs' Congressional Campaign Contributions," *IJHS* 23:1 (1993): 81–93; Kemper and Novak, "What's Blocking Health Care Reform?" 7; "Whose New Health Plan Is This Anyway?" *NYT* (15 Nov. 1992): E5; "Cash in Hand," *Wisconsin State Journal* (11 Aug. 1993): 1D; Larry Makinson, "Political Contributions from Health and Insurance Industries," *HA* 11:4 (Winter 1992): 119–34; "Health Care Lobbies" *WSJ* (27 Nov. 1992): 34; Thomas Ferguson, "The Democrats Deal for Dollars," *The Nation* (1 Apr. 1992): 476; "Medical Industry Showers Congress with Lobby Money," *NYT* (13 Dec. 1993); "Lobbyists Are Loudest in the Health Care Debate, *NYT* (16 Aug. 1994): A1, A10.

over half of the over $100 million spent in 1993 and 1994 was devoted
to political advertising—including a $20 million campaign by the Phar-
maceutical Research and Manufacturers Association and a $14 million
campaign by the HIAA. These efforts (notably the HIAA's infamous
"Harry and Louise" ads) were carefully designed to create an artificial
buzz, to generate a perception of grassroots opposition, and to encourage news coverage of the advertising campaigns themselves.[111]

The CHP collapsed not because it threatened private health interests,
but because it tried so desperately to make them all happy. The task
was to "keep the health industry divided, sector from sector and within
sectors," the task force's interest group liaison put it. "We need to both
keep the different major sectors—doctors, hospitals, insurers, pharma-
ceuticals—shooting at each other, and we need to make sure that some
players in each sector are with us." The results were disastrous. Winning
the cooperation of some only magnified the opposition of others, and
cost the administration support among its natural allies.[112] Reform and
the political compromises necessary to make reform possible seemed
increasingly incompatible:

> We must have the unions on board. The unions have objected to a tax cap . . .
> consequently a serious tax cap is not on the table. We must have the governors
> on board. Consequently , we cannot ask the states to pay any more for universal
> insurance than they are now paying for Medicaid. We must have the providers
> on board. Consequently we cannot have a significant provider tax. . . . We must
> have the big companies on board. Consequently we must allow them to oper-
> ate their own plans. We must have as many small employers on board as possi-
> ble. Consequently, we will gradually phase in employer obligations. . . . We
> must have moderate and conservative Democrats on board. Consequently we
> cannot expect to provide much more than $20 billion in new federal revenue
> for universal health insurance. Moral of the story: We cannot get so many peo-
> ple on board that our boat might sink from its own weight.

Task force advisor Walter Zelman conceded that the CHP was "a lot like
a sausage—all kinds of things thrown in, many of them not very healthy."
Senator Paul Wellstone, one of the lonely single-payer holdouts, likened

---

[111] Lehman, *A Lost Cause*, 59–60, 74; Podhorzer et al., "Unhealthy Money," 86; Darrell
West et al., "Harry and Louise Go to Washington: Political Advertising and Health Care
Reform," *JHPPL* 21:1 (Spring 1996): 35–39, 42–43.

[112] Thomas Bodenheimer, "The Major Players Start Dealing," *The Nation* (22 Mar. 1993):
373–75; interest group liaison quoted in Peterson, "The Politics of Health Policy," 191;
"Shared Sacrifice: The AMA Leadership Response to the Health Security Act," *JAMA*
271:10 (1994): 786; "Economic Dilemmas for Health Care Reform" (n.d.), Box 670, CHTF
Records; Center for Public Integrity, "Well-Healed: Inside Lobbying for Health Care Reform," *IJHS* 26:1 (1996): 19.

the CHP to rural electrification: "Of course the best way to place a power line is in a straight line. But because of the political compromises that had to be made at every step of the way, the lines end up in the shape of a snake, bending to circumvent every conceivable political barrier."[113]

After 1994 health interests continued to shape health politics and stepped up the pace of private reorganization. For-profit HMOs and hospital chains claimed more and more of the health market and encouraged a frenzy of mergers and consolidation that belied their faith in competition as a solution to the health system's troubles. It became increasingly clear that market solutions were little more than ideological cover for the efforts of some interests to wrestle resources or political advantage away from others. Indeed, market stalwarts retreated quickly when such reforms did not offer clear rewards. The AMA, which had posed as an organization of embattled entrepreneurs through much of the century, increasingly sought the professional high ground in response to the intrusion of managed care. Business interests, who celebrated competitive reforms insofar as they pared back their own health care costs and responsibilities, feared that introducing the same market discipline to Medicare and Medicaid might shuffle more of the burden their way. And HMOs, the centerpiece of political reform into the mid-1990s, became a political target as attempts to pare back benefits and monitor providers prompted state and federal interest in a patients' bill of rights and a professional backlash from doctors against "the intrusion of entrepreneurial giants."[114]

Despite their divergent stakes, health interests maintained a virtual stranglehold over post-1994 political efforts. Much of the debate shifted to the states, where the political advantages enjoyed by powerful economic interests were exaggerated by interstate competitive pressures. The Republican Congress after 1994 proved not only less interested in broad health reform (having ridden the defeat of the CHP to victory) but also quite willing to allow health interests to determine (and even draft) health legislation—a deference neatly represented by the flurry of interest in Medical Savings Accounts. And health interests continued to flood state and federal politics with money, strangling single-payer reform in California and Massachusetts, diluting or distracting various patients' rights initiatives, and ensuring that efforts to make employment-based insurance portable stopped far short of guaranteeing ac-

[113] "A Conundrum" (n.d.): Box 3210, CHTF Records; Zelman quoted in Lawrence Brown, "Looking Back on Health Care Reform," *HA* 17:6 (1998): 67; Wellstone to Hillary Clinton (15 Apr. 1993), Box 1172, CHTF Records.

[114] (Quote) James Todd, "Health System Reform: Whither or Whether?" *JAMA* 273:3 (18 Jan. 1995): 246.

cess.[115] At the same time, health care's corporate compromise was increasingly fragmented as providers and payers confronted each other over spending and medical practice, patients and payers confronted each other over the scope and stability of employment-based benefits, and various interests confronted internal tensions (general practice doctors versus specialists, small employers versus big employers, small insurers versus big insurers) over the future of private and public health care.

[115] Colleen Grogan, "Hope in Federalism? What Can the States Do and What Are They Likely to Do?" *JHPPL* 20 (1995): 479–80; Robert Kuttner, "The Kennedy-Kassebaum Bill: The Limits of Incrementalism," *NEJM* 337:1 (1997): 65; Parmet, "Regulation and Federalism," 122; Peter Dreier and Matthew Glasser, "California's Single-Payer Initiative: What Went Wrong?" *Social Policy* (Spring 1995): 11–12; Deborah Stone, "The Struggle for the Soul of Health Insurance," *JHPPL* 18 (1993): 311–12.

7

Silenced Majority: American Politics and the Dilemmas of Health Reform

THE political and ideological clout of leading health interests stood in stark contrast to the organizational struggles of health reformers. Although reformers always commanded a clear and substantial majority of public support, they only rarely made themselves heard above the cacophony of the corporate compromise and were quickly silenced when they did. In part this reflected a political system characterized by routine deference to economic interests, weak ties between reform interests and party politics, and nonprogrammatic electoral competition. And in part it reflected the peculiar politics of health care, in which private interests were well entrenched, the organization of public interests proved extraordinarily difficult, and fragmented provision fragmented reform energies as well.

This chapter traces the history of health reform—examining in turn the relative poverty of reform interests, their tenuous relationship with the Democratic Party and the labor movement, and the strategies that flowed from this material and institutional weakness. As we shall see, the resource gap was so wide that reformers were rarely able to sustain public attention or respond to their opponents. The Democratic Party, traditionally dependent upon both business patrons and its southern base, proved at best an ambivalent vehicle for reform. The labor movement's health politics were similarly uncertain, reflecting both an uneasy relationship with national politics and the Democratic Party, and the fruits of private bargaining. In turn, reform interests resorted to shortsighted strategies that often pursued provision for some at the expense of others—an ad hoc incrementalism that proved devastating to a cause whose political and actuarial logic rested on single-payer financing and universal provision.

The Resource Constraint: Confronting the Corporate Compromise

Why were advocates of national health insurance unable to translate popular support into legislative action, to match the resources commanded by their opponents, or to win the lasting allegiance of organized labor and other allies? The AALL, the principal advocate of Progressive Era health reform, was an academic organization without ties to electoral politics, the labor movement, or public health activists. It had little opportunity to build a serious constituency and little interest in doing so. AALL membership peaked at just over three thousand in 1913, and its annual budget hovered between $15,000 and $35,000. The AALL used its academic reputation and the pages of the *American Labor Legislation Review* to get its health bill on legislative calendars, but it had neither the political base nor the resources to counter organized opposition.[1] More broadly, AALL reformers "met with success," David Moss has suggested, "only when they operated within the nebulous realm of acceptability established by capital." In health politics this realm did not exist. The AALL took labor support for granted and assumed that doctors and employers would appreciate the long-term benefits of a healthy and secure working class. But without meaningful ties to the labor movement or the ability to match the political lobbying and pamphleteering of the insurance industry, the AALL could neither sustain political interest nor answer charges that its program was the product of Bolshevik social engineering rather than a response to the needs and demands of ordinary Americans.[2]

Like the AALL, the Committee on the Costs of Medical Care (1928–1932) had no popular base. The CCMC raised just over $750,000 from liberal foundations (including Milbank, Rockefeller, Carnegie, and Rosenwald), and although the funding was relatively generous, its source restrained the CCMC's research and recommendations. The foundations were dependent on private contributors or trusts that were leery of expansive reform (a point driven home by the ability of doctors to pressure the Milbank board by boycotting Borden). The foundations themselves were leery of bankrolling advocacy, and at least one (the Commonwealth Fund) refused to contribute because it assumed that the CCMC had a political agenda.[3] With the publication of the CCMC reports, reformers

[1] Paul Starr, *The Social Transformation of American Medicine* (New York, 1982), 244; Theda Skocpol, *Protecting Soldiers and Mothers: The Political Origins of Social Policy in the United States* (Cambridge, Mass., 1992), 176–85.

[2] David Moss, *Socializing Security: Progressive-Era Economists and the Origins of American Social Policy* (Cambridge, Mass., 1996), 10; "Memorandum re Doctors" (1918), reel 63, American Association for Labor Legislation [AALL] Papers (microfilm), Charles Mayo [AMA] address (1917), reel 62, AALL Papers; Testimony of Arthur Broughton before the Special Commission on Social Insurance [Mass.] (1916), reel 62, AALL Papers; "Report of the [AFL] Committees on Social Insurance" (1918), reel 63, AALL Papers; "American Association for Labor Legislation" (1940?), reel 63, AALL Papers; Isaac Rubinow, *The Quest for Security* (New York, 1934): 211–13; Alice Hamilton, "The Opposition to Health Insurance," *ALLR* 19 (Dec. 1929): 404.

[3] Minutes of a Meeting of the Executive Committee on the Costs of Medical Care (9 Mar. 1931), Box J8:6, Walton Hamilton Papers, Rare Books and Manuscripts, Tarlton Law

pressed to establish a new organization to promote its recommendations and counter the backlash of opposition. Michael Davis and others established the American Committee on Medical Costs and retained Edward Bernays, the Rockefeller public relations expert, to coordinate its activities. None of the foundations wanted anything to do with the new organization and it immediately disbanded. Davis feared that a shoestring operation might, by serving as a target for the AMA, do more harm than good: it seemed "inadvisable to form a permanent national organization, even if the means were available." A parallel effort, the Committee on Research in Medical Economics, also sought to follow up on the CCMC by "strik [ing] a balance between the activities of research on the one hand and participation in politics on the other," but raised only $35,000. Reformers were unable to make any sustained political use of the CCMC's research, while their opponents, facing few resource constraints, used the minority report as a springboard to political prominence.[4]

The New Deal afforded the opportunity to shape public policy from the inside, and reformers flocked to staff the committees charged with crafting and administering Social Security. The most important independent reform initiative in these years was the Committee of Physicians, an effort to organize liberal doctors. As doctors, committee members faced not only the AMA and its resources but also the threat of sanction or expulsion by local medical societies. Although the committee claimed between four hundred and one thousand members, all but ten or twenty active members had done little more than sign on to a vague statement of principles. And the committee had no money. Chair John Peters complained at the time that "we cannot, with safety, continue living from hand to mouth," but there seemed little prospect for any lasting institutional or material support. Again in 1940, Peters lamented that the "financial situation [was] extremely precarious" and that the committee was having difficulty even distributing material to its members. Two years later, Peters admitted that his committee had "engaged in no public activities for almost a year, but it is not entirely defunct"—a technical distinction for an organization whose bank account hovered between $300 and $500. "The 'liberal' physicians have no common program but represent

---

Library, University of Texas, Austin, Tex.; Douglas Parks, "Expert Inquiry and Health Care Reform in New Era America: Herbert Hoover, Ray Lyman Wilbur, and the Travails of the Disinterested Experts" (Ph.D. diss., University of Iowa, 1994), 220–26.

[4] Parks, "Expert Inquiry and Health Care Reform," 381–83 (Davis quoted at 383); Committee on Research in Medical Economics, Minutes of the Meeting of the Board of Directors (Feb. 1938), Box J37:9; (quote) "Minutes of a Meeting of a Special Group on the Future of Medical Economics" (Apr. 1932), Box J33:4, both in Hamilton Papers; Sydenstriker to Kingsbury (5 Dec. 1932), Box 41:178, Series I, Isidore Falk Papers, Sterling Library, Yale University, New Haven, Conn.

a variety of approaches to the general question [and] . . . have had little opportunity to clarify either their unities or their differences," one New Dealer noted, adding that "the AMA Group is united, experienced, and positive."[5]

Reformers disappointed by the New Deal put great stock in the administration's 1938 health conference. Both the Committee of Physicians and the Committee on Research in Medical Economics worked closely with the staff of the administration's Interdepartmental Committee—hoping, as I. S. Falk put it, that "the unorganized but widespread public demand for better health and sickness protection now had a positive image, a definite target, where hitherto it had only been statistical findings and professional disputes" and that "there was now organized support confronting their organized opposition." But even in such a friendly setting, reformers made little headway. Like the CCMC reports, the 1938 conference served as a lightning rod for opponents. In the aftermath, reformers were no closer to adding health insurance to Social Security than they had been in 1935. Opponents, "with the usual display of their well-known greed and self-interest," one citizen wrote the White House, were by contrast "out in full pack, baying the political rabbit, endeavoring to drive it into an obscure hole."[6]

This material weakness persisted into the 1940s. FSA administrator Oscar Ewing searched in vain for "the support of an organization that had real political power"—even floating the idea of forming an "American Patients Association." Reform voices in the 1940s, aside from the Committee of Physicians, included the Physicians Forum, group health organizations, and the Committee for the Nation's Health (CNH). Of these, the Physicians Forum was confined to New York City and was unable to either attract foundation funding or broaden its membership. Group health interests, with a growing stake in community or union-

[5] On the Committee of Physicians, see Peters to Horsely (22 Aug. 1945), Box 2:42; Draft of Principles and Proposals (1937), Box 2:50; Minutes and Agenda for 1937, Box 2:50; Peters correspondence with Hugh Cabot (1938–1940), Box 1:25–29; (quote) Peters to Osgood (18 Oct. 1938), Box 2:59; Peters to Fremont-Smith (22 Oct. 1943), Box 2:42; (quote) Peters to Osgood (1 Oct. 1940), Box 2:59; Financial Report (1952), Box 2:43, all in Series I, John Peters Papers, Sterling Library, Yale University; Oliver Garceau, *The Political Life of the AMA* (Hamden, Conn., 1961), 148; (quote) Phillips to Davis (10 July 1938), Box 12, Decimal 025, Records of the Social Security Board [SSB], Office of the Commissioner, RG 47, Social Security Administration [SSA], National Archives.

[6] (Quote) Falk to Winant (14 Mar. 1939), Falk II, 58:489; Official Report of Proceedings Before the President's Interdepartmental Committee to Coordinate Health and Welfare Activities [ICHWA] (May 1938), pp. 54–57, Box 29, ICHWA Records, Franklin D. Roosevelt Presidential Library [FDRPL], Hyde Park, N.Y.; Peters to Osgood (24 Oct. 1938), Box 2:59, Series I, Peters Papers; Davis Memo (June 1940), Box 140, Morris Cooke Papers, FDRPL; (quote) Atwood to Oleson (18 Sept. 1938), Box 1, ICWHA Records.

based plans, remained ambivalent about national reform.[7] This left the CNH. In 1944 reformers had begun looking for a means of revitalizing the AALL and its Progressive Era partner, the American Association for Social Security, and recast an exploratory Social Security Charter Committee as the CNH in 1946. The CNH initially hoped for seed money from organized labor, but was disappointed and instead relied on an endowment of $50,000 from the Rosenwald Fund and the Lasker Foundation.[8]

Financial problems plagued the CNH from its outset. Political or educational initiatives were routinely prefaced (and often overwhelmed) by the committee's meager resources. Executive Director Michael Davis conceded in 1946 that the CNH was merely "a paper organization" with 175 supporting members, of whom 7 had contributed virtually all of its funds. That year the CNH struggled to raise and spend just over $35,000—about what the AMA spent in an average week. Funding remained precarious, and only an infusion from Lasker pushed 1947 revenues above $70,000. In 1948 Davis observed that expenditures by the National Physicians Committee were running at "about ten times the budget for [our] Committee." The CNH persistently put off the task of organizing state or regional branches for financial reasons and, in an effort to increase revenues, reinvented itself by purging its membership (a "politically mixed list . . . loaded with fellow travelers and Communists") in 1948. The CNH struggled through 1948 and 1949 to decide "what changes need to be made in order to gain the support or at least divide the opposition of certain groups that are now opposed or doubtful." It even explored funding from "liberal business groups," but was still outspent almost fifteenfold through the debate over the Truman health plan—at which point the CNH and its patrons parted ways. "We get under way in 1950," announced Davis, "with the knowledge that the few large givers who have thus far supplied the major share of our budget feel they should no longer shoulder the burden." The CNH looked again to labor and to liberal doctors, but the prospects were not promising.

[7] Oscar Ewing OH, pp. 193–94, Harry S. Truman Presidential Library [HSTPL], Independence, Mo.; Jan Pacht Brickman, " 'Medical McCarthyism': The Physicians Forum and the Cold War," *Journal of the History of Medicine* 49 (1994): 390–93; Peters to Butler (22 June 1939), Box 1:24; Financial Report (1952), Box 2:43, Series I, Peters Papers; Goor to Esselstyn (7 Dec. 1960), Box 55:53, Series III, Caldwell Esselstyn Papers, Sterling Library.

[8] Davis to Hedges (19 June 1944), and "Report of January 14 1944 Meeting at the Hotel Barclay," both in reel 11, Michael Davis Papers (microfilm), HSTPL; "Report of Meeting of Informal Health Insurance Conference Group" (Sept. 1945), Box A:15, Research Files, American Federation of Labor [AFL] Papers, State Historical Society of Wisconsin [SHSW], Madison, Wis.; Monte Poen, *Harry Truman versus the Medical Lobby* (Columbia, Mo., 1979), 42–43, 83.

Revenues in 1950 fell to $37,000, leaving the CNH "with such limited funds that drastic economy was necessary."[9]

In the wake of the 1949 defeat, reformers were so marginalized that a proposal by the CNH for a poster display at the AMA's annual meeting "brought only chuckles from the AMA officers . . . it would be like the Pope bringing in the devil's advocate to the Vatican." In 1952 the CNH contemplated a wider role and a wider financial base to "unchain us from the terribly meager scale of past support" but remained in "bad shape financially": annual budgets in the mid-1950s ranged between $30,000 and $40,000, most of which went to basic staffing. In 1955 the CNH decided to forgo political activity for a more general educational program, while admitting that it "has not had the means to undertake one." As it disbanded in 1956, the CNH lamented that "today, health insurance is in the hands of powerful forces which are shaping it with only secondary regard to legislation." Other reform interests fared just as badly. The Committee of Physicians existed only on the letterhead left over in John Peters's office, and the Physicians Forum was, by 1954, in "desperate situation organizationally and economically."[10]

As health policy retreated to the goal of limited coverage for the elderly in the late 1950s and early 1960s, reformers could count on both congressional and administration support and an opposition concerned less with blocking reform outright than in shaping it to their particular interests. Organizations of the elderly suffered a familiar resource gap when confronting the AMA, but received relatively favorable treatment in the press (at one point, ABC gave the National Council of Senior Citizens free time to respond to an AMA program that had cost the latter nearly $100,000). Although hospital insurance faced little sustained op-

---

[9] CFNH Bulletin 4 (21 May 1951), Box 60, Caroline Ware Papers, FDRPL; "Report to the Executive Committee" (15 Nov. 1946); "Financial Report" (June 1947); Davis memo (23 Dec. 1947); (quote) CNH, "Considerations for 1948," reel 1; (quote) "Confidential Progress Report" (31 Mar. 1948), reel 1; Davis memo (15 Oct. 1948), reel 8; (quote) Davis Memo (27 Jan. 1950) and "CNH Activities in 1950" (Jan. 1951), reel 2, all in Davis Papers; Poen, *Truman versus the Medical Lobby,* 151–52, 177, 207; Biemiller to William (30 Nov. 1949), AFL Committee on Social Security Meeting (16 Jan. 1950), Box 16, Nelson Cruikshank Papers, SHSW.

[10] (Quote) AMA Secretary's Letter (20 June 1949), Box 43, Decimal 011.4, Federal Security Agency [FSA], Office of the Administrator (General Classified Files [GCF], 1944–1950), Records of the Department of Health, Education, and Welfare [HEW], RG 235, National Archives; [CNH], September 1955 Financial Statement, and "Conference on National Health Program" (July 1955), both in Box J49:4, Hamilton Papers; AFL Committee on Social Security Meeting (12 Nov. 1953), Box 16, Cruikshank Papers; (quote) Robin to Executive Committee (2 July 1952), reel 4, Davis Papers; (quote) CNH memo to Directors (25 Jan. 1956), Box 156:2254, Series III, Falk Papers; Poen, *Truman versus the Medical Lobby,* 177; (quote) Earnshaw to John Peters (22 Nov. 1954), Box 7:170, Series I, Peters Papers.

position, reformers continued to confront the AMA over physicians' services. Liberal doctors formed a Physicians Committee for Health Care for the Aged (PCHCA) in 1963 to counter the AMA, but made little headway. The AFL-CIO pledged $1,000 a month to support the PCHCA, but the group attracted little other support and remained a marginal organization.[11] And reformers wielded virtually no influence in the administrative frenzy that surrounded the passage of Medicare.

Reformers regrouped in the late 1960s under the auspices of the Committee for National Health Insurance, but had little impact in the debates of the early and mid-1970s. Like the congressional initiatives it supported, the CNHI was quick to beat a retreat in order to ally itself with a politically feasible plan. And like the organizations that preceded it, the CNHI was chronically broke. The CNHI was funded by a few unions (most notably AFSCME and the UAW) and the Lasker Foundation, but never approached the minimum annual budget (just over $200,000) it needed to launch a modest educational campaign. "Funds are limited," noted Walter Ruether in 1968, and barely two years later the CNHI was still "critically short of money" with pledged income "barely sufficient to support a continuation of our present level of activity." The CNHI (a nonprofit, educational organization) established the Health Security Action Coalition (HSAC) as a lobbying arm in late 1970 and did what it could to encourage grassroots organizing (in the hope that local chapters could raise their own money), but money woes persisted. CNHI officials routinely lamented, as one put it, that "our current level of funding is inadequate to mount any significant public education campaign." In mid–1971 the CNHI had to cancel a major pamphlet mailing and pull the plug on its youth program. By the standards of such organizations, the CNHI (succeeded in the mid-1970s by the HSAC) did relatively well, parlaying labor and foundation support into annual budgets of $84,000 in 1970, $217,000 in 1973, and $364,000 in 1979. But by the standards set by the AMA and other health interests, the CNHI remained a bit player.[12]

[11] "New AMA Blitzkrieg," *Senior Citizen News* clipping in White House Central File [WHCF] LE/IS 77, Lyndon Baines Johnson Papers, LBJ Presidential Library, Austin, Tex.; "Group Practice Bill" (n.d.), Box 291, Secretary's Subject Files (1955–1975), HEW Records; Richard Harris, "Annals of Legislation: Medicare," *New Yorker* (16 July 1966), 45; Mayer to Esselstyn (16 July 1962), Box 1:1; Meany to Esselstyn (22 Aug. 1963) and Cruikshank to Esseltyn (8 Apr 1963), Box 1:1; Mott to Esseltyn (1 Aug. 1962), Box 1:6, all in Records of the Physicians Committee for Health Care for the Aged, SHSW.

[12] On the CNHI, see (quote) Ruether to Altmeyer (27 Dec. 1968), Box 3, Arthur J. Altmeyer Papers (add.), SHSW; (quote) Minutes of the CNHI Executive Committee Meeting (14 Jan. 1971), Box 146:2127; CNHI financial statements 1970–1974, Box 146:2126–2130; "Budget Analysis" (May 1979), Box 146:2131; (quote) Minutes of the CNHI Executive Committee Meeting (13 Nov. 1970), Box 146:2126; "Financial Status Reports" (Oct.

By this time, the cause of national health insurance was drowned out by a chorus of business-sponsored "reform" lobbies. As the stability of employment-based care occupied political attention, reformers were often torn between the strategic attraction of mandating private benefits and the persistently powerful arguments for displacing them. Organizations such as Public Citizen, Citizen Action, and Physicians for a National Health Program (PNHP) played an important educational role—drafting single-payer legislation, documenting the inequity of managed care, and monitoring the political activities of health interests. But their reach and resources were dwarfed by those of medical, insurance, and business interests. The results were predictable: although the Clinton task force counted nearly 95 percent of the public in favor of "substantial change"— including nearly 80 percent support for "some system of national health insurance"—it dismissed the single-payer option and focused on employment-based, budget-neutral solutions. It is impossible, given the proliferation of groups on both sides and the magnitude of direct and indirect spending by opponents, to accurately gauge the resource mismatch in the 1992–94 debate. Clearly "liberal" doctors (represented by the seven-thousand-member PNHP) had little impact either within the AMA or as an alternative to it. Consumer organizations (such as Public Citizen) challenged the inequity and excesses of private insurance, but could not overcome the industry's immense political advantages.[13]

This experience—from the AALL to the PNHP—underscores both the debilitating material disadvantage faced by reformers and the absence of any meaningful political organization of the public interest. Although reformers invariably claimed a substantial plurality of public support, their efforts were overwhelmed by the willingness and ability of health

1972), Box 146:2128, all in Series III, Falk Papers; Minutes of the CNHI Executive Committee (16 Sept. 1969); Minutes of the CNHI Executive Committee (10 Dec. 1969); Minutes of the CNHI Executive Committee (13 Nov. 1970); Max Fine to [CNHI] Executive Committee Members (23 Dec. 1970); Minutes of the CNHI Executive Committee (14 Jan. 1971); Minutes of the CNHI Executive Committee (25 May 1971); Minutes of the CNHI Executive Committee (23 Sept. 1971); "Work Plan and Budget Proposal" (Jan. 1972); Joint Meeting of the CNHI and HSAC Executive Committees (26 Jan. 1972); Joint Meeting of the CNHI and HSAC Executive Committees (10 Nov. 1972); Joint Executive Committees [CNHI-HSAC] Meeting (12 Mar. 1973); Joint Meeting of the Executive Committees of the CNHI and HSAC (2 Aug. 1974), all in Box 110, Part II, Series VI, Records of the United Auto Workers Social Security Department [UAW-SSD], Archives of Labor History and Urban Affairs, Wayne State University, Detroit, Mich.; David Jacobs, "The UAW and the Committee for National Health Insurance: The Contours of Social Unionism," *Advances in Industrial and Labor Relations* 4 (1987): 123.

[13] (Quote) "Public Attitudes on National Health Insurance, 1992" in Box 1173, Records of the Clinton Health Care Task Force [CHTF], National Archives; Starr to Magaziner (16 Dec. 1992), Box 3305, CHTF Records; Peter Dreier and Matthew Glasser, "California's Single-Payer Initiative: What Went Wrong?" *Social Policy* (Spring 1995): 12.

interests to outspend them in legislative hearings, electoral campaigns, and public debate. Contesting medical conservatives on these terms, as CNH director Frederick Robins observed in the late 1940s, was "like trying to put out a forest fire with a sprinkling can."[14]

Health Care and Party Politics

The reformers' task would not have been nearly so difficult had other organizations—especially the Democratic Party—taken up their cause. But American political parties are notoriously nonprogrammatic, undisciplined, constituency-service organizations: they stand for election but little else. The existence of only two national parties (a circumstance sustained by legal and political barriers to the entry of third parties) discourages substantive programmatic distinctions. Federated political authority and regional strongholds made partisan showdowns over national public policy even more unlikely. Steadily declining voter turnout and reliance on private funding of elections encouraged interest-based political organization at the expense of programs or policies that might appeal to—let alone mobilize—a broad political base. And the Democratic Party, the most logical vehicle for reform, was restrained by its southern wing (into the 1960s) and by (especially after the 1960s) its business patrons.[15]

Neither party confronted health care as a serious issue until the middle 1930s. The Roosevelt administration was reluctant to pursue health care alongside its pension and unemployment programs and found ways—in 1935, in 1938, and after—to defer the issue to further study. The Democrats, as we have seen, hesitated for a number of reasons—including the poor fit between health coverage and social insurance, the opposition of organized medicine, and southern anxieties about social policy. The party's 1940 health platform was drafted by the AMA: it was "the most pleasing plank on health that could be gotten through for the Democratic Party," the Texas Medical Society said, "and the medical professions seem universally pleased with it." For their part, the Republicans

[14] Alan Derickson, "Health Security for All? Social Unionism and Universal Health Insurance, 1935–1958," *JAH* (Mar. 1994): 1343–44; Oscar Ewing OH, pp. 193–94, HSTPL; Robins quoted in Poen, *Truman versus the Medical Lobby,* 182.

[15] On the Democrats, see Frances Fox Piven, "Structural Constraints and Political Development: The Case of the American Democratic Party," in *Labor Parties in Postindustrial Societies,* ed. Frances Fox Piven (New York, 1992), 251–54; Ira Katznelson, Kim Geiger, and Daniel Kryder, "Limiting Liberalism: The Southern Veto in Congress, 1933–1950," *Political Science Quarterly* 108 (1993): 285–88; Joel Rogers and Thomas Ferguson, *Right Turn: The Decline of the Democrats and the Future of American Politics* (New York, 1986), 40–61.

viewed the issue as a golden political opportunity. Even those resigned to Social Security could draw the line at health care and inveigh against the threat of socialized medicine. This line of argument was bolstered in the late 1930s by the New Deal's sagging political fortunes, by organized medicine's response to the 1938 Washington Health Conference, and by the Justice Department's antitrust "vendetta" against the AMA. The GOP's 1938 health platform, as one Democratic observer noted, was composed of "complete neglect of the absolutely needy," "slurring re-marks about the present administration," and "the fear of some vague bogey labeled socialized medicine."[16]

This cut the template for the next decade of health politics: Democrats timidly pursued the possibility of adding health insurance to Social Secu-rity and Republicans used the issue as a surrogate for a broader attack on the New Deal. The Democrats, however, were equally constrained by the nature of their own party. Southern Democrats had supported the New Deal as long as it poured federal money south and shaped federal law to southern concerns. But after 1945 southerners needed the New Deal less and feared it more. The first hints of dissent came in a 1946 congressional vote over executive reorganization (widely seen as a pre-lude to health legislation), and the full-blown Dixiecrat revolt of 1948 gave Truman the license to cast his health net widely with the assurance that it would be shredded in Congress. Southerners returned to the fold, but the party remained divided and immobilized on the health issue.[17]

The southern anchor exaggerated the party's natural reluctance to establish any clear programmatic direction. "Campaign work does not consist [of] *formulating* a policy or program," Democrat Clark Clifford stressed in 1948. "Campaign work consists [of] *selling* policies and pro-grams already arrived at in public and *attacking* the enemy." The FSA labored under the burden of the most basic background research: "We need, especially, information, education, and strategy materials, and we don't seem to have any place where they are being produced." Coopera-tion among the White House, the FSA, and Senators Wagner and Murray

---

[16] FDR to Bureau of the Budget (23 Apr. 1941), President's Official File [POF] 103:1, Franklin D. Roosevelt Papers, FDRPL; State Medical Association of Texas to Oscar Chap-man (n.d), Box 5, Oscar Chapman Papers, HSTPL; (quote) comments on Republican Platform Committee, "Report on the Conference on Health Insurance" (Aug. 1938), Box 9, Decimal 025, SSB, SSA Records.

[17] William Pemberton, *Bureaucratic Politics: Executive Reorganization during the Truman Ad-ministration* (Columbia, Mo., 1979), 118; Poen, *Truman versus the Medical Lobby,* 122; Davis to CNH Executive Committee (13 May 1948), reel 1, Davis Papers, Transcript of Robins Statement (24 Aug. 1949); Welfare Legislation Luncheon (15 May 1950), Box 4, DNC Files, HSTPL; "How the National Health Program Would Serve the South" (May 1949), Box 43, Decimal 011.4, FSA, Office of the Administrator (GCF, 1944–1950), HEW Records.

was sporadic. And efforts to coordinate legislative details or strategy with Congress were frustrated by both the administration's programmatic uncertainty and its fear (in the wake of GOP investigations of SSA "propaganda") that advocacy itself posed political dangers. Some Democratic National Committee (DNC) members went so far as to blast the administration for "the misuse of the good offices of this Committee in support of the agitation for compulsory health insurance."[18]

Both parties were eager to make electoral use of health care, quite aside from (and often at the expense of) actual legislation. Through 1948, Truman's advisors recommended pushing the health issue only because they were confident that nothing would make it through the final months of the 80th Congress. As November approached, the DNC pulled back and avoided making health care a campaign issue—arguing privately that, having outflanked the Republicans on health, the Democrats would be fools to go out on a limb and actually advocate legislative solutions. Reformers, by this time, understood the limits of party politics all too well. The CNH expected the Democrats to "continue to give at least nominal advocacy to the Truman program, including national health insurance" but doubted "whether the party will really make health insurance one of its major domestic issues." The Republican National Committee (RNC) concurred, arguing that "in a clever way they are hoping it won't succeed. Then, with the 1950 election coming up they can say to the people, 'We tried but a few Republicans wouldn't let us.' " Both parties, by the RNC's estimate, were interested less in legislation than they were in "baiting the trap to catch votes in 1950." The meager Republican response encouraged the Democrats to play up partisan distinctions for public consumption while moving steadily toward the Republican position. After 1949 party officials determined that health care remained a "desirable issue" but recommended further study while that Democratic candidates "soft pedal the health issue and rely upon the record to date."[19]

<hr />

[18] "Progress of the Campaign" (unsigned, 1948), Box 23, Clark Clifford Papers, HSTPL; DNC files, POF 299A, Boxes 940–41, Truman Papers, HSTPL; CNH Executive Committee Notes (25 Nov. 1947), reel 1; Kingsley to Murray (25 Mar. 1949), reel 8, both in Davis Papers; "Public Health Insurance Legislative Proposals" (28 Mar. 1949), and Franklin to Bush (25 Apr. 1949), Box 44; Miller to Murray (22 Dec. 1948), Box 46; Statement by Robins (13 Feb. 1950), Box 45; Hayes to Thurston (28 Nov. 1949), Box 45, all in Decimal 011.4, GCF (1944–50), HEW Records; (quote) Transcript of Robins Statement (24 Aug. 1949), Welfare Legislation Luncheon (15 May 1950), Box 4, DNC Files, HSTPL.

[19] "Behind the Wagner Bill," *Medical Care* 3:3 (1943): 257; "Progress of the Campaign" (unsigned, 1948), Box 23, Clifford Papers; CNH Executive Committee Notes (25 Nov. 1947), reel 1, Davis Papers; Cruikshank to Green (14 May 1948), Box 16, Cruikshank Papers; Clifford, "Memorandum for the President" (1947), Box 23, Clifford Papers; (quote) CNH, "Considerations for 1948," reel 1, Davis Papers; RNC, "The Truth about Socialized

Health care disappeared from both party platforms until the stirrings of Medicare in the late 1950s. The tenor and timing of that debate, as we have seen, was shaped largely by the prospect of drawing sharp partisan lines on the issue in the 1960, 1962, and 1964 campaigns. Democrats saw hearings on the 1958 Forand bill and its successors as an opportunity to advertise the poverty of Republican health policy. And President-elect Kennedy's directions to HEW in 1960 put the task of highlighting the differences between Democratic and Republican policy ahead of the task of actually composing a workable bill. Although the Democrats ultimately won the passage of Medicare and Medicaid, SSA staff admitted that the legislation was distracted by electoral considerations and diluted by the absence of any clear programmatic direction—let alone serious options to the left.[20]

Into the 1970s both parties struggled with the politics of health care— a task magnified for a Democratic Party that could no longer rely on the panacea of economic growth. The congressional proposals of 1970–71 were driven largely by the presidential aspirations of Democratic legislators. Reformers backing Senator Edmund Muskie pushed for legislation in the fall of 1971, admitting "the major function should be to give the Senator a track record in health. Any legislation that may be passed (or even receive real consideration) will be a secondary gain." Kaiser officials came away from a meeting with Senator Edward Kennedy with the impression that the senator "has more on his mind than health care legislation, like maybe comments or indications of financial support for someone's presidential bid" (indeed Kennedy slowed his bill's progress in the hope of milking it through the Democrats' 1972 convention). In the wake of Nixon's reelection, congressional Democrats retreated and offered only pale variations on various bipartisan plans to stabilize employment-based care and rein in costs. In the White House after 1976, Democrats lost interest in all but narrow solutions to health inflation. The Carter White House did establish a committee to tackle health reform but its "key purpose" was "the criticism by some Democrats that 'Mr. Carter is doing nothing about National Health Insurance,'" one party member complained, adding that "Carter and HEW do not want the

Medicine" (1949), SHSW Pamphlets; Poen, *Truman versus the Medical Lobby*, 101; David Stowe, "Memorandum: Administration's Health Program" (12 Oct. 1951), Box 2, Staff Member and Office Files [SMOF] (Stowe), Truman Papers.

[20] Avery to Shephard (9 July 1959), Box 225, Decimal 900.1, Secretary's Subject Files [SSF] (1955–1975), HEW Records; "Possible Legislative Proposals in the 87th Congress" (2 Dec. 1960), Box 137, Decimal 011, SSF (1955–1975), HEW Records; Wilbur Cohen, "Random Reflections on the Great Society's Politics and Health Care Programs after Twenty Years," in *The Great Society and Its Legacy: Twenty Years of U.S. Social Policy*, ed. Marshal Kaplan and Peggy Cuciti (Durham, N.C., 1986), 118.

Committee to prepare a bill, to endorse a bill, or arrive at a consensus on an approach to national health insurance."[21]

This cynicism had been matched by the Nixon White House, whose health policy was largely animated by fear and resentment of congressional Democrats. The administration's goal, as John Erhlichman saw it through 1970 and 1971, lay in "seizing and holding the political initiative in an area where the administration is perceived by some to be hostile or disinterested" while ensuring that the White House could "hold back the Kennedy Plan," "get the credit for what he proposed and what gets passed," or "bring Long and Kennedy [to] each other's throats." Critics agreed, as one UAW official put it, that the administration's proposals were nothing more than "a device to postpone discussion of the proposal prior to the election campaign." At the same time, congressional Republicans remained firmly aligned with the AMA's do-nothing stance, and did little to help the White House win even a superficial victory. HEW's congressional relations staff "repeatedly undercut our program," Domestic Policy Advisor Patrick Moynihan complained to Nixon, "hinting to Republican Congressmen that you are not really behind these crazy New Deal measures, etc." For their part, reformers persisted with the dwindling conviction that the "next election" (the 1972 campaign, the post–Watergate congressional elections in 1974, the 1976 campaign) would provide an opening.[22]

After the mid-1970s, both parties drifted to the right in response to the ongoing economic crisis and the business anxieties that accompanied it. The Republicans abandoned any vestiges of Eisenhower-Nixon liberalism and became increasingly enamored with market solutions. For the Democrats, whose principal navigational strategy after the demise of

[21] (Quote) Notes for Muskie Election Committee (1971), Box 223:10, Wilbur Cohen Papers, SHSW; Falk to Altmeyer (23 Dec. 1970), Box 3, Altmeyer Papers (add.); (quote) Re Senator Kennedy (13 Mar. 1971), Box 162, Edgar Kaiser Papers, Bancroft Library, University of California, Berkeley; Minutes of the Meeting of the CNHI Technical Committee (5 July 1972), Box 3, Altmeyer Papers (add.); (quote) Arthur Weissman to Edgar Kaiser (23 May 1977), Box 489, Edgar Kaiser Papers.

[22] Ehrlichman to Ed Morgan (17 Dec. 1969), Box 36, File IS:1, White House Special File (Confidential Files) [WHSF], Richard M. Nixon Papers, National Archives; (quote) Ehrlichman to Nixon (10 Nov. 1970), Box IS:1, WHSF, Nixon Papers; (quote) Glasser to Jeffrey (2 July 1970), Box 105, Part II, Series VI, UAW-SSD Records; (quote) handwritten notes (11 Mar. 1971), Box HE:1, White House Central File [WHCF], Nixon Papers; (quote) Chapin to Ehrlichman (18 Feb, 1971), Box IS:1, WHSF, Nixon Papers; see Schedule proposals (1971–1972) in Box IS:2, and "Report of the Domestic Council Health Policy Review Group" (8 Dec. 1970), Box IS:1, WHSF, Nixon Papers; (quote) Cavanaugh to Harper (24 June 1971), Box IS:1, WHSF, Nixon Papers; (quote) Moynihan to Nixon (4 June 1970), Box 20, File FG 23, WHSF, Nixon Papers; CNHI Executive Committee Minutes (1974–1978); [CNHI] "Work Plan" (June 1977), all in Box 110, Part II, Series VI, UAW-SSD Records.

growth politics was to follow the GOP, health policy consisted of celebrating past achievements (such as Medicare) while doing little to check their destruction. Reformers watched the Carter administration skirt the issue and concluded glumly that it was "postponing NHI for a generation."[23] Congressional proposals in the early 1990s, ranging from a full-blown single-payer system to a "pay or play" employer mandate to "market" reform, all claimed Democratic sponsors. The Clinton plan tried to synthesize this programmatic disarray and employ the party itself as a legislative advocate. On the programmatic side, the Clinton task force simply threw everything into the pot, a reflection of both the party's lack of intellectual or political moorings and its eagerness to please a bewildering array of interested parties. The task force began by dismissing the single-payer option and marginalizing its advocates (dubbed "contrarians") by assigning them to obscure study groups or pushing them out the loop entirely.[24] Even on the limited terrain left, the administration viewed every choice as a potential landmine. In the end, the task force could do little more than pursue private support by promising different things to different interests and build public support by "locat[ing] and turn[ing] public fear." The party was so unaccustomed to such programmatic efforts that its National Health Care Campaign stumbled badly and the administration was widely criticized for using the DNC for something other than winning elections.[25]

The Last Best Hope: Labor and Health Politics

Organized labor has been the most prominent, if also the most disappointing, agent of health reform. The labor movement was both a persistent advocate of benefits for its members and the most logical organizational springboard for broader reform efforts. American unions played the same pivotal role in health politics as did workers and unions in

[23] CNHI Executive Committee Meeting (25 May 1978), Box 110, Part II, Series VI, UAW-SSD Records.

[24] See Brown to Magaziner (n.d.) ; Zelman to Magaziner (1 Mar. 1993), both in Box 3305, CHTF Records.

[25] OMB, "Report on Meeting with Ira Magaziner" (7 June 1993), Box 1097; National Health Care Campaign Materials, Box 1183; (quote) Lois Quam, handwritten notes, Box 1173; "Landmines" (n.d.), Box 670; "Message Themes" chart, Box 1172, all in CHTF Records; Theda Skocpol, *Boomerang: Clinton's Health Security Effort and the Turn against Government in U.S. Politics* (New York, 1996), 33–36, 90–95; Center for Public Integrity, "Well-Healed: Inside Lobbying for Health Care Reform," *IJHS* 26:1 (1996): 25–26.

similar efforts in other democratic capitalist settings.[26] At the same time, these efforts underscored (and contributed to) two thrusts of American exceptionalism: the failure to achieve national health insurance and the political weakness of organized labor. Given its uneasy relationship with state and national politics, its uneven organizational reach (even at its peak, the U.S. labor movement remained a low-density, decentralized outlier among its industrial democratic peers), and the ways in which private social provision narrowed its political horizons, the labor movement did little more than pursue security and benefits for its members. Over time, labor's role in the health debate undermined the prospects for universal health insurance—in part because the American labor movement (as a consequence of internal discrimination and external pressures) had few universal pretensions and in part because family-wage employment-based provision bore such little relation to the actual social and familial needs for health services.

In the Progressive Era, labor could not separate the issue of social insurance from its larger, and largely unhappy, relationship with the state. The weakness of political institutions in the late nineteenth and early twentieth centuries left the social and political status of labor largely to the judiciary—an institution predisposed to sort out social conflict on the basis of property rights. This intersection of state weakness and judicial activism discouraged collective interests and rewarded a "rights consciousness" that ultimately won some legal protections even as it eroded the mutual obligations of state and citizen. It was this experience that led the AFL to view the efforts of 1914–20 with such suspicion. While some unions and state federations worked with the AALL, AFL president Samuel Gompers famously dismissed the effort as "undemocratic," "repugnant to free-born citizens," and "at variance with our concepts of voluntary institutions and freedom for individuals." While reformers tried to cement the distinction between contractual and charitable programs, workers were less confident that the AALL plan insulated them from the stigma of the latter. "Clothe it in whatever garb you will or disguise it as you may," concluded the AFL's Committee on Social Insurance, "compulsion by legislative enactment for health insurance carries with it the stigma of the inability of the people to do for themselves."[27]

---

[26] Marie Gottschalk, "The Phantom of Public Policy: The 'Exceptional Politics' of Organized Labor and the American Welfare State" (paper presented at a meeting of the Policy History Conference, St. Louis, 1999), passim.

[27] Gompers quotes from Gompers, "Voluntary Social Insurance vs. Compulsory," and National Civic Federation, *Compulsory Health Insurance: Annual Meeting Addresses, 1917* (New York, 1917), 22; (quote) "Report of the Committee on Social Insurance" (1918), reel 63, AALL Papers; (quote) Grant Hamilton, "Proposed Legislation for Health Insurance," in

Labor's health politics through the 1920s maintained the conviction that wages won through collective bargaining constituted the best social policy. The collapse of wartime experiments in labor policy, the "open-shop" assault on collective bargaining, the widespread employment of legal injunctions, and the emergence of welfare capitalism all hardened the AFL's official commitment to voluntarist solutions. At the same time, this commitment was an increasingly hollow one. The AFL never hesitated to support state action (including pensions and restrictions on the labor of women or children) that regulated workers beyond the AFL's concerns. Individual unions and state federations mimicked the AFL's boilerplate voluntarism while advocating a wide range of social policies, including compulsory health insurance. And exhortations to individual freedom and union autonomy rang less convincingly as the Depression savaged private wages and welfare capitalism. More important, the emergence of the CIO and the New Deal dramatically expanded the political horizons of workers and their unions and recast their relationship with the state and the Democratic Party.[28]

The labor movement, or at least the northern urban working class, forged an alliance with the Democratic Party in the early 1930s as the New Deal codified basic bargaining rights and proved a relatively generous (and politically astute) source of relief. But the Democrats did not fully represent or satisfy labor's political aspirations. The southern foundation of Democratic power always qualified its relationship with the labor movement, a fact underscored by the Southern concessions written into the Wagner and Social Security acts, the collapse of Operation Dixie in 1946, and the passage of Taft-Hartley in 1947. For these reasons there seemed to be, in both the inchoate protests of 1933–35 and the emergence of the CIO after 1935, an opportunity for the emergence of a genuine labor party. But for a variety of reasons—including the persistence of legal and political obstacles to third-party competition, the resurgence of the AFL in the late 1930s, and the strategic anxieties of both CIO leaders and Popular Fronters—the CIO devoted its political ener-

U.S. Department of Labor, *Proceedings of the Conference on Social Insurance*, Bureau of Labor Statistics Bulletin 212 (Washington, D.C., 1917), 562–63; Skocpol, *Protecting Soldiers and Mothers*, 205–47; Alan Derickson, " 'Take Health from the List of Luxuries': Labor and the Right to Health Care, 1915–1949," *Labor History* 41:2 (2000): 173–78. On voluntarism, see William Forbath, *Law and the Shaping of the American Labor Movement* (Cambridge, Mass., 1991); Victoria Hattam, *Labor Visions and State Power: The Origins of Business Unionism in the United States* (Princeton, N.J., 1993); Michael Rogin, "Voluntarism: The Political Functions of an Antipolitical Doctrine," *ILRR* 26 (1961–62), 521–35.

[28] Linda Gordon, *Pitied but Not Entitled: Single Mothers and the History of Welfare* (New York, 1994), 213–15; Lizbeth Cohen, *Making a New Deal: Industrial Workers in Chicago, 1919–1939* (New York, 1990).

gies to the Democratic Party. This relationship was formalized during the war and early postwar years as the politics of mobilization, the cold war, and full employment combined to narrow labor's options.[29]

By the end of the 1940s labor stood near its organizational peak and, by design and default, vested all of its political aspirations in the Democratic Party. At the same time, labor claimed no real standing in a party that remained rooted in the "solid South" and that had traded the politics of the New Deal for the panacea of growth politics. By the early 1950s the CIO was reduced to bargaining with the Democratic Party, as CIO-PAC chair Jack Kroll complained bitterly, "much as it would with an employer." The notoriously barren marriage between the Democratic Party and organized labor was, more precisely, an abusive relationship in which labor suffered the battering of Democratic politics but had nowhere else to go.[30] The consequences for health reform were clear. Because the CIO emerged after 1935, the labor movement had little impact on the shape or scope of the original Social Security Act. The CIO stepped forward as an advocate of national and universal health programs in 1938, but by this point the administration had largely lost interest. Although the CIO remained an advocate of national health insurance through the 1940s, it could not sway the party's faith in full employment as an adequate or alternative source of social provision. Some in the CIO understood the limits of private benefits and placed them on the bargaining table as a dismal but necessary alternative to an elusive political solution. Others embraced both private benefits and the right of the AMA, as Teamster Dave Beck put it, "to protect the interests of your members and fight for the preservation of your profession . . . you doctors have a pretty good union."[31]

[29] Michael Davis, *Prisoners of the American Dream* (London, 1986), 68–91; Frances Fox Piven and Richard Cloward, *Why Americans Don't Vote* (New York, 1989), 122–38; Nelson Lichtenstein, "From Corporatism to Collective Bargaining: Organized Labor and the Eclipse of Social Democracy in the Postwar Era," in *The Rise and Fall of the New Deal Order, 1930–1980*, ed. Steve Fraser and Gary Gerstle (Princeton, N.J., 1989), 122–44; Colin Gordon, "The Lost City of Solidarity: Metropolitan Unionism in Historical Perspective," *Politics and Society* 27:4 (1999): 561–86; Stephen Kunitz, "Socialism and Social Insurance in the United States and Canada," in *Compulsory Health Insurance: The Continuing American Debate*, ed. Ronald Numbers (Westport, Conn., 1980), 112–13.

[30] Kroll quoted in James Foster, *The Union Politic: The CIO's Political Action Committee* (Columbus, Mo., 1975), 199–200; Davis, *Prisoners of the American Dream*, 82–101; Lichtenstein, "From Corporatism to Collective Bargaining," 140. The "barren marriage" is developed in Davis, *Prisoners of the American Dream*, 52–101; the idea of an "abusive relationship" is in Joel Rogers, "How Divided Progressives Might Unite," *New Left Review* 210 (1995): 29.

[31] Jennifer Klein, "Managing Security: The Business of American Social Policy, 1910s–1960," (unpublished ms.), 277–82; Lichtenstein, "From Corporatism to Collective Bargaining," 138–39; "Highlight Points for Discussion with AMA" (1949), Box 44, Henry J.

Through the 1950s and 1960s, labor remained wedded to both the Democratic Party and its deference to private health coverage. Although the mid-1960s saw a substantial expansion of social policy, the Great Society rested on a fundamental satisfaction with the performance of the private economy and a conviction that tinkering at its margins would sweep up those left behind. In turn, labor's willingness to consider universal programs faltered as health costs increased, employer-financed health plans became the norm, and large employee groups reaped the benefits of experience rating.[32] Employment-based benefits, after all, had become an important source of union security and union power. Even after 1964, when the civil rights movement loosened southern control over the party, the AFL-CIO voiced little support for health reform. Organized labor was skeptical of Medicare, and backed the bill in 1965 largely out of the conviction that public retiree coverage would lower the costs of commercial insurance.[33]

As the economy stumbled into the 1970s, the foundation of private coverage began to crumble and organized labor renewed its interest in national health insurance. By this time, both the labor movement and the Democratic Party were in disarray as well—the former bracing for an era of political backlash and concessionary bargaining, the latter scrambling to adjust its faith in growth politics to an economy in decline. After the debacle of 1972, in which the AFL-CIO declined to endorse George McGovern's candidacy, labor's influence in the party was splintered and marginal. Some progressive unions dug in behind the party's liberal wing (most closely identified with Senator Kennedy) and established independent political committees—an effort culminating in the UAW-backed Labor Clearing House in 1976. At the same time, AFL-CIO leaders briefly explored the possibility of retreating to a bipartisan posture from which they could endorse Republicans as well.[34] Labor and the Democrats were ill prepared for the dismal 1970s. In some respects, their relationship was now more important than ever; in other respects, that relationship was increasingly seen—on both sides—as an anachronism or a liability.

Kaiser Papers, Bancroft Library; (quote) Dave Beck, "Government Medicine: Danger Ahead!" (1951), Box 59, Henry J. Kaiser Papers.

[32] Minutes of the Meeting of the AFL Committee on Social Security (3 Mar. 1954), Box 16, Cruikshank Papers; Ira Katznelson, "Was the Great Society a Lost Opportunity?" in *The Rise and Fall of the New Deal Order, 1930–1980*, ed. Fraser and Gerstle, 195–205; Smith to Pollack (June 1964), Box 1, Part I, Series II, UAW-SSD Records.

[33] Danstedt to Glasser (2 Mar. 1965); "Potential Big 3 Savings with Medicare" (27 July 1964); Glasser to Bluestone (18 June 1964), all in Box 2, Part I, Series I, UAW-SSD Records. On labor and the Great Society, see Michael Brown, *Race, Money, and the American Welfare State* (Ithaca, N.Y., 1999), 277–80; Harris, "Annals of Legislation: Medicare," 51.

[34] See Davis, *Prisoners of the American Dream*, 100–1; and, for a more optimistic account, Taylor Dark, *The Unions and the Democrats: An Enduring Alliance* (Ithaca, N.Y., 1999).

Progressive unions supported the Health Security Act of the early 1970s, but for many in the labor movement, reform threatened to erase the substantial advantages (favorable tax treatment, expansive benefits, and experience-rated commercial premiums) enjoyed by employment-based plans.[35] This investment in private coverage was especially apparent surrounding the passage of the Employment Retirement and Income Security Act in 1974. Although ERISA created a regulatory vacuum that ultimately allowed employers to duck state insurance regulation and federal standards, labor lobbied for the law in order to protect nationally bargained benefits from state taxation.[36] Labor hesitated even to raise money for the Committee for National Health Insurance lest it open a political and strategic rift between national leadership and the more progressive UAW faction. And by 1974 labor and its congressional allies had retreated to proposals that resembled the Nixon position of 1970–71.[37] The labor movement fell in behind Jimmy Carter in the 1976 campaign, although many did so reluctantly and only after his nomination was assured. Some progressive unions went so far as to make the candidate's support of national health insurance a condition of their support and worked closely with the Carter campaign on its health platform. But the administration was quick to disappoint, both in its lukewarm support of labor law reform in 1977–78 and in its retreat on health insurance. Yet the UAW and others had few other options. An effort to build a Progressive Alliance in late 1978 fizzled, and even the most disenchanted supported Carter as the party's nominee in 1980.[38]

After 1980 labor's status in the Democratic Party grew more desperate and more complicated. More than ever, the AFL-CIO needed a sustained political presence. Yet as its own membership crumbled and the Demo-

---

[35] Joint Meeting of the Executive Committees of the CNHI and HSAC (2 Aug. 1974); Glasser to Woodcock (27 Nov. 1974), both in Box 110, Part I, Series VI, UAW-SSD Records.

[36] See Margaret Farrell, "ERISA Preemption and Regulation of Managed Care: The Case for Managed Federalism," *American Journal of Law and Medicine* 23:2/3 (1997): 256–58, 265–76; Daniel M. Fox and Daniel C. Schaffer, "Health Policy and ERISA: Interest Groups and Semipreemption," *JHPPL* 14 (1989): 239–60; Mary Ann Chirba-Martin and Troyen Brennan, "The Critical Role of ERISA in State Health Reform," *HA* 13 (1994): 144; *Nation's Business* (Mar. 1996): 17–18.

[37] Fine to Glasser (13 Nov. 1974); Glasser to Woodcock (6 Dec. 1972); Glasser to Woodcock (25 Mar. 1974); and Fine to Glasser (28 Mar. 1974), all in Box 105, Part II, Series VI, UAW-SSD Records; Jacobs, "The UAW and the Committee for National Health Insurance," 120–21.

[38] Martin Halpern, "Jimmy Carter and the UAW: Failure of an Alliance," *Presidential Studies Quarterly* 26:3 (1996): 755–57, 759–64, 768–70; Gary Fink, "Fragile Alliance: Jimmy Carter and the American Labor Movement," in *The Presidency and Domestic Politics of Jimmy Carter*, ed. Herbert Rosenbaum and Alexuj Ugrinsky (Westport, Conn., 1994), 786–89; Glasser to Woodcock (3 July 1974), Box 105, Part II, Series VI, UAW-SSD Records.

crats acquiesced to the fundamental premises of Reaganomics, labor leadership saw little choice but to line up behind a congressional delegation and a succession of presidential candidates who made no bones about rethinking their traditional relationship with the labor movement. Serious health reform disappeared from the agenda, while labor leaders and party regulars neither offered serious objections to Reagan's assault on social programs nor supported the efforts of Jesse Jackson's 1988 presidential run to mobilize candidates and voters around a national health program.[39]

Although Clinton's nomination and election represented the culmination of the party's drift to the right, partisan inertia and horror at the Republican alternatives threw the labor movement behind the new administration. Labor's dilemma was neatly underscored through 1993 by the parallel debates over NAFTA and health reform. The AFL-CIO faced off against both business lobbyists and the White House in the NAFTA fight, while essentially deferring to both in the development of a health program. The AFL-CIO funneled almost $10 million to the DNC in support of the health bill, although its constituent unions disagreed sharply over its key provisions—some fearing displacement of existing private plans, some holding out for a single-payer system, some merely supporting whichever version the administration was currently proposing. This was accompanied by a studied indifference to the single-payer option floated by congressional Democrats. In the end, labor would be disappointed by both the watered-down health plan and the administration's support for NAFTA (after the passage of NAFTA in November 1993, the AFL-CIO "turned off the spigot" to the DNC and its National Health Care Campaign).[40]

Just as labor's health politics were constrained by its relationship with the Democratic Party, they were also constrained by the relationship of workers, unions, and union leaders to the system of private benefits that emerged after the late 1930s. As we have seen, there was little question that labor would pursue private benefits, and it did so, quite self-consciously, as a short-term response to the political failures of the 1930s and 1940s. Over time, however, labor developed a vested material and political interest in the private welfare state. At best, this distracted and fragmented the labor movement's political attentions and, at worst,

[39] Ferguson and Rogers, *Right Turn*, 138–93; Vicente Navarro, *The Politics of Health Policy: The U.S. Reforms, 1980–1994* (Cambridge, Mass., 1994), 78–110; Gottschalk, "The Phantom of Public Policy," 28–32.

[40] Marie Gottschalk, "The Missing Millions: Organized Labor, Business, and the Defeat of Clinton's Health Security Act," *JHPPL* 24:3 (1999): 506–9; Lawrence Weil, "Organized Labor and Health Reform: Unions Interests and the Clinton Plan," *Journal of Public Health Policy* 18:1 (1997): 30.

made labor unions a willing partner in the corporate compromise. Labor's pursuit of private benefits was always a necessary strategy against a background of persistent political failure. But the strategy also contributed to the failure as labor's scattered successes fragmented its interest in reform and gave it a tangible stake in the institutions of employment-based coverage.

Success at the bargaining table invariably eroded support for political alternatives. In the wake of the UMW's landmark agreement to an industrywide health and welfare fund in 1946, *The Nation* worried that such industry-specific coverage "may in time form a network of vested interests which would tend to block the kind of complete public provision for medical services which is so badly needed." By the early 1950s, the CNH noted an increasingly prevalent "vested interest in a voluntary system," and "a tendency on the part of many unions to lose effective interest in national health legislation even though they may continue to give it verbal support in convention resolutions."[41] As private benefits spread through the 1940s and 1950s, unions increasingly argued that universal coverage might actually come at their expense, especially if it meant a retreat from the experience-rated premiums they had won from commercial insurers and the employer funding they had won from management. Labor support for public health insurance in California, for example, evaporated as unions "concluded that they could obtain all the benefits of Warren's bills as fringe benefits in their labor contracts and impose the entire cost of the system on employers." Various formulae for sharing the costs of a payroll-funded national health plan floated in 1948 and 1949 threatened to fix a cost to workers that most major unions were working to impose on employers alone.[42] "Health insurance plans developed by many unions through collective bargaining are working in the direction of a limited and costly commercial type of insurance," the CNH conceded, "and at cross purposes with the legislative program for national health insurance."[43]

[41] (Quote) *The Nation* 162 (25 May 1946), 616; (quote) "Developments, Trends, and Outlook in Collective-Bargaining Welfare Plans" (Nov. 1949), Box 77:839, Series II, Falk Papers; Davis, "Subjects for Meeting" (15 Apr. 1948), reel 1, Davis Papers.

[42] Lichtenstein, "From Corporatism to Collective Bargaining," 128–29; Labor File, Box 55, PCHNN Records; Alan Derickson, "The United Steelworkers of America and Health Insurance, 1937–1962," in *American Labor in the Era of World War I*, ed. Daniel Cornford and Sally Miller (Westport, Conn., 1995), 72–73; "United Action for Health," *Economic Outlook* [CIO] (Apr. 1953); (quote) Byrl Salsman OH in *Earl Warren and Health Insurance, 1943–1949* (Berkeley, Calif., 1971), 12; "The Relationship of Collective Bargaining Contracts to NHI" (2 Nov. 1949), Box 65:622, Series II, Falk Papers; Ruether to Senator Lehman (1 Feb. 1951), Box 211, Edwin Witte Papers, SHSW.

[43] John Brumm [CNH], "Some Issues Raised by Union Health and Welfare Plans" (Oct. 1954), Box 67:655, Series II, Falk Papers.

Postwar bargaining also enmeshed organized labor in a particular form of group-based indemnity coverage that made the leap to universal coverage even less likely. Unions' efforts to offer health coverage always depended upon their ability to assemble a stable and substantial actuarial pool. The tension between group coverage and community coverage was magnified by the ascendance of collectively bargained and commercially insured health plans. Postwar bargaining erected "silos of solidarity" around some industries and eroded both multi-union community organization and any sense that organized labor might represent a broader consumer interest. "[Union] health funds are expended without the guidance of a prevailing overall philosophy or policy," lamented one observer in the early 1950s. "Plans set up by individual unions have tended to stay 'single,' and new health centers often spring up next door to old ones. . . . To date only one multi-union plan on a partial community basis has been established and has prospered."[44] Labor saw local multiunion cooperation as either administratively impossible or an invitation to a lowest common denominator of benefits. CIO unions routinely argued that community health plans would dilute benefits already won, that their costs would be borne by union members, and that employment-based indemnity plans were unsuited for community pooling. By the 1960s labor only rarely looked beyond the horizon of employment-based benefits. "Unions are becoming the most potent force furthering the development of voluntary plans," noted one observer. "They are in the same camp with management."[45]

A large part of the dilemma, for labor and its allies, was the specter of "double taxation." Payroll-based care invariably undermined support for residual public programs. Indigent care "should not be loaded into the subscription rate of subscribers who are already paying taxes and otherwise contributing to support of local hospitals," argued one UAW official

[44] Jerome Pollack, "A Labor View of Health Security," (3 May 1954), Box 67:654, Series II, Falk Papers; Green to HST (14 Jan. 1952), Official File 103G, Box 577, Truman Papers; E. R. Brown, "Consumers' Cooperatives and Labor Unions" (1940), Box 103, Papers of the Cooperative League; Goor to Esselstyn (7 Dec. 1960), Box 55:53, Series III, Esselstyn Papers; (quote) John Brumm, "Relating Cooperative and Community Prepaid Group Practice Health Plans to Labor Health Programs" (July 1955), reel 5, Davis Papers; "Preliminary Proposals for a Labor-Federal Government Partnership for Improving Health Care" (1966), Box 38:229, Series II, Lorin Kerr Papers, Sterling Library; CNH Bulletin (Sept. 1954), Box 67:655, Series II, Falk Papers; Derickson, "Health Security for All?" 1336–37, 1351–52; CNH Bulletin (Sept. 1954), Box 67:655, Series II, Falk Papers. I owe the "silos of solidarity" metaphor to Joel Rogers.

[45] Background materials and clippings in Box 110, Series II, Falk Papers; Address of Frederick Mott to the Economic Club of Detroit (10 Feb. 1958), Box 4 (Mss 400), Altmeyer Papers; Lane Kirkland Memo (6 July 1967), Box 10:250, Series I, Esselstyn Papers; (quote) Franz Goldmann, "Labor's Attitude toward Health Insurance," ILRR 13:4 (July 1960): 92.

in 1958. "We are willing to pay once for this service, maybe twice, not three times." "The great bulk of workers, who are covered compulsorily," a Social Security official added in 1962, "might feel that it is unfair to give identical protection from general revenues—to which they also contribute—to those not in the [contributory] system." During the early 1970s, reformers pondered not only the political perils of departing from the contributory logic of private and public social insurance but the inequity of asking workers to underwrite both the private welfare state (through payroll contributions) and the public welfare state (through taxes). "I think we may have difficulty in convincing workers that they should pay a tax on their earnings to help finance health benefits to persons who have paid no such tax and are not 'medically needy,' " argued Arthur Altmeyer. "It is no answer to say that health benefits for such persons are paid out of general revenues because workers, like everybody else, have to pay taxes included in general revenues in addition to paying the health security tax based on their wages."[46]

The political costs of labor's dependence upon and commitment to private benefits became starkly apparent in the 1970s. The emerging health crisis sparked labor's interest in national health insurance, which many saw as a means of sandbagging existing benefits, restraining their costs, and dumping the "absolute albatross" (as the UAW's Douglas Fraser put it) of negotiating them. At the same time, however, many unions were unwilling to risk existing benefits (often paid for exclusively by employers) or the tax haven offered by ERISA. As a result, "the labor groups who could be expected to be most active in promoting NHI are most concerned about their collective bargaining activities . . . which diminishes or negates the likelihood of their making NHI a critical issue." The UAW's Walter Reuther had agreed to spearhead a Committee of 100 (what later became the CNHI) to lobby for national health insurance in the late 1960s, but neither the UAW nor the broader labor movement devoted serious attention to the issue. Instead, the AFL-CIO drifted away from universalism and toward mandated employment-based care.[47]

[46] (Quote) Statement by Emanuel Mann [UAW] before the Insurance Department of the Commonwealth of Pennsylvania (13 Nov. 1958), Box 1, Part I, Series II, UAW-SSD Records; (quote) Robert Ball to the Secretary (20 June 1962), Box 166, Decimal 056.1, SSC (1956–1974), HEW Records; (quote) Altmeyer to Falk (8 Feb. 1970), Box 3, Altmeyer Papers (add.); "The Alienated Rank and File," *The Nation* 209 (17 Nov. 1969): 527–30.

[47] "Statement of AFL-CIO Executive Council on Medical Costs" (13 May 1968), Box 109:4, Cohen Papers; Fraser quoted in *BW* (4 Sept. 1978): 65–66; "Note on Tax Provisions" (12 Nov. 1972), Box 150:2178, Series III, Falk Papers; Farrell, "ERISA Preemption and Regulation of Managed Care," 256–58; (quote) Altmeyer to Falk (9 May 1970), Falk to Altmeyer (15 May 1970), Box 3, Altmeyer Papers (add.); "Correspondence Re: 1971 contract" (1971) Box 11:191, Series I, Kerr Papers. After Ruether's death, Altmeyer conceded, "I really know nothing of what plans Walter had for mobilizing support for NHI." See

Labor's dilemmas and anxieties were replayed in 1992–94. Although the late 1970s and 1980s had eroded private benefits even further, labor's interests remained shortsighted and fragmented. Attentive as always to the fiscal, political, and social promise of national health insurance, the labor movement nevertheless confronted the Clinton plan with diverse and often contradictory interests. Many large unions and multiunion "Taft-Hartley" plans joined their employers in pressing for the right to maintain experience-rated premiums by opting out of public insurance pools. Most unions dug in against the taxation of employment benefits and any changes in ERISA, including waivers designed to nurture single-payer at the state level. Most unions viewed the Clinton plan not as an opportunity to make the leap to single-payer reform but as an occasion to defend their diverse stakes in private provision. In effect, labor turned its back on consumer groups and single-payer advocates and threw its lot in with private employers, many of whom—at least in the early months of the debate— also seemed willing to accept federal reforms that stabilized and standardized employment-based coverage. Labor, of course, was quickly disappointed. Business bailed out as soon as it became clear that mandates and cost control could not be reconciled. The administration paid little heed, passing NAFTA in late 1993 and paring back its health plan in a vain effort to keep insurers and employers on board. And the single—payer alternative withered in the absence of serious labor support.[48]

Half a Loaf? Dilemmas of Incremental Reform

Across the twentieth century, the likelihood of serious reform—given the enormous resource disadvantage faced by reformers, the programmatic limits of the party system, and labor's political ambivalence—remained dim. In response, reformers and legislators routinely retreated to, and often preferred, some combination of incremental reform and deference to the states. Given the enormous constraints facing health reformers, stopgap or partial solutions often presented themselves as the only "realistic" or practical goals. Yet given the logic of social insurance generally and of health care particularly, such solutions tended to make things worse by fragmenting care, distracting reform energies, and undermining future appeals to universal coverage. In turn, uneven economic de-

Altmeyer to Falk (9 May 1970), Falk to Altmeyer (15 May 1970), Box 3, Altmeyer Papers (add.); Marie Gottschalk, *The Shadow Welfare State: Labor, Business, and the Politics of Health Care in the United States* (Ithaca, N.Y., 2000), 75–82, 86–101, 149–52.

[48] Weil, "Organized Labor and Health Reform," 31–41; Gottschalk, "The Missing Millions," 491, 496–500, 508–10, 514–16.

velopment and federated responsibility discouraged national political solutions, encouraged states to compete against one another, exaggerated the political influence of economic interests, and sheltered stark regional inequities. This has been especially true in the case of health reform, an issue for which national solutions are both uniquely important and peculiarly elusive.

American federalism made the states both a logical first step for reformers and a convenient refuge for opponents. The politics of the insurance industry, as we have seen, were animated largely by fear of federal intrusion (although some large insurers came to resent the burden of "sitting down with fifty governments")[49] and the states retained regulatory responsibility even as increasingly expansive definitions of the commerce clause brought much of the rest of the economy under the federal wing. Other interests had different stakes in federalism: employers had little interest in state or federal health reform—at least until some firms began to see mandated employment-based care as a means of socializing existing costs and responsibilities. Most employers viewed state regulation not as a haven from federal interference but as an administrative nightmare that put "fifty hands on fifty triggers."[50] State responsibility, in turn, slowed and shaped the progress of a wide range of public and private health policies. Group health plans were shaped by state laws that exempted some from regulation as insurers and confined others to medical society (Blue Shield) control.[51] Federal indigent care programs (including Kerr-Mills, Medicaid, and SCHIP) tolerated a wide range of standards, a tack that reflected deference to state insurance regulation and racially and regionally charged measures of "health and decency."[52] ERISA established some federal benefit standards but also encouraged employers to escape not only state but federal scrutiny through self-insurance.[53]

---

[49] Grahame to Bates (24 Oct. 1946), Box 17, Grahame Papers.

[50] "Some Legal Problems" (21 Aug. 1954), Box 849:1; H.M.W. to R.N.G. (21 Apr. 1955), Box 849:9; file on Indiana Lawsuit against Health and Benefits Plan, Box 850:8, Pennsylvania Railroad Papers, Hagley Museum and Library, Wilmington, Del.; (quote) " 'Medicare,' the Cure That Could Cause a Setback," *Fortune* 67:5 (May 1963), 167.

[51] C. Rufus Rorem, "Enabling Legislation for Non-Profit Hospital Service Plans," *Law and Contemporary Problems* 6:4 (Winter 1939): 529–31; Franz Goldmann, "Public Policy in Organizing Medical Care," *AAAPSS* 273 (1951): 64; Draft of Proceedings, Association of Labor Health Administrators (28 Mar. 1957), Box 37:212, Series II, Kerr Papers.

[52] "Briefing Paper on Federal and State Roles" (n.d.), Box 4001, CHTF Records; Letter to Zelman (5 Mar. 1993), Box 4000, CHTF Records; Children's Defense Fund, "CHIP Checkup: A Mid-term Report on the State Children's Health Insurance Program" (27 May 1998), archived at www.childrensdefense.org.

[53] Colleen Grogan, "Hope in Federalism? What Can the States Do and What Are They Likely to Do?" *JHPPL* 20 (1995): 478–79.

All of this distracted and fragmented the efforts of reformers who (especially once private insurance had a foothold) often had to replicate their efforts in many jurisdictions. Before the 1930s, health reform proceeded on the assumption that constitutional prohibitions made federal solutions impossible. After the 1930s, reform proceeded on the assumption that political considerations (the Democratic South) made federal solutions difficult and deference to the states necessary. Health reformers routinely argued that it was politically prudent and programmatically pointless to follow the New Deal's lead in allowing individual states to determine standards of provision and participation—a practice that was at once "unavoidable and inevitable on political grounds" and a guarantee that the results "at best, would be a patchwork of programs not unlike grandmother's quilt in appearance."[54] Such disparities persisted as the first flurry of state participation in Medicare and Medicaid was followed, in short order, by fiscal pressures that encouraged the federal government to push much of the burden back to the states.[55]

Much of the timidity and futility of state health policy, in turn, reflected the fact that the background political advantages enjoyed by economic interests were magnified in local and regional settings. Local interests routinely stifled local innovation by raising the flag of competitive disadvantage. During the AALL debate, some manufacturers complained that costs "would not be uniform between the States. It is not difficult to conceive of such legislation increasing [labor costs] to the extent of compelling manufacturers to move their works out of state." In the 1940s, both opponents of state plans and advocates of national reform raised the problem—the former in arguing that reform would put the state in question at a competitive disadvantage, the latter in arguing that only national coverage could avoid "exposing [employers] to potential disadvantages as against their competitors in other states." Such dilemmas arose again in the 1990s as some states pursued reform in response to both the ongoing crisis of costs and coverage and the failure of the Clinton plan. In this flurry, only Hawaii (insulated from interstate

[54] (Quote) Harry Becker, "What Labor Wants in a Disability Benefit Program" (Dec. 1949), Box 201, Witte Papers; Barkev Sanders to Falk (8 Nov. 1945), Box 63:587, Series II, Falk Papers; HEW, "Medical Care for the Aged Under MAA and OAA" (1964), Box 133:5, Cohen Papers.

[55] Special Committee on Aging, "Performance of the States: Eighteen Months of Assistance with the Medical Assistance for the Aged Program" (Washington, D.C., 1962); "Recommendations of the Medical Cost Study" (25 Nov. 1966), 109:4, Cohen Papers; Frank Thompson, "New Federalism and Health Care Policy: States and Old Questions," *JHPPL* 11 (1986): 650–52; "Presidential Briefing Book: Access for Underserved and Vulnerable Populations," Box 3292, and "Briefing Book on Low Income Coverage," Box 3296, CHTF Records.

competition) made any progress, while efforts to mandate employment-based care elsewhere (notably Washington, Florida, and Massachusetts) foundered.[56]

Given their competitive anxieties, their acute sensitivity to local interests, and their importance in sustaining regional economic strategies, states demonstrated little utility as "laboratories" for health policy. During each flurry of state interest in compulsory or mandated health insurance, serious legislative attention was confined to those states in which private or voluntary plans were most developed. State policy, in other words, tended to magnify interstate disparities and make national reform even less likely.[57] While reformers often retreated reluctantly to state solutions, opponents saw state responsibility as a means of undermining national or universal programs. In many respects, American social policy embraced the very regional inequities it should have been addressing. "What is so biblical about these state lines . . . what are the so-called diversifications in local needs?" CIO counsel Lee Pressman asked in 1938, adding that such arguments were "too frequently used by the reactionary forces that simply try to prevent us from having any program."[58]

Just as federalism fragmented and frustrated reform, the monotonous strategy of incremental reform offered the illusion of progress while making the goal of national health insurance more elusive. Time and time again, settling for less—whether this meant putting off reform for another round of study, deferring to the states, championing categorical coverage, or supplementing and subsidizing employment-based care—failed to bring reformers any closer to universal national health insurance and made it harder to argue for such a system next time around. Each retreat to discrete coverage of mothers or children or the elderly implicitly argued that those left behind were less deserving. Each concession to private health insurance inflated the political and ideological and economic investment in contributory, job-based coverage. And each plan for "staging" or staggering the introduction of new programs invariably stumbled over new political or budgetary circumstances. Reformers did not, as some have suggested, move too far too quickly and sacrifice prog-

[56] Thompson, "New Federalism and Health Care Policy," 648–49; Wendy Parmet, "Regulation and Federalism: Legal Impediments to State Health Care Reform," *American Journal of Law and Medicine* 191 (1993): 122; *Iron Age* cited in Moss, *Socializing Security,* 142; Geraldine Sartain, "California's Health Insurance Drama," *Survey Graphic* 34:11 (Nov. 1945): 44; (quote) "Draft Report on S. 1679" (21 June 1949), Box 65:616, Series II, Falk Papers.

[57] Andrews, "Progress towards Health Insurance" (1917), reel 62, AALL Papers; Robertson, "The Bias of American Federalism," 280–85.

[58] Draft copy: "The Nation's Health" (1938), Box 10, ICHWA Records; (quote) Pressman in Official Report of Proceedings before the President's Interdepartmental Committee (18 July 1938), p. 385, Box 29, ICHWA Records.

ress through their unwillingness to compromise.[59] Indeed, it was the pragmatic conviction, as expressed by Wilbur Cohen and others, that "it is both desirable and practical to improve our health system on an incremental basis" that enabled opponents to consistently delay and distract reform.[60]

Perhaps the most persistent and debilitating commitment to incremental reform was the embrace—enthusiastic for some, grudging for others—of employment-based insurance. In the 1930s and 1940s, conservatives viewed private plans as the best defense against state intervention and trumpeted their potential and their virtues. Many reformers accepted the full-employment, family-wage logic of job-based coverage, and even those who understood the political and actuarial menace of discrete group coverage nevertheless supported it—because dismal access to basic services made any innovations welcome, because the larger Social Security debate granted such cultural and political resonance to the idea of contributory social insurance, and because they hoped that employment-based coverage would prove an administratively and politically convenient springboard for universal coverage. By the early 1950s reform proposals routinely incorporated both paeans to the autonomy of medical professionals and provision that any public plan "not invade a field of any substantial interest to the voluntaries."[61]

But concessions to private coverage had a way of becoming commitments, and it became harder and riskier to consider displacing private insurance. As the Truman plan collapsed, reformers retreated to the goal of "rounding out" private plans with public coverage for elderly and the indigent. The passage of Medicare and Medicaid, in this respect, was a modest and incremental reform in an otherwise expansive liberal moment. By this time private coverage was deeply entrenched and political attention was confined largely to "the shortcomings, inequities, and inefficiencies of the present system." Not surprisingly, reform measures of the 1970s and after abandoned any pretense of displacing employment-based care as health inflation amid chronic budgetary anxieties made

[59] See, for example, Daniel M. Fox, *Health Policies, Health Politics: The British and American Experience, 1911–1965* (Princeton, N.J., 1986), 11–14, 47–51, 79–83, 89–93.

[60] Cohen to Ribicoff (25 Sept. 1973), Box 223:1, Cohen Papers.

[61] Minutes of the Conference on Medical Care (15 Nov. 1937), Box 43, and Hugh Cabot, "The Case against Compulsory Health Insurance" (July 1938), Box 8, both in ICHWA Records; "The Voluntary Prepayment Medical Care Agency: Its Place in a National Health Program" (Oct. 1946), Box 46, Decimal 011.4, GCF (1944–1950), RG 235, HEW Records; Edward Berkowitz and Kim McQuaid, "Social Security and the American Welfare State," *Research in Economic History,* supp. 6 (1991): 169–90; Altmeyer to Ewing (31 Oct. 1947), Box 4, Altmeyer Papers; (quote) Ewing to HST (22 Jan. 1952), Box 33, Ewing Papers.

regulating or mandating private coverage an attractive political option.[62] After a decade of Reaganism, few questioned either the political necessity or the fiscal propriety of basing reform on the existing structure of job-based insurance.

These incremental responses not only fragmented the larger reform movement but also fragmented its access to, and relationship with, the state. By the middle of the twentieth century, advocates of maternal health, children's health, veterans' health, public health, and rural health all claimed administrative beachheads. The progress of national health insurance was slowed not by a poverty of administrative capacity or experience, but by the tremendous variety of federal approaches and interests—including the Women's Bureau, the Children's Bureau, the Veterans Administration and its predecessors, the Public Health Service, and various incarnations or fragments of Social Security. Tellingly, national health insurance proposals, especially in the 1940s, were often linked to complex and contentious executive reorganization plans. At crucial junctures, this administrative patchwork discouraged cooperation as various reform interests battled each other for federal attention and resources and found themselves (as one reformer noted) "at different stages of readiness to break with the AMA if necessary."[63]

Time and time again, reformers retreated to "realistic" and incremental alternatives, only to find that those alternatives reified distinctions between the deserving and the undeserving, narrowed the acceptable options for the next round of debate, and exacerbated the underlying crisis. In some instances, reformers beat a quick retreat because they never viewed universal coverage as anything but a legislative bargaining chip. The goal, as HEW staffers acknowledged in the late 1950s, was to

[62] Milton Roemer, "I. S. Falk, the Committee on the Costs of Medical Care, and the Drive for National Health Insurance," *American Journal of Public Health* 75 (1985): 847; CNH, "Considerations for 1948," reel 1, Davis Papers; (quote) Altmeyer to Falk (24 Dec. 1970), Box 3, Altmeyer add.; Falk memo Re: Executive Committee (9 Sept. 1978), Box 146:2131, Series III, Falk Papers; Falk to Altmeyer (7 Feb. 1971), Box 3, Altmeyer Papers (add.); Falk, "Report to the Executive Committee," (4 Jan. 1974), Box 146:2130, Series III, Falk Papers; Minutes of the Meeting of the CNHI Technical Committee (5 July 1972), Box 3, Altmeyer Papers (add.).

[63] Poen, *Truman versus the Medical Lobby,* 75–82, 163–64; Oscar Ewing OH, p. 174, HSTPL; Michael Davis to Hugh Cabot (21 Mar. 1938), Box 5, ICHWA Records; William Carleton, "Government and Health before the New Deal," *Current History* 45:264 (1963): 75–76; Cohen to LBJ (14 June 1968), Box 122:3, and House Subcommittee on Investigation of the Department of Health, Education, and Welfare, *Investigation of HEW,* Box 122:7, Cohen Papers; (quote) Falk to Winant (14 Mar. 1939), Falk II, 58:489; "Proposal for Department of National Health" (13 Aug. 1945), Official File 103C, Box 576, Truman Papers; Gordon, *Pitied but Not Entitled,* 269–71; Starr, *Transformation of American Medicine,* 275.

"ask for the moon and settle for cheese." In some instances, reformers supported pale alternatives (such as the 1960 Kerr-Mills bill) in the hope that any progress amounted to an entering wedge or a foot in the door. But a less-than-universal welfare state tended to get smaller rather than larger. "Is it worth getting the foot in the door at all costs," *The Nation* asked in 1962, "—or, in the course of further legislative compromises, will the opening become so small that wisdom dictates remaining outside?" By the late 1980s the strategy of incremental reform had almost entirely given way to more desperate attempts to maintain existing public coverage and private insurance. And as cost control trumped increased coverage, "reform" often meant little more than further deference to the market as a means of organizing coverage and provision.[64]

The dismal logic of incremental reform is readily apparent in the experience of various fragments of the health reform movement. Consider the trajectory of maternal reform. Maternalism was a complex and diverse political stance, united by its attention to children but divided by attitudes about women, race, class, and the role of the state. Maternalists sanctified the sexual division of labor even as they attended to its consequences and were never clear as to whether they were interested in protecting women at work or in protecting women from work. In health care, this ambivalence was reflected in debates over the provision of maternity benefits to working women and in the categorical focus of public programs for women and children. Each posed intractable dilemmas. Attending to the immediate conditions of working women invariably raised the larger issue of whether women should be working at all. Unlike "protective" wage and hours legislation, which often had the intended effect of discouraging women's employment, maternal benefits seemed, to many, a direct public subsidy of a social ill. Well-meaning (and often strategic) attention to provision for children and mothers tended to undermine the political or ethical case for covering anyone else.[65]

Over time, maternalists grew leery of losing either hard-won political acceptance of maternal and children's health programs or the institu-

[64] (Quote) Memorandum for Grahame (4 Nov. 1958), Box 18, Grahame Papers; Memorandum: Alternative Policy Positions (20 Mar. 1961), Box 20, Grahame Papers; (quote) "Criteria for a Good Bill," *The Nation* 194 (17 Feb. 1962): 136; Theodore Marmor, *America's Misunderstood Welfare State* (New York, 1990), 183.

[65] Gwendolyn Mink, *The Wages of Motherhood: Inequality in the Welfare State* (Ithaca, N.Y., 1995), 5–15; Sonya Michel and Robyn Rosen, "The Paradox of Maternalism: Elizabeth Lowell Putnam and the American Welfare State," *Gender and History* 4:3 (1992): 364–83; Robyn Muncy, *Creating a Female Dominion in American Reform, 1890–1935* (New York, 1991), passim; Molly Ladd-Taylor, *Mother-Work: Women, Child Welfare, and the State, 1890–1930* (Urbana, Ill., 1994), 17–134; Linda Gordon, "Putting Children First: Women, Maternalism, and Welfare in the Early Twentieth Century," in *U.S. History as Women's History: New Feminist*

tional stronghold afforded by the Children's Bureau. The bureau's anxieties reflected both its conviction that a broad synthetic set of programs for mothers and children was more important than a universal health program alone, and the ongoing assault on the legitimacy and authority of maternalist reform. The AMA had been unrelenting in its attacks on the bureau during the tenure of Sheppard-Towner and spearheaded efforts in 1930 and after to undermine lay control over maternal and children's health programs.[66] As a consequence, the early debate over health and social security found the nation's strongest public health advocates (the Children's Bureau and state health officers aligned with the PHS) at loggerheads. In 1930 Grace Abbot feared that maternal and children's health programs would be "greatly neglected if required only as a by-product of [a] general health program." Four years later, Katherine Lenroot of the Children's Bureau advised the CES to consider only a health program "directed primarily toward education of mothers in health care of children and in standards of maternity care, and education of communities as to the child health resources which should be provided."[67] Into the 1940s, maternalists continued to argue for the expansion of discretionary programs and offered only lukewarm support for the Truman plan—in part because they feared that maternal and children's programs would lose their special status and in part because they feared that any accompanying administrative reorganization would swallow the bureau. Much to the dismay of other reformers, the Children's Bureau insisted on retaining "the complete unity of a maternity and child care program" even if it meant "the potential sacrifice of unified services for whole families under the insurance programs."[68]

Essays, ed. Linda Kerber, Alice Kessler-Harris, and Kathryn Kish Sklar (Chapel Hill, N.C., 1995), 71, 80–82, 85; Gordon, *Pitied but Not Entitled,* 105, 258.

[66] Poen, *Truman versus the Medical Lobby,* 90–91; Parks, "Expert Inquiry and Health Care Reform," 126–29, 130–32; Haines to Baker (1 Feb. 1928), Box 279, Central File, 1925–1929, RG 102, Records of the Children's Bureau; Gordon, *Pitied but Not Entitled,* 94–95, 200–201; Grace Abbott, "Memorandum for the President" (5 Feb. 1930), Box 422, Central File, 1929–1932, RG 102, Records of the Children's Bureau.

[67] Parks, "Expert Inquiry and Health Care Reform," 129; (quote) Abbot to Hutchcraft (22 May 1930), Box 422, Central File, 1929–1932, RG 102, Records of the Children's Bureau; (quote) Katherine Lenroot, "Preliminary and Confidential Suggestions for Development of a Children's Program as Part of the Federal Security Program" (Aug. 1934), Box 5, CES Records; Gordon, *Pitied but Not Entitled,* 256–57; FDR to Perkins (13 Nov. 1934), POF 103:1, FDR Papers.

[68] Lenroot to Wayne Coy (16 Dec. 1946); Martha Eliot, "Services to Children in Defense Industry Centers" (1940), both in Box 30, Decimal 045.2, Records of the FSA, Office of the Administrator, GCF (1939–1944), HEW Records; Secretary of Labor to Truman (15 Mar. 1946), Box 46, Decimal 011.4, FSA, Office of the Administrator, GCF (1944–1950), HEW Records; Pemberton, *Bureaucratic Politics,* 54–55; Underwood to Harrison (3 Jan. 1939), Box 834, Central File, 1937–1940, RG 102, Records of the Children's Bureau;

Consider the trajectory of the group health movement. Driven by the poverty of basic medical services in rural and remote industrial settings, the development of patient-based plans was uneven and often depended on relations with local medical societies and the willingness of state legislatures to nurture cooperatives. The growth of group practice, trumpeted by the CCMC in the early 1930s, pressed medical societies and hospitals to develop the fledgling Blue Cross/Blue Shield system. Through this flurry of innovation, most group health advocates supported national health insurance, because the benefits offered by group plans were quite meager, because group plans still faced political and professional opposition, and because fragmented group coverage remained an actuarial nightmare.[69] Increasingly, however, group health advocates viewed broad political solutions as a threat rather than as an opportunity. This was a pragmatic and anxious response to persistent opposition from professional associations and medical societies. Group health plans needed stable contractual relationships with doctors and hospitals. The price of such a relationship, time and time again, was deference to the professional interests and political horizons of medical conservatives.[70]

In turn, the group practice movement was distracted by the health politics of the labor movement. Through its first flush of success, the CIO saw local cooperative and consumer organizing as an important complement to collective bargaining. But as the major CIO unions settled into pattern bargaining after the war, they devoted fewer organizational and financial resources to such efforts.[71] By the 1940s the Cooperative Health

---

Health Insurance and Medical Care files, Boxes 136 and 196, Central File, 1945–1948, RG 102, Records of the Children's Bureau; (quote) Falk, "Conference with Dr. Eliot" (28 Feb. 1946), Box 3, Decimal 11.1, Division of Research and Statistics, SSA Records.

[69] See co-op histories in Box 103; Cooperative League Press Release (24 Jan. 1946), Box 96; Testimony of Harry Becker (24 June 1946), Box 96; Cooperative Health Federation Press Release (6 May 1948), Box 95; Group Health files, Box 96, all in Papers of the Cooperative League of the United States of America, HSTPL; Prospectus of the Health Insurance Plan of Greater New York (1945), Box 33, Henry J. Kaiser Papers; Klein, "Managing Security," 237–40, 249–58.

[70] "The Story of One Health Cooperative" typescript in Box 96, Papers of the Cooperative League; Statement of George Jacobson, Box 57, PCHNN Records; Sidney Garfield, Report on Trip to New York (9 June 1944); Prospectus of the Health Insurance Plan of Greater New York (1945); Report of the HIP Medical Directory (27 May 1947); Report of the HIP Medical Director (18 May 1948) all in Box 33, Henry J. Kaiser Papers; Baehr to Rawls (6 Dec. 1944), Box 5, George Baehr Papers, Sterling Library; George Baehr address (17 June 1954), Box 209, Witte Papers; William Hard, "Medicine and Monopoly" (Dec. 1938) clipping in Raymond Zimmerman, SMOF 18, Truman Papers.

[71] J. P. Harbasse, "Labor and Cooperation in the United States" (n.d.), Box 103, Papers of the Cooperative League; "Preliminary Proposals for a Labor-Federal Government Partnership for Improving Health Care" (1966), Box 38:229, Series II, Kerr Papers; Margaret Klem, "Voluntary Medical Care Insurance," *Annals of the American Academy of Political and*

Federation was focusing most of its attention on labor, an institution that represented the largest critical mass of health consumers, whom it was willing and able to deliver in actuarially stable groups. But labor's interest was largely confined to the best coverage it could win for its members in discrete bargaining struggles. Sometimes this meant supporting local group health efforts, but increasingly it meant joining employers in negotiating with commercial insurers. By the time group health advocates pulled together the new Group Health Association of America (GHAA) in 1959, labor support had vanished almost entirely.[72] Increasingly, the politics of group health echoed those of the labor movement, as group health interests looked merely to augment or stabilize existing patterns of group practice. With the emergence of managed competition and its variants, the group health movement also became increasingly tangled up in efforts to recast group coverage around the HMO model. As early as the mid-1960s it was clear that the largest group plans such as Kaiser were, as one critic noted, "in fact if not in theory, proprietary in nature and about as 'consumer sponsored' as Metropolitan Life."[73]

Consider the intersection of health politics and civil rights. In many respects, African-American civil rights and public health activists were the most persistent advocates of truly universal social programs, and understood the perils of deferring public policy to states or labor markets. Even mainstream civil rights organizations like the NAACP consistently supported national health insurance, scored legislative solutions that failed to "scotch all discrimination before it even gets started," and recognized the racial implications and motives of professional opposition.[74]

Social Science 273 (1951): 101; "Report on UAW-CIO Cooperative Activities" (1945), Box 106, Papers of the Cooperative League; Lane Kirkland Memo (6 July 1967), Box 10:250, Series I, Esselstyn Papers.

[72] "Plans for Council of Cooperative Development" (1945?), Box 106, Papers of the Cooperative League; Taylor to Cooke (26 Sept. 1940), Box 149 Morris Cooke Papers, FDRPL; Address of Lane Kirkland to California State Chamber of Commerce (29 Nov. 1956), Box 207, Witte Papers; Esselstyn to Nelson Cruikshank (2 June 1965), Box 13:306, Series I; misc. GHAA correspondence, Boxes 55:52–57, Series III; Esselstyn to MacColl (21 Dec. 1960), Box 55:53, Series III; Goor to Esselstyn (7 Dec. 1960), Box 55:53, Series III, all in Esselstyn Papers.

[73] James Doherty [GHA] to Falk (26 July 1974), Box 144:2090; Leonard Woodcock, "Health Security, Prepaid Group Practice, and HMOs" (1975?), Box 145:2116, Series III, Falk Papers; (quote) Carroll to Shoemaker (24 Oct. 1966), Box 38:229, Series II, Kerr Papers; (quote) Cole to Garrison (9 July 1971), Box 23, John Wiley Papers, SHSW; Medical Committee for Human Rights, "A Radical Alternative to National Health Insurance" (July 1971), Box 23, Wiley Papers.

[74] Gordon, *Pitied but Not Entitled,* 116, 141–42; (quote) Address of Louis Wright (1939), Part 1, reel 10:0512, Papers of the NAACP (microfilm); Walter White to FDR (24 Sept. 1934), President's Official File 121:1, FDR Papers; W. Montague Cobb, "The National Health Program of the NAACP," *JNMA* 45:5 (1953), 334–35; Gary Orfield, "Race and the

But while all decried inequity and segregation in health provision, civil rights activists and black professional organizations often disagreed sharply over the best means of addressing them. For most of its history, the National Medical Association promoted accommodation, racial "uplift," and incremental progress against segregation—and was willing to countenance professional and institutional segregation if it meant opportunities for black professionals. In their pursuit of professional recognition, NMA leaders also proved willing to echo the AMA's fears of socialization as early as the 1930s, in the hope that a united defense of professional autonomy might help erase the color line in medical education, licensing, and organization.[75] After 1945 the NMA was more willing to battle health segregation and worked closely with the NAACP on a range of issues, but its primary concern remained professional desegregation; it joined the AMA in opposing national health insurance in 1948 in exchange for the latter's commitment to opening up state and national medical societies. By the 1960s federal programs and the rapid expansion of the health care industry had given black professionals a substantial stake in the patchwork of private health insurance, federally financed hospitals, and means-tested medical assistance programs. The NMA joined the AMA in defending a "free enterprise system of health care" and routinely opposed a "monolithic, government controlled program" that would not necessarily "address itself to the socioeconomic aspect of the poor and other minority groups," and called instead for an expansion of Medicare and Medicaid.[76]

Liberal Agenda: The Loss of the Integrationist Dream, 1965–1974," in *The Politics of Social Policy in the United States,* ed. Margaret Weir, Ann Orloff, and Theda Skocpol (Princeton, N.J., 1988), 312–15; Brown, *Race, Money, and the American Welfare State,* 263–92; James Shepperd, "Minority Perspective on National Health Insurance," *JNMA* 68:4 (1976): 287; "National Health Insurance: A Position Paper by the National Medical Association," *JNMA* 70:7 (1978): 538–41; Richard Cooper, "Is the United States Entering a Period of Retrogression in Public Health?" *JNMA* 75:8 (1983): 741–44; Albert Vann, "Health Care Delivery in America: Major Concerns," *JNMA* 72:7 (1980): 721–22; Robert Dawson, "Equal Access to Health Care Delivery for Blacks," *JNMA* 73:1 (1981): 53–55.

[75] Vanessa Gamble, *Making a Place for Ourselves: The Black Hospital Movement, 1920–1945* (New York, 1995), 4–14, 153–69; "Health Insurance," *JNMA* 26:4 (1934): 174–75; Edward Beardsley, *A History of Neglect: Health Care for Blacks and Mill Workers in the Twentieth-Century South* (Knoxville, Tenn., 1987), 89–90, 117–21; Gamble, "Black Autonomy versus White Control: Black Hospitals and the Dilemmas of White Philanthropy, 1920–1940," *Minerva* 35 (1997): 251–65; G. Hamilton Francis, "The Negro Doctor and the Threatened Socialization of Medicine," *JNMA* 25:1 (1933): 20–22; C. E. Walker, "The National Health Program," *JNMA* 30:4 (1938): 147–49; Martha Eliot to Katherine Lenroot (20 Nov. 1939), Box 834, Central File, 1937–1940, RG 102, Records of the Children's Bureau, National Archives; NMA, Report of the Committee on Medical Economics (1938), POF 511:2, FDRPL.

[76] Gamble, *Making a Place for Ourselves,* 182–84; Beardsley, *A History of Neglect,* 247, 249–51; Special Committee of the NMA (Nov. 1938), Box 5, Chapman Papers; Address of Louis

The NMA's politics were not simply shortsighted and selfish but, like those of some maternal reformers, reflected the immediate urgency of delivering services where none were available—even at the expense of universal or integrated provision. Such concerns were largely shared by local health activists, for whom the distant promise of federal policy paled beside the task of providing the most basic public health programs in the Jim Crow South. Through the 1920s, 1930s, and 1940s, local activists maintained a wide range of clinical and educational programs, focusing on tuberculosis, venereal disease, and infant and maternal mortality. Between 1932 and 1950 these programs were sustained and coordinated, in part, by the Public Health Service's Office of Negro Health Work. By the 1950s, however, such efforts were distracted by the broader emphasis on desegregation and the promise of private coverage in the postwar economy. As southern health care became more a civil rights issue and less a public health issue, the black community traded the distinct problems of southern or segregated medicine for the broader problems of American health care. As Michael Brown has suggested, the Great Society both trafficked in the universal logic of civil rights and threatened the future of social policy by identifying African Americans and African-American organizations so closely with the welfare state. Increasingly, public health programs were isolated (and stigmatized) as accessories to means-tested welfare medicine.[77]

In all, reformers faced a tangle of intertwined obstacles. Perhaps most starkly, their efforts were always constrained by an enormous resource disadvantage. Given both the natural resources skew in American electoral and legislative politics and the tremendous stake claimed by medical and insurance and business interests, substantial health reform only rarely broke the surface of national debate. Reformers, in turn, claimed only tenuous footing in party politics. The labor movement—in a context of dismal political options, managerial hostility, and fragmented

---

Wright (1939), Part 1, reel 10:0512, Papers of the NAACP; Poen, *Truman versus the Medical Lobby*, 162; Wright to Oppenheimer (18 Dec. 1943), Part 15B, reel 14:430, Papers of the NAACP; George Cannon, "Adequate Medical Care of the Individual and Family," *JNMA* 41:1 (1949), 19; Report of the Committee on the Sydenham Hospital (1944), Part 15B, reel 14:516, Papers of the NAACP; New York Urban League, "The Struggle for a Voluntary Hospital in Harlem" (1944), Part 15B, reel 14:0534–0536, Papers of the NAACP; (quote) Charles Bookert, "President's Column," *JNMA* 69:11 (1977): 777; (quote) Arthur Coleman, "National Health Insurance and President Carter," *JNMA* 69:1 (1977), 1; David McBride, "Black America: From Community Health Care to Crisis Medicine," *JHPPL* 18:2 (1993), 325–26.

[77] Brown, *Race, Money, and the American Welfare State*, 272–75; Susan Smith, *Sick and Tired of Being Sick and Tired: Black Women's Health Activism in America, 1910–1950* (Philadelphia, 1995), 17–40, 58–82; Beardsley, *A History of Neglect*, 102–14; Gamble, *Making a Place for Ourselves*, 188.

private bargaining—was unable and unwilling to exert any natural leadership in the health reform fight. And all of these constraints confronted (and continue to confront) fragments of the reform movement with strategic dilemmas in which immediate or incremental progress—the proverbial foot in the door—almost invariably comes at the expense of universal programs.

Conclusion

The Past and Future of Health Politics

A T the root of our current situation, and of the historic failure of national health insurance in the United States, lies the persistent mismatch between the political resources commanded by health interests
and those commanded by reformers. Though increasingly at odds over
the costs or implications of political solutions, the parties to health care's
corporate compromise have at least shared the ability and the willingness to deflect reform whenever their stakes in the private health market
have been threatened. And these stakes have increased markedly in recent years, as the costs of private health coverage continue to outpace
inflation and the health industry stumbles through a market revolution.
By the end of the 1990s HMOs and their variants claimed nearly 80
percent of the health insurance market. While the numbers in HMOs
grew steadily, the number of HMOs shrank almost as dramatically as
insurers and hospitals bought and sold each other at a frenzied pace.
Through the early 1990s major mergers and acquisitions in health care
numbered about 20 a year; this figure ballooned to over 500 in 1995 and
over 650 in 1996—a year in which fully 10 percent of all for-profit hospitals were involved in a corporate reorganization of some order. "The top
ten for-profit hospital firms have been coupling like rabbits," noted one
observer, "though unlike rabbits, each liaison leaves fewer firms not
more." Although such corporatization reshapes health politics and medical practice, it has meant only sporadic returns for the HMOs themselves, whose impressive profit margins of the mid-1990s have all but
evaporated.[1]

Reformers, by contrast, enjoy none of the political advantages claimed
by economic interests in the United States or by reform interests in other
national settings. This disadvantage has been compounded in the decade
since the Clinton health initiative, an episode that managed to discredit
health reform even as it disappointed most health reformers. Although

[1] Gail Jensen et al., "The New Dominance of Managed Care: Insurance Trends in the
1990s," *HA* 16:1 (1997): 125; "The Patient Is Stable—For Now," *BW* (8 Jan. 1996): 102;
Sandy Lutz, "Let's Make a Deal," *Modern Healthcare* (Dec. 1994): 29–32; (quote) David
Himmelstein and Steffie Woolhander, "Giant HMO A or Giant HMO B?" *The Nation* (19
Sept. 1994): 312; Steffie Woolhander and David Himmelstein, "Costs of Care and Administration at For-Profit and Other Hospitals in the United States," *NEJM* 336:11 (13 Mar.
1997): 769–74.

advocates of single-payer, national health insurance soldier bravely on, serious political attention is increasingly confined to a narrow range of piecemeal and incremental reforms: prescription drug coverage for Medicare patients, tax credits for the purchase of private insurance, lower age or income-eligibility thresholds for existing public programs such as Medicare, and the regulation of HMOs to protect patient rights. Even at the state level, to which many reformers retreated after 1994, arguments for broader coverage typically hope that modest reform of existing programs (SCHIP expansion, COBRA subsidies, Medicaid waivers) can continue to mop up around the edges of a leaky system of employment-based provision.[2]

One consequence of this, in both the history of health reform and current health politics, has been the demobilization of the labor movement as a voice for reform. Through the formative years of the private welfare state, the core CIO unions chose security over solidarity and increasingly viewed universal health programs as a threat to the experience rates, preferential tax treatment, and employer-financing enjoyed by job-based group insurance. By any measure, labor bet on the wrong horse. Employer provision has proved uneven and fickle, especially as deindustrialization eroded the actuarial logic of group insurance, and self-insurance, coinsurance, and managed care became the rule in the group plans that survived. Just as important, labor accomplished little of the security it hoped would accompany collectively bargained benefits. As growth in private coverage flattened in the late 1960s, labor's fortunes tumbled: by 2000, union density (at 14 percent of the workforce and only 9 percent of the private workforce) had fallen to barely a third of its postwar peak. In politics and private bargaining, the labor movement helped to determine the balance between private and public provision. But that balance also shaped the labor movement by inflating the stakes of private bargaining without, in the long run, conceding much security to either unions or the workers they represented.

What is remarkable, through all of this, is how fascinated we remain with the promise of private provision—although that fascination now rests less on the promise that private insurance will eventually reach us all than on the political obstacles to displacing it. Employment-based health insurance, floated as an alternative to public insurance in the middle years of the century, is now little more than a leaky life raft for

---

[2] Marcia Angell, "Placebo Politics," *American Prospect* 11:23 (6 Nov. 2000). For examples of state-level efforts, see Maryland Budget and Tax Policy Institute, "Working but Not Insured: A New Opportunity to Provide Health Insurance to Working Parents" (Feb. 2000); Maryland Citizen's Health Initiative, "A Proposed Plan for Universal Health Insurance Coverage in the State of Maryland" (Sept. 2001).

politicians clinging to budget-neutral solutions and workers with no-where else to swim. Private coverage, in turn, reflects the larger confu-sion over the place of health care in an American tradition of social insurance. Not only is it difficult to pursue national health insurance in the contemporary political climate but, after nearly a century of political discourse championing private alternatives and demonizing public ones, it is difficult to even talk about it. In the wake of the Clinton failure, efforts to combine the old idea of an "earned right" with the new politics of fiscal restraint yielded the individual Medical Savings Account (MSA). Proponents argued that the combination of MSAs and catastrophic cov-erage was the only way to salvage both the risk basis of commercial insur-ance and the contributory principle of social insurance—as one insurer put it, such a combination was the only way to both sustain "individual freedom and personal responsibility" and "break the mentality that in-surance is 'free' and that the goal is to maximize usage." The 1996 Health Insurance Portability and Accountability Act, which opened the door for MSA pilot programs and made some effort to ensure that workers could maintain group coverage from one job to the next, captured the dilem-mas of contributory health care: the "portability" provisions sought to spread risk across broader employment groups; the MSA provision, by contrast, carried risk segmentation and contributory care to their logical extreme—"the healthy," MSA enthusiasts argued, "need not subsidize the sick."[3]

Not surprisingly, given the gap between the promise and the perfor-mance of private health insurance, the three-pronged health crisis—high costs, uneven coverage, and inadequate care—persists. Aggregate growth in national health expenditures slowed somewhat after 1994 (settling in at just over 13 percent of GDP) but remained nearly 60 percent ahead of the general inflation rate. By 2000 per capita health spending (at just under $4,000) had more than doubled since 1987. Medicaid spending ballooned even more dramatically and swallowed nearly a quarter of some states' budgets—just as many states collapsed into recession and fiscal troubles in late 2001.[4] At the same time, the scope and security of health

[3] Lee Tooman in House Committee on Ways and Means, *Hearing: Private Health Insurance Reform Legislation* 102:2 (Mar. 1992), 249; "Who Will Jump into the MSA Pond?" *Business and Health* (Oct. 1996): 47–56.

[4] Costs calculated from Health Care Financing Administration [HCFA], "National Health Expenditures by Type of Service and Source of Funds: Calendar Years, 1960–97"; HCFA, "National Health Expenditures Aggregate, per Capita, Percent Distribution, and Annual Percent Change by Source of Funds: Calendar Years 1960–97"; see also Eli Ginz-berg, "Managed Care and the Competitive Market in Health Care," *JAMA* 277:22 (11 June 1997): 1812–13; Teresa Coughlin et al., "The Medicaid Spending Crisis, 1988–1992," *JHPPL* 19:4 (1994): 837–58; Henry Aaron and Robert Reischauer, "The Medicare Reform Debate: What Is the Next Step?' *HA* 14:4 (1995): 10.

coverage continued to slip. Private insurance coverage, which had pla-
teaued at around 75 percent in the late 1970s, dipped back to barely 70
percent—an unprecedented decline in an otherwise stable labor market.
The share of national health spending met by private insurance, never
much more than one-third, also began to slip in the middle 1990s—the
slack taken up by individual workers and public programs (the employee
share of premiums in employment-based plans grew at an annual rate of
over 13 percent, more than double the rate of health care inflation, as
deductibles and exemptions and coinsurance became the norm). Since
1994, in turn, the number of uninsured and underinsured has continued
to grow: 18 percent (forty-four million) were uninsured at any one time,
while over 30 percent went without insurance for at least one month in
2000.[5] And all of this has been accompanied by an unprecedented crisis
in the quality of care for those lucky enough to remain insured—underscored by provider and patient reaction to HMO practices.

Finally, the health care crises have attenuated the persistent inequity
of the American health care system. At the intersection of employment-
based insurance, stigmatized public programs, and uneven access to
basic care, citizenship in the welfare state remains tenuous for the poor,
for women (and their children), and for people of color. Fully 85 percent
of the uninsured are low- and moderate-income families and individuals
whose employers do not offer health insurance but who do not qualify
for Medicaid (in the wake of the 1996 welfare reforms and a frenzy of
state-level reforms, eligibility for Medicaid ranged from 60 percent of
those whose incomes fell below the federal poverty line in the District of
Columbia to less than 30 percent in Nevada). Although private coverage
rests near 70 percent for the population as a whole, rates of coverage are
slightly worse for women and dramatically worse for African Americans
(51 percent in 1999) and Hispanics (just over 40 percent). This racially
uneven coverage reflects the traditional weight of discrimination in private insurance and private employment, and the fact that the pattern of
uninsurance for agricultural workers has shifted from the South to the
Southwest in recent decades. Indeed, rates of uninsurance ranged wildly,
from under 10 percent in some upper midwestern states to almost 25
percent in some southwestern states.[6]

[5] Barbara Smith, "Trends in Health Care Coverage," *NEJM* 337:14 (1997): 1000; HCFA,
"National Health Expenditures by Type of Service and Source of Funds: Calendar Years,
1960–97"; HCFA, "National Health Expenditures Aggregate, per Capita, Percent Distribution, and Annual Percent Change by Source of Funds: Calendar Years 1960–97"; Steven
Schroeder, "The Medically Uninsured—Will They Always Be with Us?" *NEJM* 334:17
(1996), 1130; "Second-Class Medicine," *Consumer Reports* 65:9 (Sept. 2000): 42–43.

[6] On coverage rates, see www.census.gov/hhes/hlthins/: Bureau of the Census, "Health
Insurance Coverage Status and Type of Coverage by Sex, Race, and Hispanic Origins,

There is, unfortunately, little prospect that such problems will attract serious political attention—let alone the sort of universalist intervention demanded by the political and actuarial logic of health care—in the near future. Each lost opportunity (1918, 1935, 1949, 1965, 1971, 1994) fragmented provision, lowered the sights of reformers, underscored the clout of health interests, and made subsequent reform both more difficult and less urgent. Through the middle decades of the twentieth century, a conspiracy of factors (the racial and gendered limits of New Deal democracy, the postwar promise of private provision, the political culture of social insurance, the political clout of organized medicine and its allies, the political ambivalence of the labor movement and its allies) left the United States—alone among its democratic peers—without a national health system. Through the last decades of the century, the weight of this failure was compounded by ongoing inflationary, competitive, and fiscal crises that simultaneously made private insurance less stable and public solutions less likely. Into the new century, health care will, in all likelihood, remain a compelling public concern but an elusive political target.

1987–1999"; Helen Schauffler and Richard Brown, "The State of Health Insurance in California, 1998" (University of California, Berkeley, Center for Health and Public Policy Studies, 1998), 1.

Archival Sources

Archives of Labor History and Urban Affairs, Wayne State University, Detroit, Mich.
Records of the United Auto Workers, Social Security Department

Bancroft Library, University of California, Berkeley, Calif.
Edgar Kaiser
Henry Kaiser

Hagley Museum and Library, Wilmington, Del.
Chamber of Commerce
DuPont Papers
Willis Harrington
Imprints Collection
National Association of Manufacturers
National Industrial Conference Board
Pennsylvania Railroad
Westmoreland Coal

Lyndon Baines Johnson Presidential Library, Austin, Tex.
Lyndon Johnson Papers
   Office Files of Horace Busby
   Office Files of Douglas Cater
   Office Files of Joseph Califano
   Office Files of James Gaither
   Office Files of Mike Manatos
   Office Files of Henry Wilson
   Robson-Ross Office Files
   White House Central Files
Administrative Histories
Joseph Califano Papers
DNC Records
Oral Histories
   Wilbur Cohen
   Elizabeth Wickenden Goldschmidt
   Robert Ball
Task Force Reports

Microfilmed Collections
American Association for Labor Legislation
Civil Rights during the Johnson Administration, 1963–1969
NAACP Papers

National Archives, College Park, Md.
Nixon Presidential Materials, White House Central Files
RG 47, Records of the Social Security Administration
RG 86, Records of the Women's Bureau
RG 102, Records of the Children's Bureau
RG 235, Records of the Department of Health, Education, and Welfare
Records of the Interdepartmental Working Group on Health (Clinton task
    force)

National Archives, Washington, D.C.
RG 46, Records of the United States Congress, Senate
    Records of the Senate Committee on Finance
    Records of the Senate Committee on Labor and Public Works
RG 233, Records of the United States Congress, House of Representatives
    Records of the House Committee on Education and Labor
    Records of the House Committee on Interstate and Domestic Commerce
    Records of the House Committee on Ways and Means

Franklin D. Roosevelt Presidential Library, Hyde Park, N.Y.
Morris Cooke
Cooperative League of America
Harry Hopkins
President's Interdepartmental Committee to Coordinate Health and Welfare
    Activities (ICHWA)
Franklin D. Roosevelt
Alexander Sachs
Caroline Ware

State Historical Society of Wisconsin, Madison, Wis.
American Federation of Hosiery Workers
American Federation of Labor
Arthur J. Altmeyer
Wilbur Cohen
Nelson Hale Cruikshank
Imprints and Pamphlets Collection
Frank Kuehl
William Leiserson
Physicians Committee for Health Care for the Aged
John Wiley
Edwin E. Witte

Sterling Library, Yale University, New Haven, Conn.
George Baehr
Caldwell Esslestyne
Isidore Falk

Lorin Kerr
Goldie Krantz
John Peters

Tarlton Law Library, University of Texas, Austin, Tex.
Walton Hamilton Papers

Harry S. Truman Presidential Library, Independence, Mo.
Oscar Chapman
Clark Clifford
Michael Davis (microfilm)
Democratic National Committee
Oscar Ewing
Howard McGrath
Papers of the Cooperative League of the United States of America
President's Commission on the Health Needs of the Nation
Harry Truman

University of Iowa Special Collections, Iowa City, Iowa
Orville Grahame
Donovan Ward

Index

National Medical Association (NMA), 189,
 294–95
National Physician's Committee (NPC):
 on example of German health system,
 140–41; history of, 221–22
National Resources Planning Board, 123
National War Labor Board (NWLB), 57–
 59
New Deal: African Americans discrimi-
 nated against by programs of, 190–91;
 deferring to AMA on policy, 218; and
 family-wage assumptions, 155; health
 care and, 16–19; premise of insuring income, 123; southerners' relationship to,
 182. *See also* Roosevelt administration
NICB (National Industrial Conference
 Board), 61
Nixon administration: and close ties with
 AMA, 247; health policy of, 32–36, 120,
 124, 152, 247–48, 273; and view of Medicare and Medicaid, 119
NPC. *See* National Physician's Committee
 (NPC)

Old Age Security Income (OASI), 24
organized labor, 11; and alliance with Democratic Party, 276–80; and attitude toward Clinton Health Plan, 284; and the
 Blues, 73–76; and health reform, 274–
 84; and NAFTA, 280; no longer a voice
 of reform, 298; and postwar attitude towards private insurance, 63–64; and private benefits, 280–84; relationship of,
 with insurers, doctors, employers in the
 1950s, 230–31. *See also* health care bargaining; *and under individual union
 names*

Parran, Thomas, 115
party politics and health reform, 269–74
"Patient's Bill of Rights," 171
patients' rights laws, 45
Pennsylvania Railroad: and membership in
 MBA, 52; segregated MBA in, 50
Physicians for a National Health Program
 (PNHP), 268
Pittston strike, 86
Piven, Francis Fox, 175
pluralist view. *See* liberal or pluralist view
 (on lack of national health insurance)
political culture of health care debate,
 136–71

poor, as target of health care assistance,
 127–28
Powell, Adam Clayton, 198
President's Committee on the Health Needs
 of the Nation (PCHNN) (1952), 22
Pressman, Lee, 287
private health insurance: before the New
 Deal, 47–57; as enjoyed by upper tiers of
 labor market, 46; and failures as alternative to national health insurance, 46;
 and limitations of private coverage, 77–
 78; and public policy, 46–89; rapid postwar growth of, 60; as result of insistence
 on contributory programs and confusion on how to pay, 122. *See also* insurance industry
private interests. *See* American Medical Association (AMA); economic interests;
 employers; insurance industry
private welfare state, 9, 85, 89; foundations
 laid for (1941-1945), 57; 1945–1950
 building of the, 60–67; consolidation of
 (1950–1965), 67–76; in crisis (1965-
 2000), 82–89. *See also* welfare state
Progressives. *See* American Association for
 Labor Legislation
Puccini, Art, 252

race, and health care provision: from 1946
 to 1970, 193–202; agricultural labor as
 factor in, 183–84, 191–92; American welfare state as a Jim Crow welfare state,
 172; before the the New Deal, 177–82;
 Civil Rights and health reform, 293–95;
 current crisis for minorities in, 300; discrimination against African American
 health professionals in, 173; during the
 New Deal, 182–92; and economic discrimination in health care, 174–75; and
 establishment of western European and
 American welfare states, 176; from 1946
 to 1970, 193–202; and health care distinctions 1980–2000, 85; history of
 health care in relation to, 172–209; and
 hospital desegregation, 193–202, 205–7;
 implications of Sheppard-Towner Act regarding, 180–81; and infant mortality
 and and life expectancy rates: whites v.
 Latino Americans and blacks and Latino
 Americans, 177; as influence in health
 policy, 6–7, 8, 10; and legitimacy of welfare state, 204; and local administration
 of programs, 186–87; and maternal

POLITICS AND SOCIETY IN TWENTIETH-CENTURY AMERICA